Experiencing Politics

California/Milbank Books on Health and the Public

Experiencing Politics

A Legislator's Stories of
Government and Health Care

John E. McDonough

UNIVERSITY OF CALIFORNIA PRESS
Berkeley   Los Angeles   London

THE MILBANK MEMORIAL FUND
New York

Photographs by John Swan, with permission.
Illustrations by Kathy Stern, with permission.
Cartoon by Brian Savage, with permission from
the Cartoon Bank.

University of California Press
Berkeley and Los Angeles, California

University of California Press, Ltd.
London, England

Library of Congress Cataloging-in-Publication Data

McDonough, John E. (John Edward)
    Experiencing politics : a legislator's stories of
government and health care / John E. McDonough.
        p.   cm.—(California/Milbank series
on health and the public ; 2)
    Includes bibliographical references and index.
    ISBN 0-520-22410-8 (cloth : acid-free paper)—
ISBN 0-520-22411-6 (pbk. : acid-free paper)
    1. Massachusetts. General Court. House of
Representatives.   2. Legislators—Massachusetts.
3. Political planning—Massachusetts.   4. Medical
policy—Massachusetts. I. Title. II. Series.
JK3166.M34   2000
328.744'092—dc21   99-056844

Printed in the United States of America
08 07 06 05 04 03 02
10 9 8 7 6 5 4 3 2

The paper used in this publication meets the minimum
requirements of ANSI/NISO Z39.48–1992 (R 1997)
(*Permanence of Paper*).

To Father Jack Roussin
whose memory touches all who knew him
and
to Devlin, Amy, and Jax

Contents

Foreword

The Milbank Memorial Fund is an endowed national foundation that engages in nonpartisan analysis, study, research, and communication on significant issues in health care and public health. The Fund makes available the results of its work in meetings with decision-makers, reports, articles, and books.

The purpose of the Fund's publishing partnership with the University of California Press is to encourage the synthesis and communication of findings from research that could contribute to more effective health policy. John McDonough's book achieves this goal in a special way.

McDonough integrates political life with the academic study of politics. His experience as a legislator and a scholar gives him unusual insights and memorable stories. The Fund and the Press solicited reviews of McDonough's manuscript from persons experienced in practical politics as well as from political scientists, and then convened the reviewers to discuss the manuscript with the author. These reviewers concurred in praising McDonough for communicating his delight in both the theory and practice of politics.

This book contributes to public understanding of politics and policy making by demonstrating that experience, theory, and analysis can be mutually enhancing. It also demonstrates the inseparability of the health of the public from the health of the republic.

Daniel M. Fox
President

Samuel L. Milbank
Chairman

Acknowledgments

Writing this book has been in my mind since 1994 when I sat in John Tierney's policy and politics class at the University of Michigan School of Public Health. I started searching for a publisher in mid-1996 and received a string of rejections. At a meeting of the Reforming States Group, a project of the Milbank Memorial Fund, I told my idea to the Fund's president, Dr. Dan Fox. "Let me help you," he instantly offered. This book would not have been written without the incredible support of Dr. Fox, Gail Cambridge, and the Fund.

The University of California Press has been exceptionally supportive and helpful throughout this process, particularly editor Lynne Withey.

Because of the Fund's support, I was privileged to have an earlier version of this book read by a distinguished review panel: former Massachusetts Representative Carmen Buell, John Colmers, Pamela Dickson, Minnesota State Representative Lee Greenfield, Dr. Richard Hall, former California Assemblyman Phil Isenberg, Dr. Larry Jacobs, Judy Meredith, Dr. Mark Peterson, Kansas Senator Sandy Praeger, Dr. Jeff Prottas, Dr. Alan Rosenthal, Dr. John Tierney, and Lincoln, Nebraska, Mayor Don Wesely.

Several friends and associates who were involved in the case stories read one or more chapters for accuracy: Ray Ausrotas, Margaret Blood, David Cortiella, Steve Long, Representative Jim Marzilli, Joseph McDonagh and Matt McDonough, Michael Miller, Rob Restuccia, Paul Romary, Brian Rosman, and David Sullivan. Thanks to them and to many more who shared their memories, stories, and perceptions with me.

Thanks also to colleagues and associates at the Heller School at Brandeis University who supported this project, especially Jack Shonkoff, Stan Wallack, Stuart Altman, Scott Sahagian, Chris Hager, Mike Doonan, David Breakstone, and Michele King. Special thanks to the School of Public Health at the University of the Michigan and the many people who helped me through: Catherine McLaughlin, Barry Rabe, John Tierney, Bill Weissert, Leon Wyszewianski, David Perlman, and others. Thanks to students at the Heller School at Brandeis University, the Harvard School of Public Health, and the Boston University School of Public Health who have helped to sharpen my thinking about the policy models and health policy in our courses together.

I will always be indebted to the people of Jamaica Plain, Roxbury, Roslindale, and Dorchester for the opportunity they gave me seven times to serve as their state representative in the Massachusetts legislature. While there are far too many to mention, I am especially indebted to Lee Ash, Bernie Doherty and Karen Caplan, Barbara Burnham, Rosa Clark, Dave Curtis, Diane Duggan, Steve Gag and Laura Gang, Eva Gerena, my successor Representative Liz Malia and Rita Kantarowski, Bob McDonnell, Sue Minter, Tom Morin, Margaret Noce, Neal-dra Osgood, Ruth Parker, Marcia Peters, Mirna and Jaime Rodriguez, Alvin Shiggs and Maria Quiroga, Ric and Dianne Quiroga, Sandra Storey and John Swan, Marie Turley, and many others.

Thanks to Massachusetts House Speakers George Keverian, Charles Flaherty, and Tom Finneran who helped me in so many ways to advance my policy priorities and who gave much advice and support through the years. Thanks also to the many hundreds of men and women with whom I served, schemed, plotted, fought, complained, confided, and celebrated through thirteen years. *Illegitimi non carborundum!*

Thanks to those across the nation who work through government to improve health and health care and who have inspired me for many years: colleagues with the Reforming States Group; associates at the National Conference of State Legislatures, Dick Merritt, Shelly Gehshan, Kala Ladenheim, Tracy Hooker, and Martha King; and friends at the National Academy for State Health Policy.

Finally, most special thanks and love to Janice Furlong, who supported me in immeasurable ways through every step of this long process.

Introduction

*Seeing Politics through
Different Lenses*

The real act of discovery consists not in finding new lands
but in seeing with new eyes.

Marcel Proust

A long-serving member of the Massachusetts House of Representatives gingerly seated himself in the vacant black leather chair next to me in the cavernous and historic House chamber. A district border in southwest Boston was all we really shared in common. Prior to this moment, my most vivid memory of him had occurred during a meeting of the Boston legislative delegation in my first year as a rep, as I awkwardly made conversation by remarking that he always seemed to face difficult reelection fights that attracted multiple serious opponents. "Don't worry about me," he smiled. "My perception of vulnerability is my greatest strength." He most often could be observed seated at the far back of the chamber reading books connected with his two compelling passions: the right-to-life movement and the Catholic cause in Northern Ireland. Today, however, he wanted to be my friend. "John," he said in a voice cracking from years of tobacco smoke, "do you have any precincts near me that you would be willing to let me take?" He was referring to the upcoming redrawing of legislative districts, always an intense game of who gets what. "Gee, I don't know," I demurred. "I've worked them really hard. The people there know and like me. And why would you want them anyway when no one there knows you?" "Well," he said, "I find that I always do better in places where people don't know who I am."

It's a fact that most Americans don't know their elected officials, personally or from a distance.[1] Whether we know them or not, little seems to counteract the dispiriting cynicism that infects large portions of our public life at the turn of the century. It is not difficult to understand why politics and public affairs are held in such low esteem. The constant, vituperative combat between Republicans and Democrats in Washington, D.C., and in state capitals, the imbroglios involving campaign cash, ugly and pervasive negative political advertising, and numerous and seemingly unending political scandals all combine to confirm the public's worst fear: that something is pathetically awry in our nation's civic and political culture. Briefly, in early 1997, signals were sent from both sides of the political aisle in Washington that a cooling of passions was in order. Some members of Congress from both parties even went on a retreat to Hershey, Pennsylvania, to try to establish a more collegial atmosphere (the trip was repeated in 1999). Not surprisingly, the cease-fire didn't last.

The cease-fire didn't last because it can't. The stakes are too high in public politics for both sides to sit complacently at the same time: the side that's out of power always wants to get in. Moreover, the issues under discussion are of such public consequence that no side can afford to appear passive. The media and the public contribute to this dynamic; they are always drawn to conflict, the more intense the better, and most often regard with boredom or skepticism occasional shows of unity and agreement. Even more basic, the structure of American government was consciously designed to ensure continuous conflict, rivalry, and egotism. "Ambition must be made to counteract ambition," Madison wrote in *The Federalist Papers,* No. 51, defending the structure of the proposed U.S. Constitution as one that would best protect the liberty of citizens. Nonetheless, Americans most commonly accept the view that our public institutions somehow have lost their way and strayed from the founders' vision.

At the same time, we invest enormous authority and trust in our government, and especially in our legislative institutions—federal, state, county, and local. We give our legislatures remarkable powers to pass laws that govern our own behaviors, from the trivial to the profound. In these bodies, we always find a striking range of talents, personalities, experiences, values, ideas, strategies, and energies. Those who have not worked in direct contact with legislatures—the vast majority of Americans—have little or no understanding of what really goes on, and how decisions really get made. And yet the decisions made in these bodies become laws that affect every aspect of our lives. We need to find ways to bring the realities of these institutions—good and bad—closer to the public's consciousness.

This book's premise is that a large portion of the public's cynicism is rooted in misunderstanding of essential features of our public institutions, the policymaking process, and the much-maligned dynamic of politics in all its varied forms. Watching or participating in public affairs in a poorly understood way can be as vexing and confusing as trying to play or watch a sports contest or a card game with no knowledge of the basic principles and rules. The result usually is frustration, throwing one's hands up, and walking away. Yet, because of the system's openness and media coverage, many seem to assume that in politics they should automatically "get" what's going on without making the effort to learn the system or the rules.

Participating in politics and public affairs with a genuine understanding of the process, the dynamics, the pacing, and the "game" can be an enriching, liberating, and joyful experience that few appreciate who have not done it. The neophyte activist savoring his or her first political win (electoral or issue-based) can experience a high equal to any athletic achievement. The more who participate, the more exciting and satisfying the results can be. My purpose in writing this book is to give readers an understanding and appreciation of the real workings of politics and policymaking—a view from the ground where the battles are fought and the passions are most deeply felt. While most of my examples and case stories are drawn from the public policymaking sphere—primarily state, but also federal and local—the lessons and ideas presented here can help to make sense of politics in the private sphere as well, at work, in the community, with the family. Because being political is a core human attribute, many of the essential dynamics of politics are the same in both the public and the private spheres.

MODELS FOR POLITICAL LIFE

To explain and illustrate important dynamics in the political arena, this volume presents a series of ways to understand politics and the policy process that I have found useful in the course of my public political career. For thirteen years, between 1985 and 1997, I served as a state legislator in the Massachusetts House of Representatives representing several diverse neighborhoods in the city of Boston: Jamaica Plain, Roslindale, Roxbury, and Dorchester. As a legislator, I became involved in such issues as health care policy, public safety, housing and urban development, and criminal justice, and in tax and spending debates. As a community leader, I was caught up in issues of community and economic development, affordable housing, crime, and much more. Though I had spent most of my life involved in politics in many ways, I had never been exposed to any organized, systematic ways of understanding political phenomena. Like most political activists, elected or not, I spent most of my time focused on the *what* of politics—the guts of issues—and little of my time focused on the *how*.

Between 1992 and 1996, while still in the legislature, I pursued a doctorate in public health at the School of Public Health of the University of Michigan and studied health care politics and policy with Dr. John Tierney of Boston College. He exposed me and my fellow students to many of the political models which form the core of this book. Because of my years as an elected official, I had a rare opportunity to engage in what is sometimes called "learning backward"—first engaging fully in a particular activity and later studying it, a process which greatly enhances and intensifies the learning experience. I brought to this learning process a sharp frame of reference to evaluate the relevance of these models and ideas—whether or not they made sense in the context of my own political involvement. (Aristotle complained: "The young man is not a proper audience for political science. He has no experience of life, and because he still follows his emotions, he will only listen to no purpose, uselessly."[2] This observation may not be true for others, but it certainly was for me.)

I began to employ some of the more intriguing policy tools in my work in the Massachusetts State House and in the community. I found them to be extraordinarily valuable, not just to understand something that had already happened, but to plan future activities and campaigns. I began to incorporate features of these models and ideas in my speaking engagements before a wide variety of audiences—from poor, minority women in a subsidized housing development in Roxbury looking to get better services, to national groups of physicians seeking to exert greater influence on health policy. In a course I taught on health policy and politics at the Boston University School of Public Health, I began to teach these models, asking students to apply them to their own experiences. I found intense interest and enthusiasm in learning these ways of viewing political phenomena. A common reaction I received was: "Why haven't I ever heard any of this before?" I remember having the same feeling. The truth is that while the models and concepts included in this volume are well known to political and policy science academics, they are completely unfamiliar to the vast majority of Americans, even those most actively involved in policymaking every day. I came to believe that if more people understood these concepts, some significant portion of the public's distaste for politics would diminish and be more productively channeled. The writer Robert Kuttner has observed that Americans love democracy and hate politics, failing to make the connection that politics is the practice of democracy. Those of us from across the ideological spectrum who *love* politics—as I surely do—have a common stake in working together to create better public understanding of its essential features and nuances.

The models and concepts presented in this book can be thought of as lenses helping us to perceive key features of a politicized situation that could not have been seen without looking through them. Not every lens is effective in every situation. No one lens does it all. Each has limitations. But all can be useful in a wide array of circumstances. Graham Allison presented the best-known use of this approach in his book *The Essence of Decision*.[3] He used three different conceptual lenses or "maps," as he called them—the rational actor theory, the administrative operating systems theory, and the bureaucratic politics theory—to tell three entirely different stories about what happened in the 1962 Cuban missile crisis, each true yet each highlighting a different aspect of this crucial Cold War event. As Barbara Nelson describes the approach, "Each version has a different character as the protagonist, and a different interpretation and causation of events."[4] Allison powerfully demonstrates that even when we can agree on the basic facts of a situation, the search for meaning in politics—of events, data, statements, and decisions—is contested terrain. This volume seeks to help readers with the search.

Frequently I am asked to rank the various models in terms of their relative importance. While I have my personal favorites (Deborah Stone's ideas in chapter 2 and John Kingdon's model in chapter 7), I usually refuse the request. Instead, I liken the various models to tools in a carpenter's toolbox. Which of these—the hammer, the saw, the screwdriver, among others—is most important for the carpenter? It depends on the nature of the job. Similarly, the usefulness and applicability of these various structures depend on the nature of the political conflict and the challenges facing the various actors. Different models will be more or less useful depending on what one is seeking to accomplish or to understand. To aid readers, I have grouped the models and chapters into three sections: basic ideas, key themes, and integrative models. Certainly, other writers would choose other models to include, leave some of my choices out, and create different groupings. I don't claim my choices are the best; I only hope readers find them useful.

Readers should also understand that while I portray the various models in ways that emphasize their usefulness, they are *just* models, with limitations as well as advantages. Usually, political or policy scientists focus all or most of their attention on a single model in their books. By presenting about a dozen—one or two per chapter—I hope to convey a sense of their limitations, and also of their complementary features. While they are presented in separate chapters, some of the best insights can be obtained by applying them in an infinite variety of combinations and concentrations. The integrative models in part 3 perform best on this score.

STORIES FROM A POLITICAL LIFE

I structured and wrote this book to be unlike any other about politics and policy I have read. A series of models or ways of understanding politics are presented in separate chapters that describe and discuss each particular construct. Paired with each model are one or more case stories from my own political life, taken mostly from my thirteen years as a member of the Massachusetts House of Representatives. The stories are written to provide readers with an in-depth, inside look at real-life politics and policymaking in one state legislature and, equally important, to illustrate the particular model under discussion.

I use the term *case story* instead of the more familiar expression *case study* to emphasize the personal aspect of these examples. From over one hundred possible cases, I chose ten that I found compelling and helpful illustrations of each conceptual model. The stories are told from my own perspective, which was central to each. I am acutely aware that other participants could—as in Allison—tell vastly different and equally valid stories about the same episodes from their distinctive vantage points. All chapters have been read for accuracy and authenticity by at least one person directly involved in the episode. Nonetheless, each is told to a significant degree from my personal perspective.

Half memoir and half guide to useful political and policy models, this book seeks to do something different from the vast majority of books that can be found in bookstores under the category of "current affairs" or "politics." Most of these books are either memoirs that relate "war stories" from an individual's career or ideological discussions that seek to define and shape current thinking, left, right, or center. There is not a lot in them that seeks to explain what politics is, how it really works, and how it feels to be in the middle of high-stakes political conflict. That's my aim. In the process, I hope to provide tools readers can learn to use themselves to become more effective political players. This book is also different from two other kinds of political books and sources. Journalistic accounts of political controversies and academic political science studies, because of their necessary and appropriate requirements for distance and objectivity, most often miss the *passion* that political activists experience and bring to their practice of politics. I'm not dismissing these efforts, just recognizing inherent limitations that leave many hungry for more.

As noted, the stories in this book are all taken from my own political life. Throughout my life, I have been unabashedly and without apology on the left of the political spectrum. The stories and my roles in them thus lean in that direction: health care access reform, tenants' rights, campaign finance reform, anti-death penalty. It is not my intention to proselytize readers or to convince them of the correctness of my positions or actions. My views on many of these issues have shifted over time. I hope readers with different beliefs and ideologies will not be repelled and will find value in exploring the models and learning about some of the realities of political and legislative life. The stories are presented to bring to life the conceptual models and to provide a real-life, inside look into the political and legislative arenas, no more and no less.

Readers will notice in the case stories and in the descriptions of various models a disproportionate reference to health care policy. That is because health policy was my area of specialization—and love—throughout my years in the House. Not all legislators choose to specialize, though many do, in areas such as criminal justice, environment, social services, transportation, insurance, housing, economic development, and education. I was widely recognized as a health policy specialist, and so I hope others interested and involved in health policy derive inordinate usefulness from this volume.

ORGANIZATION OF THE BOOK

Part 1, including chapters 1 and 2, presents the "Basics," several core ideas that permeate every successive chapter: first, a definition of politics, and second, a discussion of the ways language shapes political meaning.

Chapter 1 provides an answer to a question I ask frequently that stumps most people: what is politics? I find most people from all walks of life—including professional politicians—have great difficulty defining a term so commonly used that is such a universal dynamic affecting all our lives. Offering a definition seems a useful starting point. In describing a distinct and emblematic form of politics—electoral—I relate two stories of personal campaigns for elective office, one my race for class president in the sixth grade and the other my first race for state representative in 1984. We are never too young or too old to learn.

Chapter 2 presents less a specific model and more a method of understanding politics by examining how we talk with—or at—each other in the political world. In this chapter, I draw on the work of Deborah Stone, who presents a compelling analysis of how we use and misuse words, metaphors, numbers, and other rhetorical devices to create shared meanings to achieve political goals. Sometimes, creative use of these devices enhances understanding and smoothes the path to progress; at other times, they confuse and impede, deliberately or inadvertently. The case story in this chapter relates my involvement in 1990 with a street gang whose members called themselves the "X-Men" and who sought to control a part of my district called Egleston Square. Their story illustrates the striking ways language and perspective shape vastly differing political meanings.

Part 2, "Themes," includes three chapters, each presenting a set of concepts that infuse a substantial proportion of political life. The first discusses the central role of conflict in political life; the second explores the ever-present tension between public interest and self-interest; and the third examines the critical dynamics of representation and/versus relationships in politics.

Chapter 3 presents ways to think about the role of conflict in politics and policymaking. Many of us are taught that conflict is bad and something "nice people" avoid. Often, we wonder why our elected officials fight with each other so much instead of just working things out. Drawing on writings of Niccolò Machiavelli, E. E. Schattschneider, and others, I outline a structured way to think about conflict in the political realm. Two related case stories involve two groups who fight with each other nearly all the time—tenants and landlords—and two legislative battles over rent control and condominium conversion protections.

Chapter 4 discusses interests, large and small, organized and unorganized, and seeks to answer a controversial question: are we all just looking out for our own individual self-interest, or are we instead motivated by ideas and the "public good"? Is there such a thing as the "public interest," or is it, instead, just a cover for collective greed? The chapter explores the growth of "rational choice" models and the competition between them and other approaches emphasizing the power of public ideas. The case story describes intense and excruciating battles during a severe state fiscal crisis in 1989 and 1990, as well as a fierce dispute over the rights of elderly citizens who shelter their assets to avoid paying the state for their nursing home costs.

Chapter 5 explores two related concepts, representation and relationships. Representation presents a challenge nearly all elected officials face at some point: do I represent my own beliefs and conscience, or do I follow the will of my district? Writings of Hannah Pitkin and others provide useful guidance. I also use the representation dilemma to explore an equally important dynamic, the role of relationships. While it is easy just to say, "Relationships matter," I also explore a construct known as "agency theory" to understand them more concretely. The case story examines two related and vexing issues facing federal and state legislative bodies today, campaign finance and ethics reform. In the process, I explore the roles of representation and relationships, asking which, in the final analysis, matters more.

Part 3, "Models," presents two ways to understand key dynamics in politics and policy that combine many of the insights embedded in the previous chapters. The punctuated equilibrium model in chapter 6—as obscure as the name sounds—makes it easier to see when broad-based reform versus incremental change is possible. Chapter 7's agenda-setting model is an invaluable tool activists can use to chart and win political reforms.

Chapter 6 tackles the big picture, describing the nature of those brief, electric moments when broad-scale change—positive or negative—not only becomes possible but actually happens. The punctuated equilibrium model of policy change, developed by Frank Baumgartner and Bryan Jones, explains how this happens. Sometimes the only viable path is incremental, step-by-step change, whereas seeking reform too extensive can lead to nothing happening at all. Sometimes, though, major change is possible, and seeking modest reform wastes a historic opportunity. Deciding between these two scenarios is crucially important in politics. The punctuated equilibrium theory is a significant help. The case story involves big-picture change in Massachusetts hospital regulation in 1991. Three choices were presented: incremental tinkering with the existing structure, a huge governmental health expansion by establishing a "single-payer–Canadian" financing scheme, or deregulation and a sharp turn toward the market as the controller of the state's health future. Was this an opportunity for major, systemic change, and, if so, of what kind? When, why, and how a big change sometimes happens is the theme.

Chapter 7 explains why some issues get on the public agenda and receive speedy and favorable action, others get on the agenda but go nowhere, and still others never reach the public agenda at all. The answer can be found in Kingdon's agenda-setting model. I show how Kingdon's model explains the failure of President Bill Clinton's campaign for national health reform in 1993 and 1994 better than any explanation I have encountered. The case story illustrates my use of this model prospectively in 1995 and 1996 to seek passage of a major health care access law, a fight that required winning enough votes to override the veto of a popular incumbent governor.

Part 4, "Endings," wraps up the journey of this book with a simple and elegant dualism in chapter 8 that, to me, captures the essence of the political. Chapter 9 attempts the impossible: bringing it all together.

Chapter 8 presents one final way to understand politics by discussing two competing metaphors always in play, the conversation and the game. Which one better captures the essence of American politics at the opening of the twenty-first century? The case story relates my final legislative battle as a member of the Massachusetts House. This was a bitter dispute over whether to reinstitute capital punishment in the wake of a grisly and horrific murder—a dispute in which the dynamics of the conversation and of the game are both quite active.

Finally, in chapter 9, I pull these models and ideas together to provide some insights developed during my years in politics. I also present concluding perspectives on the role of legislatures and legislators, as well as my thoughts about the future of U.S. health care policy.

THE LEGISLATIVE CONTEXT

Because the case stories in this book focus primarily on the legislative portion of public policymaking, it will be helpful for some to understand the broader context of which legislating is only one part. Those who took social studies in high school are familiar with the tripartite division of labor in federal and state policymaking in the United States among the executive, legislative, and judicial functions.

A different and useful model provided by Beaufort Longest describes two distinct and consecutive policy phases, each with two separate parts. The first phase, "Policy Formulation," contains the first step, "agenda setting," by which issues/problems reach the public policy agenda for discussion and potential action, and the second step, "development of legislation," where issues that reach the public agenda are either addressed by enactment of statutes or laid aside. Issues that successfully navigate the first phase move to the second, "Policy Implementation" (sometimes referred to as the "bureaucratization of policy"), which contains the third step, "rule or regulation making," and the fourth step, "operation," where policies are put into action.[5] Policy implementation always creates consequences, outcomes, and perceptions resulting in feedback that often triggers a third, "Policy Modification," phase. Once triggered, policies often need to be modified at any one of the four prior steps, resetting the process in motion. The Longest framework is presented in schematic form below:

Phase I: Policy Formulation
Step One: Agenda Setting
Step Two: Development of Legislation

bridged by enactment of legislation, leads to

Phase II: Policy Implementation
Step Three: Rule or Regulation Making
Step Four: Operation

creating consequences, outcomes, perceptions
creating feedback that can trigger

Phase III: Policy Modification

Legislators often will be key players in step one, the agenda-setting stage, though just as often they are not, and other officials or interests play that role. (Agenda setting is the central model in chapter 7.) Legislators normally, though not always, will be less involved in steps three and four, the rule-making and operation phases. Legislators will often be involved in triggering the policy modification phase. Legislators and legislatures always are indispensably and centrally involved in the second step, the development of legislation. A policy proposal moves forward or dies, most of the time, depending on the actions of legislative bodies. While their role in the overall policy process is not all-encompassing, it is crucial.

It must be noted that this volume is not intended as a guide to state legislatures as institutions or to the behavior of legislators as a group. That work has been performed admirably by others, most notably, Alan Rosenthal of Rutgers University, who tracks the historical evolution of state legislatures in the modern era and wonderfully captures their essence in the 1990s.[6] Tom Loftus, former Speaker of the Wisconsin State Assembly, provides an enlightening view of his institution in *The Art of Legislative Politics*.[7]

A NOTE ABOUT MASSACHUSETTS

Though the themes and ideas of this book are intended to be helpful to anyone, all of the case stories focus on Massachusetts state government, and its House of Representatives in particular. Accordingly, a little background information is in order.

Massachusetts, with more than six million residents, is the nation's thirteenth-largest state (one of four called a "commonwealth") and among its most reliably liberal-progressive (though its voters did choose Ronald Reagan in 1980 and 1984 as well as Republican governors in the three state elections in the 1990s). Governors play a major role in politics and policy, and four of them loom large in various chapters of this book. Liberal Democrat Michael Dukakis served between 1975 and 1978, and then again between 1983 and 1990. His nemesis, conservative Democrat (later turned Republican) Edward J. King, served between 1979 and 1982. Libertarian Republican William Weld served between 1991 and 1997, and moderate Republican Argeo Paul Cellucci filled out the remainder of Weld's second term beginning in August 1997 and was elected to the office in his own right in 1998.

The Massachusetts Senate and House of Representatives are known collectively as the General Court. The Senate includes 40 members with districts of about 150,000 persons, and the House includes 160 with districts including about 36,000 persons. Both have been overwhelmingly dominated by Democrats since the late 1950s, with Senate Republicans numbering between 7 and 16 during the course of this book, and House Republicans numbering between 27 and 36. The two key members in the Senate are the presiding officer—the President—and the chairman of the Senate Committee on Ways and Means, which initiates all spending bills. In the House, the presiding officer is the Speaker, and the chairman of the House Committee on Ways and Means also exercises huge influence. During the course of this volume, I interacted with four Speakers, each strikingly different from the others: Thomas McGee of Lynn (1975 to 1984), George Keverian of Everett (1985 to 1990), Charles Flaherty of Cambridge (1991 to 1996), and Thomas Finneran of Boston (1996 to the present). They will be introduced in greater detail during the course of the book.

Except for the committees on ways and means and a few others, the vast majority of legislative committees in the Massachusetts General Court are joint House-Senate bodies, each with six senators and eleven representatives. All bills—with the exception of budget appropriations bills, which go directly to House Ways and Means—are first referred to a joint committee for a public hearing and consideration. Each committee is cochaired by a senator (named by the President) and a representative (named by the Speaker). After the two top leaders in each branch, the committee chairs wield the greatest amount of influence, particularly over the fate of legislation that emerges from each one's respective joint committee. While party caucuses in each branch ratify the President's/Speaker's nominees for chairmanships, it was always done pro forma during my years in the House. Because chairs have greater influence and prestige, and because they receive a salary hike of between $7,500 and $15,000, selection as a chair has great consequence for each individual legislator (at the time of this book's writing, the base salary for all senators and representatives was about $46,000). Because of the President's/Speaker's near-complete control over the selection process, they both hold enormous power over their respective chambers. Each individual who becomes President or Speaker makes a different choice as to how to exercise that power—as will be evident throughout the book.

Proposed legislation—called a bill—that emerges from a joint committee travels sequentially through the House and then the Senate, or vice versa. If one chamber refuses to act on a bill, the other can do nothing formally to pry that matter loose. Appropriations (budget) bills must always go through the House first. Once released from committee, non-budget bills cannot be amended on the floor "beyond the scope" of the original bill; however, appropriations bills can be amended on the floor to include virtually anything, budget-related or not.

Prior to 1995, each session lasted for one year, from the first Wednesday in January to Tuesday midnight prior to the successive first Wednesday in January. Any bill not sent to the governor's desk prior to the midnight deadline died. Changes to the joint rules in 1995 created two-year sessions that permit bills to carry over from the odd-numbered to the even-numbered year, 1995–96 and 1997–98. Formal sessions are required now to conclude on July 31 of the even-numbered year, though both chambers may continue to meet until the end of the year in "informal" sessions where unanimous consent is required for all matters acted upon. While these procedural points may seem arcane, they are mentioned here because each has key relevance to several of the case stories. They are repeated at appropriate points.

FINAL POINTS

In writing this book, I was acutely aware that most of the men and women with whom I served in the Massachusetts legislature between 1985 and 1997 could have written a book full of stories at least as interesting and compelling as mine. Then again, the same could be said for the thousands of men and women serving in the other forty-nine state legislatures, not to mention the U.S. Congress. Any member who serves any length of time in any legislative body in the nation (federal, state, county, or local) has stories that reveal truths not just about legislating but also about human frailty and courage, humor and tragedy, honor and dishonor, growth and regression, challenges and change. Their stories are everywhere.

That begs a question: what is so special, then, about my stories? Not a whole lot. I simply had the idea, the time, and the energy to put them together in this volume in a way that, I hope, will inform and enlighten readers. I also hope pairing my stories with the models gives each story more relevance, power, and value. I have the modest ambition that telling these stories will help to create better understanding of government, policymaking, and politics in ways that will lead to the improvement of all three. I tell stories involving my own political work and my distinctive role because those are the ones I can truly tell from the point of view of an inside participant. I hope this volume will encourage other legislators and political actors to come forward with their stories. So many I have heard richly deserve telling to wide audiences.

Throughout this book, I reject the negative, cynical view of politics so pervasive in our society and culture. It is not my contention that politics is always good. Politics itself is neither good nor bad. It is a neutral force everyone of us uses in some way in all of our lives. Whether the practice of politics turns out for good or evil depends very much on the values we bring to our political engagements and on our personal perspectives about the appropriate uses of power. Politics is inherently neither bad nor good—it's what we choose to make of it. Many people— liberal, conservative, or whatever—get involved in political activity and leave dispirited and disgusted. They assume that the right of everyone to participate should somehow guarantee their right to win. But the best political actors know losses are as common as wins, and the only real losers are those who abandon the field to others.

Another cultural theme suggests politics is about "them": cigar-smoking pols who inhabit the lobbies and dark-paneled offices of Congress, state capitols, and city and town halls. In this thinking, politics is about what "they" do to "us," how they take advantage of us to feather their nests and to satisfy their constant needs for ego gratification, cash, and reelection. This volume suggests, instead, politics is about "us," about the needs of ordinary people and how they get translated effectively or poorly into policies. How much politics is about "them" is heavily determined by the degree to which the political arena is abandoned or neglected by "us." My challenge and hope are to help readers become more familiar and comfortable with life in the arena so that you will want to join.

PART ONE

Basics

Politics does not come easy to many people. It is commonly seen as an external, threatening force that undermines fair play and rewards the undeserving by favoring connections over merit. Political talk is often regarded either as unreal discourse that disguises genuine and serious disagreement for a self-interested and false sense of unity or as rhetoric that needlessly polarizes to achieve selfish advantage.

O.K., it's true! But is that all there is to politics?

These first two chapters place the political in a more neutral context, first by defining our essential term and second by describing the various uses of language in political life. The themes of these two chapters set the stage for all that follows. The definition of politics presented in chapter 1 and the discussion of political language in chapter 2 resonate inside every subsequent model and in each case story. The stories are also introductory—introducing readers to my early political experience in the sixth grade, to my first campaign for state representative, and to the streets of my district.

CHAPTER ONE

Politics Is . . .
and Debating Points

Politics is show business for ugly people.

Jay Leno

When speaking with groups, I often begin by asking if anyone can give me a definition for the word *politics*. Because nearly everyone has used the word, most often in a pejorative sense, it is always intriguing to watch people struggle for an answer to a question they have never before been asked.

"'Poli' is from the Greek, and that means 'many,' and tics are bloodsucking insects," said one respondent. I liked that one so much, I usually repeat it up front.

"Republicans and Democrats" is a frequent reply. They are both very much a part of politics, I answer, but so is a lot else that has nothing to do with either or any political party.

"Working for compromise," says another. Sometimes politics is about compromise, consensus, and negotiation—some refer to these as the basic tools of politics, like the carpenter's hammer, saw, and screwdriver—but sometimes politics is about imposing one's will on a recalcitrant individual, about confrontation, government shutdowns, threats of war, and brinkmanship.

"Government and taxes," suggests one. Most certainly there are politics in government; and tax policy is *always* political. But politics happens outside of government—the office, the family, the church—as well as inside.

"People," says someone, thinking expansively. Hmmm, I respond. One of former U.S. House Speaker Newt Gingrich's favorite books is called

Chimpanzee Politics [1] (required reading for first-year House Republicans
in 1995), which discusses in absorbing detail political conflict and power
struggles among primates. Besides, while politics is a major dynamic in
human society, there is also a lot more going on in our lives than just the
political—something politicians and political scientists need to remind
themselves of often.

It is instructive that nearly everyone—from highly educated professionals to regular working folks—has difficulty defining what we mean
by something as universal as politics. Thus, it makes sense to begin by
offering the definition I find most helpful and providing a series of illustrations that bring it to life. Discussion of two key stories from my deep
political past follows to illustrate two common and key facets of politics: elections and debates.

POLITICS IS . . .

Politics is the way people decide who gets what, when, where, how,
and why—without resorting to violence. Political scientist Harold
Lasswell came up with the core of this definition in the 1930s, the "who
gets what . . ." part.[2] I borrowed the secondary phrase from Hannah
Arendt. No other definition I have encountered is as easily accessible and
comes as close to capturing the broad essence of political phenomena.

"Who" refers to the winner-loser-contestant in a political conflict, for
example, Al Gore versus George Bush in an electoral contest, senior citizens versus hospitals in a Medicare budget fight, two or more aspiring
managers in a match of office politics, or a neighborhood civic group
versus a real estate developer in a community zoning dispute.

"What" relates to the stakes in the battle, for example, preservation
of an endangered species in an environmental politics fight, creation of
a voting district designed to empower a particular group in a redistricting process, or custody of the family dog in the personal politics surrounding a contested divorce.

"When" suggests that timing often can be a critical element in determining the achievement of a political goal. For example, passing the federal line-item veto was considered an impossibility before Republicans
took control of both houses of the U.S. Congress in 1995 but an easy
legislative win thereafter (until it was overturned by the U.S. Supreme

Court); maneuvering one's boss for a pay raise will be a lot more difficult after an unfavorable earnings report; promoting passage of a death penalty statute may be substantially more successful after a grisly and callous murder.

"Where" indicates that political possibilities may differ from one terrain to the next. For example, passing gay rights legislation in liberal Massachusetts will be easier than in conservative Alabama; locating a halfway house for substance abusers in a highly organized and affluent suburb can be much more difficult than in a poorly organized and disadvantaged neighborhood; paying hospitals for providing the same service will result in different levels of payment for urban teaching versus rural community institutions; getting one's spouse to spend time with the in-laws may be easier if those relatives live in the same geographic area as opposed to an island in the Caribbean. Another lively example of the "where" in politics involves the strenuous efforts of state and city governments to lure professional sports teams to their vicinities.

"How" explains the way strategies and tactics influence political outcomes. For example, one nation offers favorable trade status in exchange for the adoption of various human rights protections; the federal government convinces states to provide health insurance to uninsured children by offering new and generous financial incentives; a young groom convinces his bride-to-be to take his last name after getting his friends and family members to pressure her to agree.

"Why" synthesizes all of the above to explain why some person, group, or other entity (1) got what they wanted, (2) did not get what they wanted, (3) got what they did not want, or (4) did not get what they did not want.

The phrase "without resorting to violence" places politics on a continuum of methods by which rights and resources within a society are distributed. At one end of the continuum is democratic political action in a civil society; at the other end are violence, dictatorship, and war where normal civic functions have been eliminated or have lost their capacity to work. In other words, political action is the principal alternative to violence in figuring out how to deal with the disparate needs, desires, and values in society. Hannah Arendt describes this in *The Human Condition*: "To be political, to be *in polis* meant that everything was decided through words and persuasion and not through force and violence."[3]

This definition is not meant to suggest that political issues are necessarily decided in a democratic or fair manner. Most often, the way that rules and processes are established—for example, the process leading to the creation and ratification of the U.S. Constitution—is a highly charged political exercise. The result may be inclusive or exclusive, democratic or authoritarian, open or closed, equitable or highly unfair, or any mix of the above. Once the process is set, people act politically to get the best result they can through that process. If people are unable to get what they want out of the process—be it a rule, regulation, statute, or constitution— they often will attempt to change the rules governing the process, or the process itself, which sets off yet another exercise in politics. Recent attempts to change the U.S. Constitution to require a balanced federal budget or to limit the number of terms that senators and representatives can serve are examples of efforts to change the process by groups dissatisfied with the results of their political activities under the prevailing rules.

Generally, Americans have a negative impression of politics, and that impression has grown steadily worse over the past fifty years. This assertion is supported by surveys that have asked whether people trust the federal government. In the 1950s and 1960s, more than 70 percent of Americans said they "always" or "most of the time" trusted the federal government to do the right thing; by the mid-1990s, the percentage had dropped consistently to the low–20 percent range.[4] But as I observed in my introduction, politics inherently is neither good nor bad. It is a neutral force. Whether it turns out to be good or bad depends heavily on the values one brings to the exercise of politics. Of course, just because one person's values suggest that his or her political activity is high minded and ethical does not mean that others have to agree.

While politics, itself, is a neutral force, the absence or collapse of politics may be quite harmful. Politics is the way that individuals and groups in a society—fairly or not—figure out how to distribute rights and privileges as well as duties and obligations. When some groups decide that the political deck is unfairly stacked against them and feel that their ability to change the system is rigged, they may resort to violence—witness Yugoslavia, Lebanon, Eritrea, Rwanda, and others of the world's contemporary hot spots where civil political processes have broken down in recent decades. South Africa and Northern Ireland, on the other hand, are examples of the potential for politics to resolve conflict and avoid violence. Both dynamics, politics and war, are at their core about "who gets what . . . ." In civil society, we try to do this through politics, and it is in our collective self-interest to see that our political processes work as fairly and effectively as possible.

The absence of politics is not necessarily good and in fact can mark an unhealthy situation. A drought of political activity may mean that certain disadvantaged groups have been shut out of an ability to participate and to claim a fair share of society's resources. One can think of the pre-1960s southern states where African Americans were systematically excluded from the political process through legal restrictions, intimidation, and violence. Machiavelli noted that the ability of citizens to create civil conflict to press their political demands is an essential element of a healthy society: "Nothing makes a republic so stable and strong as organizing it in such a way that the agitation of the hatreds which excite it has a means of expressing itself provided for by the laws."[5] The cacophony of loud voices raised to make selfish or selfless political demands, operating within a system that gives them the guaranteed ability to press their demands—though not the guaranteed right to win—is a healthy sign of a strong and vibrant society.

Some suggest that politics and violence/war are not opposites but instead simply alternative mechanisms to achieve one's ends, to get whatever one wants. The Chinese Communist leader Mao Tse-tung wrote, "Politics is war without bloodshed, while war is politics with bloodshed."[6] And the Prussian General Karl von Clausewitz wrote, "War is nothing but a continuation of politics with the admixture of other means."[7] Indeed, even within a totalitarian regime held together by the threat of violence or even in an armed conflict, politics will also be at play in innumerable ways all the time. While the relationship between the two is often quite close, there is a world of difference between political and violent means to achieve one's objectives. But recognizing how close these two essential human dynamics are to each other should elevate our appreciation for the importance of a healthy and robust politics in our societies and lives.

Some criticize the definition of politics as "who gets what . . ." as selfish and demeaning. Politics, they argue, should be about more than self-interest and the desire to acquire. This criticism views the definition of politics too narrowly. While "who gets what . . ." frequently refers to money or other self-interested claims, the definition easily encompasses the advocacy of highly moral and ethical demands, for example, the struggles by African Americans in the 1960s for voting rights, by Indians for independence from Great Britain in the 1940s, and by disabled Americans in the 1990s for access to services most of us take for granted. These were all blatant political struggles over "who gets what . . ." In these examples, the "what" refers to basic rights most of us take for granted.

These are three of many examples showing how political conflict can transform societies in highly moral ways.

The practice of politics involves both science and art. Political science is the academic study of who gets what, when, where, how, and why. Through an array of theories and models, rigorous and otherwise, political science helps us to understand political phenomena in a systematic way. Politics can be studied as a science because there are behaviors and patterns in politics that repeat. Political scientists can pose and test hypotheses that seek to explain political behavior. Other political scientists can test these same ideas and find similar results or find dissimilar results that disprove the theories. But politics is also an art because each individual engaged in political conflict can bring a personal perspective that may substantially alter outcomes in ways no empirical model can fully capture or predict. While the same combinations of paints mixed together in precisely the same way produce the same new colors, each artist can use these raw materials to produce a distinctive result and statement. So it is in politics.

Most people associate politics with the activities of government, public elected officials, and political parties. This is a traditional and accepted view of politics, and some theorists contend that our sense of the "political realm" should go no further. Substantial attention is paid to political activities in government at all levels because when public officials make decisions about who gets what, they are generally talking about the public's rights and resources. Governments pass laws that compel behaviors by all individuals within their respective jurisdictions. Governments collect money in numerous ways from individuals and firms and then redistribute these resources in even more numerous ways to individuals, firms, and other levels of government. It is entirely appropriate for the public and the media to display an aggressive and disproportionate interest in watching, analyzing, and influencing the political activities and decisions of public officials.

But politics is not confined to the public sphere. Wherever one looks in human society, we find politics—in private businesses, churches, schools, schoolyards, hospitals, families, and elsewhere. Frequently, new students will say to me, "I don't know anything about politics." I reply that they may not know a lot about the structures of politics in the public sector, but if they are alive and breathing, and interacting with other humans, they know a lot more about politics than they give themselves credit for.

In the 1960s, first the civil rights movement and then the feminist

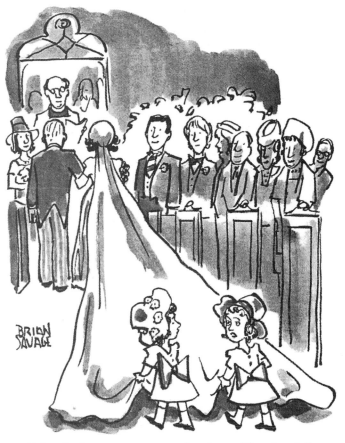

"It's all about power—getting it and keeping it."

movement opened our understanding toward this broader scope of politics. The feminist slogan "the personal is political" altered our political consciousness with profound implications for society. Matters that previously had been considered beyond the appropriate purview of public policy—domestic violence and child abuse, for example—became accepted topics for political discourse. Who gets what—in divorce, custody, control of one's body, and so on—changed and continues to change in dramatic ways as society broadens its sense of the "political." Today, some worry that we have taken our concept of the political too far, and into too many spheres. It is difficult to imagine, though, how the clock could be turned back.

Others challenge my preferred definition of politics by asserting that the law is another way that we decide who gets what in society short of violence. While it is true that countless decisions over who gets what are decided in our courts, we can see that the ways the legal system is structured and managed are inherently political. For example, all judges are either elected in their own right or else nominated and confirmed by elected politicians; who gets what fits quite appropriately into judicial selection and screening. Even more basic, all the statutes and regulations that courts interpret and enforce are created and revised by elected political bodies or by appointed officials under the control of elected politicians. The law, for better or worse, is an extension and instrument of our political systems.

One helpful way to test the usefulness of a definition is to try it out with familiar categories. Following are some recognizable categories of politics presented here to test the definition of politics as the way people decide who gets what, when, where, how and why—without resorting to violence.

→ELECTORAL POLITICS

Who gets the office, be it U.S. president, senator, city councillor, alderman, school committee member, ward committee chairman, student council president, labor union secretary treasurer, condominium association president, chair of a local gay rights organization, minister, or thousands and thousands of other positions—public or private—chosen by vote?

⇝ BUDGET POLITICS

Who gets what levels of resources from federal, state, county, municipal, or private budgets, for what purposes, and from whom? Governments obtain their revenues from a variety of sources and then pursue a political process to determine how those funds will be allocated. In state government, for example, choices are made among uses such as education, municipal aid, prisons, health needs, environmental programs, transportation and public works, tax cuts, public assistance, courts, and much more. Each one of these uses has a host of interest groups, lobbyists, and activists determined to get the largest possible share of the pie.

HEALTH CARE POLITICS

How much money is allocated for health purposes, and how are those funds distributed to, for example, hospitals, physicians, health plans, home health programs, public health initiatives, and community health centers? Within each of these categories, controversies also emerge concerning who gets what: teaching versus community versus rural versus public hospitals; primary-care physicians versus specialists; inpatient versus outpatient services; home and community versus institutional services. Who gets what rights when they belong to a managed-care organization? Who gets the right to have physician-assisted suicide?

REDISTRICTING POLITICS

Who gets what populations and borders when the time comes to redraw political district boundaries? Officeholders will seek to get and hold onto as many like-minded voters as possible and to minimize concentrations of voters who may not be as supportive. A familiar subtheme of this topic involves racial and ethnic issues, namely, who gets how many African Americans and/or Hispanics drawn into their districts? In the politics of the year 2000 U.S. census, another fight involves who gets or does not get statistically sampled as an alternative to the traditional mail and door-to-door methods.

CIVIL RIGHTS POLITICS

Who gets what protections written into law to guard against discriminatory treatment? Who gets special consideration to mitigate the effects of past discrimination? Who, if anyone, gets preferential treatment for jobs and educational admissions? In this political arena, as in many others, we can observe both internal politics—among and within various organizations for dominance and influence (that is, National Association for the Advancement of Colored People versus Urban League versus Southern Christian Leadership Conference)—and external politics involving these groups and non–civil rights groups opposed to or supportive of their goals and activities.

→ EDUCATIONAL POLITICS

Who gets to teach evolution versus creationism? Who gets a new school building in their community, and who pays for it? Who gets tenure, and who does not? Who gets public education resources: the traditional public school system or quasi-public charter schools? Who gets public dollars to promote higher education: the state university system or scholarship programs to help students attend private universities?

→ GAY AND LESBIAN POLITICS

Who gets legal protection against discrimination based on sexual preference? Who gets to determine what issues the gay rights agenda will include in the coming year? Who gets the right to marry? Who gets the right to take care of foster children?

→ OFFICE POLITICS

Who gets the best office, the one with the corner window? Who gets the job title, the promotion, the raise? Who gets the burden of having to sit next to the copier machine? Who gets access to other employees' E-mail folders?

→ NEIGHBORHOOD POLITICS

Who gets public permission via zoning approval to build an extension onto his or her house? Whose neighborhood gets the new subsidized housing for mentally ill individuals? How late will the corner tavern be permitted to stay open? Who gets to be (or gets stuck as) the leader of the local block association?

→ FAMILY POLITICS

Who takes care of the kids on the weekend? Who gets what household chores? Who gets to watch their favorite television program when there's a conflict in scheduling? Who gets the kids or the house or the car in a marital separation? Who gets to have Thanksgiving dinner at their house?

While we can observe politics nearly everywhere, it is also important to state that not everything is about politics. This is especially valuable for practicing politicians and political scientists to remember. They can easily get carried away and assume that nearly everything is political, in the same way that economists, psychologists, and other social scientists can overemphasize the influence and importance of their own specialized domains. There *is* more to life than politics; it's just that sometimes it doesn't seem that way to many of us.

Following are two case stories from my political life that are examples of who gets what, when, where, how, and why in electoral politics. The first is about my sixth-grade election for class president, and the second is about my first race for state representative in 1984.

✗DEBATING POINTS

→"Should the United States of America annex Canada?"

That was the discussion question of the hour in our sixth-grade modern U.S. history course. It was a question, unknown to me at the time, that would launch my lifelong involvement in electoral politics. The time was the fall of 1964, when Lyndon Johnson and Barry Goldwater were battling for the U.S. presidency in the wake of John F. Kennedy's assassination, the civil rights movement was operating at a fever pitch, and the Beatles were most constantly on the minds of the nation's youth. The place was St. Luke's Catholic grammar school in Belmont, Massachusetts, the original home of the resolutely anticommunist John Birch Society. I recall a grammar workbook we used in English class that taught proper language usage by having us diagram sentences that doubled as anticommunist and anti-Soviet messages ("Joseph Stalin, the hangman of the Ukraine, and Nikita Khrushchev, the butcher of Budapest, were two dictators of the Soviet Union"). Dominican sisters with names such as Sister Francis de Sales, Sister Mary Ona, and Sister Veracunda (yes, *Veracunda*) ran the school with firm discipline in their black hoods and full-length white habits. Their thick black rosary beads reached from the waist to the ankle and could be swung at us with menacing effect. My Irish immigrant mother, when asked by friends how she liked our school, would always answer in her sweet brogue, "Well, I like the nuns, because they're *tough*." She displayed an innate sense of politics by delivering in person, with her four children in tow, several fruitcakes per year to the sisters' plain brick convent.

My class consisted of thirty-five boys and girls, born in the bulge of the baby boom in 1953, coming exclusively from local Irish and Italian American families. Our teacher, a youngish Italian American nun named Sister Mary Thomasine, had unusual and distinctly liberal proclivities, beseeching us to watch the NBC evening news every night with Chet Huntley and David Brinkley and leading us to ask critical questions about matters such as U.S. involvement in South Vietnam and changing practices in the post–Vatican II Roman Catholic Church that reflected her own ambivalent feelings. By 1964, the shades of 1950s-style McCarthyism and conservatism were lifting. The Kennedy assassination was a deep blow but was eclipsed by the optimism of rock and roll, space exploration, the civil rights movement, a growing economy, and a burgeoning and maturing youth population.

On this fall day, the topic was geopolitical, the United States versus the Soviet Union, and the Cold War struggle for world dominance. In that context, one of the discussion questions at the end of the history textbook chapter was "Should the United States annex Canada?"

"What do you think?" asked Sister Mary Thomasine.

"It would give us strategic access to the polar ice cap," said Guy Oliva, leading off a parade of comments about how beneficial it would be for American interests to capture all the resources and wealth the Canadians had to offer.

Something about the tenor of the conversation irritated me enough to raise my hand. When finally recognized, I flamed: "Who are we to think that the Canadians would want to be a part of us? Don't they have anything to say about this? They have their own history, traditions, and culture, and lots of pride in who they are already. How would we feel if they just assumed that we would become a part of them? We have no more right to tell them that they should want to be a part of us than they should say that to us."

My comment set off a collective light bulb over the class: "Oh, yeah, guess that wouldn't be such a neat idea." Sister Mary Thomasine, pleased that someone saw the question as she did, wrapped up the discussion reminding us to respect the culture and integrity of others, and not to assume that what's good for us is good for the rest of the world.

As the class ended, Sister told us that she wanted to make an announcement. "We will be holding an election for class president in the next few weeks; anyone who wants to run should nominate him or herself in the next few days."

Instantly, every one of the thirty-four or so heads in the room turned to look at me in the back of the room where I sat at my desk. I had no idea what a class president was and had never given a second's thought to being one. If the election had been held at that moment, based on my prescient geopolitical comments, my fellow students would have elected me by a near-unanimous margin. Outside in the schoolyard during recess, my classmates smelled a winner and came up to me in droves to tell me I should run. My closest friends—Chris McDonald, Michael Cullen, and Steve Dolan—quickly organized themselves as my campaign committee, though their duties, and mine, remained thoroughly imprecise. They herded me to Sister Mary Thomasine, who kept a watchful eye on us in the playground.

"Sister," I told her, "I would like to run for class president."

Over the next week, the shape of the field became clear as four others joined the race. Mary Ellen McElroy was, I felt, a real threat, the only girl in the race, smart, and the one with the clearest shot at winning if she only could rally her gender, which slightly outnumbered the boys. I had known and liked Guy Oliva and John Roth since first grade, and both had outside shots at winning. One final surprise entrant did not seem particularly fearsome: Tom Loftus had joined our sixth-grade class only several months earlier, an extremely rare occurrence in our school. While he was evidently bright and likable, no one knew him well enough for me to give him a realistic shot. Thus I was more amused than concerned when he approached me and my campaign cohorts in the schoolyard during recess later that week.

"John, I would like to challenge you to a debate on who should be class president. Are you willing to debate me?" he asked earnestly.

"Sure," I half laughed. "Why not?"

Why—the more appropriate question should have been—would I agree to debate only one of my opponents, and not all of them? But political and campaign strategy were unknown concepts to me at the time, and we went together to Sister Mary Thomasine to request a one-on-one debate. Sensing that her experiment in juvenile democracy was bearing fruit, she readily agreed.

Several days later, two desks at the front of the room were turned to face the class, with Tom and I seated at them. On the basis of a coin flip, Tom got to make a statement first, followed by me, and then we could ask each other questions. Unlike me, and much to my shocked surprise, Tom actually had something to say: "If I am elected president, I will set up a series of committees made up of all of you so that everyone can participate and have a role to play in the class."

This was startling to me. Not only did he have something to say, he actually had an idea. And my turn was coming up next. I had better think of something to say, and something fast. Why did I ever agree to debate this kid? Is there any way I can get out of this? Darn, it's too late now! Uh oh, it's my turn . . . what to say?

"Well, I also think that we should set up committees," I began. "I want to get everyone involved. But I think it's important that we not set up too many committees. Especially at the start. Because if we set up too many, then if something really important comes up, all the smart kids will already be on other committees, and all we'll have left for something that may be real important are the dumb ones . . ."

A silence fell over the room. I could read the minds of my thirty-four classmates: "Did he *really* say that?" I could read my own mind: "Did I *really* just say that?"

". . . and that . . . would be . . . too bad," I concluded.

Unable to recover, unsure what to do, I sat down, awaiting Tom's opportunity to ask me a question.

"John," he said, grabbing the metaphorical knife I had just stuck in my back and pushing it in further to make sure that it would not slip out, "would you be so good as to tell us *who* you mean by 'the dumb ones'?"

Ouch! What to say? "Of course not," I stammered. "Would you?"

"I," he demurred, "would not refer to any of our classmates as 'the dumb ones.'"

Except maybe me, I thought.

With a week left until the vote, I had instantly become the political equivalent of a "dead man walking." My campaign committee tried valiantly to cheer me up, but the damage was done. My older brother, Gerry, a budding cartoonist, drew clever cartoons on index cards to promote my candidacy. After I placed them on my classmates' desks one morning before classes began, my secret crush walked over to me and ripped up the card in my face. A wounded puppy, I could only stand there and stare blankly at her.

When the votes were counted, I came in last, with four votes out of thirty-five, and knowing each one of them. Tom Loftus came in first, the hands-down winner. I learned how to be a good loser and congratulate a winner. Except I could not help noticing that over the course of the school year, he never set up any committees. I didn't care, being so relieved that my embarrassing ordeal was over. I slunk back into my pre-Canadian anonymity and vowed never to run for anything again.

·   ·   ·

Twenty years later, in 1984, I was back on the campaign trail. This time the office was Massachusetts state representative for the Twelfth Suffolk District, which included parts of the Boston neighborhoods of Jamaica Plain, Roxbury, and Roslindale. I had moved to Jamaica Plain in 1976, fulfilling a longing I had had since my early youth to live in the neighborhood of the legendary Irish American political figure James Michael Curley, former Boston mayor, U.S. congressman, and governor, who was immortalized in the 1950s novel and film *The Last Hurrah*. Curley enjoyed the reputation of urban populist and rascal and used his city connections to finance construction of a gorgeous Georgian-style mansion near the shores of Jamaica Pond, with shamrocks carved into the window shutters so no one would confuse his home with that of his more prosperous Brahmin neighbors.

For about ten years before she married, my mother lived in that mansion as maid and cook to the Curley family. The youngest of thirteen children born in the poor village of Knock in Ireland's County Mayo— the village in which the Blessed Virgin Mary is purported to have appeared to a group of young children in 1879—she had come to the United States at age twenty in 1938, shortly after Curley gave up his hold on the governor's office in an unsuccessful run for a United State Senate seat, a gambit similar to one that failed sixty years later for his Brahmin successor William Weld. Nellie Morley just happened to be looking for a housekeeping position at an employment agency when Curley was looking to fill an opening in his household. She became an integral part of the Curley family, especially to "the governor," as he was always called, who regarded her as a daughter. Curley's raucous political life was laced with tragedy as he endured the early deaths of his first wife and seven of his nine children, two on the same day, and one of those discovered by my mother.

My mother was most honored when the governor asked to be the host of her wedding, scheduled for October 1947 at Our Lady of Lourdes Church on Montebello Road in Jamaica Plain. But it became difficult to arrange when Curley was sentenced at the same time to serve a prison term for mail fraud in a Danbury, Connecticut, federal penitentiary. Nellie readily agreed to delay her marriage ceremony until June 1948 when the governor would be freed. My father, Joseph, a grocery store manager and immigrant from Galway, Ireland, raised no objections and patiently waited. The governor realized his wish and hosted the joyous wedding party.

By the time I had begun my campaign to run for state rep in early

1984, few of my base supporters had any particular memory or feeling about James Michael Curley beyond the twin statues of him standing and seated between downtown Boston's City and Faneuil Halls. The African Americans, Hispanics, young professionals, and neighborhood progressives that formed my political core were not part of his natural base. But for the older, conservative Irish establishment, whose numbers were still substantial in Jamaica Plain, the connection was meaningful and gave them a sense that—whatever their misgivings—I was one of them.

The most important question for this latter group was whether I was a worthy successor to another Jamaica Plain institution, James (Jimmy) J. Craven, Jr., who had served as state representative for nearly thirty years, who wanted to keep going, and who was both legendary and notorious in the community and in the State House on Beacon Hill. Like Curley, Craven had worked his way up from urban poverty and tough streets to respectability and power. And like Curley, he epitomized a generation of politicians who defined themselves by naming and taunting their enemies and by their robust delight in scrapping with them. Craven had nurtured and developed a strong base of working-class, church-centered Irish support and held onto it by constantly referring to the many wolves at the door who threatened the residents' security and values: liberals, carpetbaggers, abortionists, communists, homosexuals, church haters, to name a few. It was "us against them" politics, and he left no doubt that he would provide protection as well as the jobs and other favors that came with powerful State House connections.

Craven's combative style always reached its zenith during campaign seasons, when opponents would find themselves swamped on the ballot by "straw" candidates whose sole purpose was to split up the anti-incumbent vote. Late-night, last-minute, anonymous leaflet drops would hurl accusations that candidates had little time to counter. One candidate who had taken a Chinese history course at Harvard found himself labeled a "Red Chinese Communist." Tricks to throw opponents off balance were also common. An anonymous flyer advised readers to call a certain telephone number for "a free camera," only to tie up telephone lines at an opponent's campaign headquarters during election day. A Craven campaign was a reminder and relic of a lost era—before television and other diversions—when politics was entertainment and sport mixed into one.

At the State House, Craven was nicknamed "the silver fox" for both his full head of silver, combed-back hair and his legendary skill in maneuvering benefits and largesse for his favored projects and groups. Having served longer in the House than any other member, he proudly advertised his honorary title, "dean of the House of Representatives," with delight. Though he was never entrusted with the chairmanship of any committee, he long held onto a seat on the key budget-writing House Committee on Ways and Means and played that position skillfully to extract his legislative wins.

But Craven's hardball tactics could also backfire. In 1978, he threatened officials in the state's Executive Office of Communities and Development with budget retaliation if they failed to award a state grant to a favored neighborhood group. The agency fearfully complied. But when it came out that the group rented space in a building owned by his family's realty trust, the newly formed State Ethics Commission made him its test case of an official to be charged with misconduct and conflict of interest. Rather than pay a fine and accept the commission's token slap, he fought—and lost—at every step, up to and including the State Supreme Judicial Court in 1983. When the House Ethics Committee recommended a formal reprimand, Craven took the floor of the House to decry its actions as "supine, dishonorable, shameful, cowardly, and an appeasement." Nonetheless, in December 1983 the House voted 96 to 52 to reprimand him, the first such action in that body since 1962.

Many politicians had survived far worse embarrassments, but Craven had the added disadvantage of representing a district that had undergone major demographic changes over the years. By 1984, African Americans and Hispanics totaled about 40 percent of the voting base, while a burgeoning population of young professionals and newcomers held no allegiance to their representative's beliefs or tactics. In the late 1960s, this growing population of newcomers worked with the native population to defeat an already approved plan to build an eight-lane superhighway through the middle of Jamaica Plain—a feat widely thought impossible that spurred both newfound confidence and the development of new neighborhood revitalization and social service organizations. Then, in the mid-1970s, court-mandated integration of the Boston public school system precipitated a massive "white flight" from many Boston neighborhoods, including Jamaica Plain, a phenomenon that further eroded Craven's historic base.

In 1980 and 1982, Craven faced a strong, organized challenge from a feisty, lifelong resident named Edwina "Winkie" Cloherty, a veteran of the highway and other community development battles. Her outspoken, fiery manner garnered her a share of opponents, but her deep roots and active church participation made her a serious threat. The campaigns against her were noteworthy for their share of Black-Jew-carpetbagger-red baiting, with occasional acts of vandalism. The pastor at Cloherty's church sent out a notorious preelection letter challenging her faith and faithful attendance. For her part, she took Craven head-on regarding his ethics problems and lackadaisical voting record. In their first match, Craven bested Cloherty by 318 out of 4,491 votes, with four "straw" candidates drawing 102 votes. In 1982, Craven won again, this time by a mere 72 votes from 6,582 ballots, with two straws attracting 279 votes. Cloherty made it clear on a deeply disappointing election night in 1982 that she would take a third stab at the race, and I was ready to support her as I had during her first two runs.

My first political involvement in Boston had come in 1979 when I joined the mayoral campaign of Mel King, a longtime African American activist and state representative. His campaign epitomized early efforts to move beyond the racial divides created by the school busing crisis. While King had no chance to win—he finished third out of four—Jamaica Plain was a hotbed of support, and his campaign brought together a hungry cadre of new activists. In the euphoric wake of his surprisingly strong showing, I led an effort to wrest control of the two Jamaica Plain Democratic Party ward committees (Wards 11 and 19) from Jimmy Craven, who controlled both. The campaign leading up to the March 1980 ward committee election was seen by us as a dry run for Winkie's first fight, which would culminate in the September 1980 Democratic primary election. While we couldn't generate enough support to win control of the Ward 19 committee, we won all fifteen seats to take control of the Ward 11 committee. It was my first electoral win. I was chosen as the new chairman.

We used the ward committee to support Cloherty in her two runs against Craven. Though she had initially planned to make a third run, a 1983 illness led her to reconsider and to decide against a third race. I spent about three months thinking and talking to friends about the race and decided in the fall of 1983 to jump in. Since graduating from Boston College in 1975, I had spent the bulk of my work life as an organizer, first for a labor union, the Amalgamated Clothing and Textile Workers Union, and then for a statewide tenants' organization I had helped to found in 1980, the Massachusetts Tenants Organization. At MTO, I organized tenants all over the state, from groups in large cities to organizations of mobile home tenants in tiny villages and hamlets. I became MTO's legislative director and coordinated its campaign in the State

House for passage of a law to protect tenants facing the conversion of their apartments to condominiums. It was a bitter, three-year fight that taught me important lessons about legislative and political dynamics and gave me a strong appetite for more.

To me, a race to defeat Jimmy Craven in September 1984 would be primarily an organizing challenge. Some state rep elections occur at the same time as other, more prominent contests, such as those for president, governor, mayor, or major ballot questions. In September 1982, a knockdown primary fight between former Governor Michael Dukakis and the man who defeated him in 1978, incumbent Governor Edward King, had attracted a huge turnout which gave Craven a total of 2,762 votes in his race against Cloherty's 2,690 votes. But in 1980, with no other contested fight on the ballot, Craven got only 1,971 votes to Cloherty's 1,653. In September 1984, it was already clear that there would be no other contested race on the ballot to draw voters to the polls.

Craven's Twelfth Suffolk District contained about 35,000 people, of whom about 18,000 were of voting age and citizenship, and about 12,000 of them registered to vote. My research suggested there was no way Craven could top more than 2,500 votes in the upcoming September 1984 contest. If I could identify, convince, and deliver to the polls at least 3,000 other votes on election day, it didn't matter what he would throw at me, he was finished. Some friends with political campaign experience advised me to be mentally prepared to run at least twice to win. I silently rejected their advice. I knew it was doable.

Over the course of the campaign, I learned that success required lots of several things: hard work, smart moves, and luck. Early on, I learned to appreciate the importance of the third element. Key to winning the election would be having a clean shot at Craven with no other strong challengers on the ballot. That seemed to be a major problem at the start of 1984 as a lifelong Jamaica Plainer named Mike O'Connor decided that this was his chance as well. O'Connor was my age, a moderate conservative, an active church member, involved in community athletics, and able to mine political bases that would be far off-limits to me. I visited him at his home several times. While we liked each other, we were both committed to the race. I knew that if he stayed in, we would split the anti-Craven vote down the middle, assuring the incumbent's reelection. But there was nothing to do. Then, in a mid-January surprise announcement, U.S. Senator Paul Tsongas announced that he would not run for reelection in 1984 in order to spend more time with his family and battle his recently diagnosed cancer. "I've never heard anyone complain at the end of his life that he wished he had spent more time at work," he said. The remark hit home with Mike who had one young child, with another on the way. He pulled out of the race, giving me the clear shot I had wanted. Luck gave me a big break!

A friend of mine, Tom Gallagher, who had run successfully against another incumbent representative in 1980, advised me that it was considered good form for a challenger to visit the incumbent at his or her home to communicate an intention to run. Jimmy Craven was considered by his opponents to be an intimidating and severe character. Challengers to him in the past had not made this ceremonial visit and had not congratulated him after his successful and bitter campaigns. I decided to go by the book for several purposes: one, to demonstrate to my supporters that I was up to the job and would not be intimidated; two, to try to establish a different tone to the race that might minimize the antics that had been known to occur; and, three, to begin to establish a less confrontational political climate in a badly fractured community.

On a cold February weekday evening, I approached Craven's door on St. John Street and rang the bell. He came to the door in a white shirt and tie, surprised to see me. God, I thought to myself, in many ways he resembles my father. This is so weird. I couldn't tell whether my shivers came from the cold or from nervousness when I said: "Good evening, representative. My name is John McDonough and I came by to tell you that I will be running in the Democratic primary for your seat."

"Come in, come in," he said warmly and with a smile. He led me into the living room where he had a guest sitting on the couch. He called, "Olivia, come in here," to his wife, who entered smiling and wearing an apron, with a dish towel in her hand. Her smile vanished when Jimmy laughingly said, "This is the guy who wants to knock me off the block!" And they all stared at me.

"Thank you for seeing me, and I'm sorry to bother you like this," I said. "I just wanted to come by to let you know that I will be running in the Democratic primary for your seat. I have lived in the community for a number of years now, and feel that I have a record of accomplishment. I wanted to introduce myself to let you know that I have nothing against you personally. I will be running a campaign based on issues and my own accomplishments. I will not be talking about your record at all. If there is anything that happens that you think is unfair or inappropriate, I hope that you will call me directly." I handed him a small piece of paper with my address and telephone number.

I understood immediately that this was atypical behavior on the part of his opponents and he was enjoying my discomfort immensely. "Thanks for coming by and good luck," he offered. I left and wondered only if I had made a partial or complete ass of myself. But within days, I knew that it was neither. Word of my evening visit spread quickly throughout my growing organization of volunteers, and the verdict was, I had balls.

With the primary in September, spring involved putting the organization together, finding the right volunteers for the right positions, raising money in any way possible—fund-raisers, house parties, mail solicitation, meetings and phone calls with potential donors—reaching out to potential support groups, and getting ready for door-to-door canvassing.

On April 1, I began spending about ten to twelve hours every day knocking on doors—not just the targeted doors of good voters but every door. I had the city's street register, which gave me the resident's name, sex, year of birth, height, party affiliation, occupation, and voting record for the past six elections. Before anyone answered the door, I had enough information to wedge myself into at least a brief conversation. If a household did not have any registered voters, I still knocked, wanting to take a shot at convincing them to register. Every night, after a day of door knocking, I would sit at home at my old IBM Selectric typewriter and type brief messages on postcards to everyone I had met, usually between thirty and fifty a day. I would drop the cards in a mailbox the next morning before starting that day's knocking. With fifteen voting precincts, I started in the ones where I was least known—in the neighborhood of Roslindale and then in Roxbury—to gain familiarity and name recognition.

I detested some parts of campaigning, such as raising money and walking in parades, which made me feel awfully silly. Door knocking, though, was different. Meeting people one or two at a time, in a nonpressured context, was actually a wonderful experience. Most people were surprised to see a real live candidate at the door. They would tell me what was going on in their neighborhood, a little bit about their lives, and which issues were of most concern to them. The process would always leave me with an indelible impression of a street and a neighborhood: what makes it tick, who are the key people who make things happen and bring folks together, what are the key issues of concern, what is the history. When the visit was topped off by a personal postcard that arrived a few days later, a card mentioning a particular aspect of my visit, a bond formed between me and that voter, one that I hoped could survive a heavy negative assault from a well-organized opponent.

The official campaign began in early May with the filing of signatures at the Election Department in Boston City Hall to win a place on the ballot. Once the city election officials certified enough valid signatures, the candidate was required to bring the signatures to the secretary of state's Elections Division bureau. All that was required to qualify was obtaining the signatures of 150 registered Democrat or independent voters who lived within the boundaries of the district. This would also be the opportunity to discover the other names besides mine and Craven's that would appear on the primary ballot. Remembering that straw candidates gathered more votes than the margin of difference between Craven and Winkie Cloherty in 1982, I waited anxiously for the filing deadline.

In the final hours, five other candidates had papers filed on their behalf, none of whom had done anything public before that moment to indicate their desire to challenge the incumbent. Two of them had names similar to mine, Joseph A. MacDonald and John T. McLaughlin, both of Jamaica Plain. Local newspaper reporters immediately dubbed the three of us "the Mac Pack" and discovered that one had an unlisted telephone number and the other refused to make any public statements. The use of straw candidates with similar names was not unknown in Jamaica Plain as a way to confuse voters. In 1976, another Jamaica Plain state rep challenger, Richard L. Walsh, defeated another incumbent by only 15 out of 4,567 votes, on a ballot where a straw candidate named Robert Walsh drew 235 votes. Our campaign strategy to deal with the threat was twofold: first, to decry at every opportunity the "dirty tricks" which occurred in every race against Craven; and second, to emphasize the "E" in John E. McDonough. That meant that every campaign flyer had the "E" in boldface and different colors. It meant that all telephone canvassers reminded voters to "remember the 'E', because John stands for everybody." It meant that on election day, every one of my several hundred poll workers wore large blue paper badges bearing nothing more than a huge black letter "E."

Three other candidates also had nominating petitions filed for the September primary. Michael Campbell had run as a straw candidate several times before and never did any campaigning. Paul Lozier was a local insurance agent whom I unsuccessfully challenged before the State Ballot Commission on the basis of his recent change of address. I had thought he was yet another straw but changed my mind as he waged a genuine though ineffective campaign. One final candidate was especially troubling. Rosemarie Celester was an African American woman who lived in a subsidized housing development in the Roxbury portion of the district. She had never been politically active and had no organization, though she was the ex-sister-in-law of the Roxbury district police commander. I could not prove how, but I firmly believed that Craven had found a connection to convince her to run. Though it was one of the most uncomfortable experiences of the race for me, I talked with her several times and urged her not to allow herself to be used by Craven to draw African American votes away from me. She denied being used by him, saying that she got into the race through her membership in the women's branch of the Black Masons. The final time I went to see her, she refused to open the door but told me that she had decided not to file her papers with the secretary of state. It was a great relief, and extremely discomfiting.

With the field set, my campaign organization and I continued the hard work of organizing, raising money, and door knocking. In the summer heat, I began to pick up the first of numerous street rumors being circulated about me by the Craven camp. At several doors in one of my opponent's strongholds, I was asked if it was true that at my first fundraiser in March at the Jamaica Plain Knights of Columbus Hall, my workers had ripped a crucifix off the wall and flung it on the floor along with other religious items in a kind of ritualistic pagan orgy. The truth was that the chair of my fund-raising committee, fearful that a crucifix on the wall behind the rock band might be damaged, carefully took it down and wrapped it, handing it to the hall's bartender who, unbeknownst to us, was a loyal Craven lieutenant. Not the smartest move, by any measure, but hardly a pagan ritual. The story followed me for the remainder of the campaign, providing a good example of how difficult it can be to stop a rumor.

Matters got uglier over house signs—posters boosting my name recognition and candidacy. Craven always succeeded in blanketing the district with large signs, though holding back the launch until Labor Day. My organization began posting large numbers of signs in early June to make up for my name recognition deficit. One volunteer, Dave Curtis, spent a good portion of each day churning out signs. He needed to because, in some neighborhoods, our signs were torn down almost as quickly as we posted them. Door knocking in one Roslindale precinct in late August, I noticed a slightly trodden path leading into a small wooded area that I climbed out of curiosity. In a little clearing, I saw about fifty of my signs torn into thousands of tiny pieces, with the sticks broken and crushed. And they accused me of pagan rituals, I thought!

Numerous organizations invited all the candidates to participate in public debates before the primary. Craven's refusal to participate turned them all into nonevents. He responded favorably to only one group, the Roslindale Civic Association, located in the most conservative, church-oriented part of the district. With the primary election scheduled for September 18, the August 27 evening debate would occur with plenty of time to be covered in the weekly community newspapers and to influence the final outcome. I remembered my sixth-grade debate with Tom Loftus and resolved that I would not be caught flat-footed again.

A crowd of several hundred (composed almost exclusively of supporters from various political camps) filled the well-lit auditorium of the Roslindale Knights of Columbus Hall that evening. Candidates from several other local races went first, as the sponsors saved the evening's main event for last. Both Craven and I had filled the audience with our supporters. I prepped mine with questions for the incumbent—about his ethics violations, straw candidates, lack of presence in the district, low voting record in the House, and more. I wore a light brown suit, white shirt, and dark blue tie and felt sweat from the warm temperatures and the anticipation. When our turn came, we went to the front of the hall and sat in folding metal chairs at the front table. I deliberately sat right next to Craven, and he did not respond to my greeting, "Good evening, representative," simply staring out into the rapt audience.

We were each permitted a brief opening statement, to be followed by questions from the audience. As the incumbent, Craven spoke first. He stood up from his chair, facing the audience: "Throughout this campaign, I have been repeatedly asked by my constituents, 'Jim, what has been your greatest accomplishment throughout all your long years of service as state representative?' And I have to answer them this way—I don't know what my greatest accomplishment has been, *because there have been so many!*" On and on he went for several more minutes, describing how certain carpetbagger agitators wanted to ruin the community and turn certain parts of the community into red-light districts. Then he went for the wrap-up: "I am so happy that you all came here tonight. I wish very much that I could stay with you and answer your questions. But unfortunately, I have a cold and must go home to take care of it. Thank you and good evening." With that he walked through the hall and out the front door to jeers and catcalls from my supporters and others, and to the stunned silence and astonished faces of his own backers. The general had just walked out on his own troops, leaving them in disarray.

This was too delicious! How could I be so lucky? Maybe he'll realize the incredible blunder he's made and come back? How could anything from here on match that performance? The debate went on: Paul Lozier, Linda Cornell, the Republican candidate , and I (MacDonald, McLaughlin and Campbell, all invited, did not show). I was good, but it was not terribly inspiring until the question-and-answer period. Craven's sister-in-law stood up, without identifying herself, and asked a question of me: "I just want to say that I could never support anyone who would condone the taking of innocent young lives through abortion. I don't know how you can seek to represent this community and support such an awful thing."

Just like me in the sixth grade, Jimmy Craven had pushed the knife into his own back. It was my turn to twist: "There are some issues, like abortion and capital punishment, when people's opinions are too opposite to each other and there is no way that you can hope to represent everyone's point of view. I have to speak to my own conscience on these matters, just as I respect yours and other's views. That's the most we can do on issues such as these.

"But there's one more thing that I have to say," I continued. "Whatever your views, wherever you come from, if I am elected your next state representative, *I will NEVER* [pause and point] *walk out that door on you!*" Standing ovation [from my supporters, of course]. Slam dunk. All the community newspaper accounts highlighted Craven's walkout and my response to him.

The debate only helped to solidify the lead we had already built. We already had identified more than 3,000 favorable votes, with more coming in daily. By early August, I had door-knocked the entire district once, and immediately began a second trip around. In early September, Craven began his expected series of attacks on me, including a letter to conservative parts of the district attacking me for supporting abortion rights, gay rights, and more. But by the time he began his fiercest assaults, I had already established a reputation and relationship with most of the district that he found difficult to undermine. He had waited too long to start the assault and now found it ineffective because I had got to the voters before he did. On the final few nights before the primary, flyers resembling my own campaign literature were dropped in several of my stronger precincts, but with the name and face of John T. McLaughlin in place of my own. It was the final gasp of a dirty-tricks machine that had run out of time.

On September 18, I beat Jimmy Craven by a margin of 3,184 to 2,189. McLaughlin pulled 210 votes, Lozier 97, MacDonald 63, and Campbell 61. Craven never called me or sent any message of concession or congratulations. When he gave his farewell speech to the House of Representatives in December, his most memorable words came at the end: "I am leaving you [pause] for now."

But his own actions ended any chance of a return engagement. Craven resigned his representative seat several days before the official end of his term. In a move known to only a few, he was hired at the very end of December as a special aide to Speaker of the House Tom McGee, who was himself locked in a losing battle to hold onto the Speaker's gavel. McGee was toppled on January 2, 1985, the day I was sworn in as representative. Because Craven's new position paid a much greater salary than a representative's, he had seemingly locked himself into a substantially higher pension on the basis of just several days of work over two years (Massachusetts pension payments are calculated by taking the average of the highest three salary levels reached in any three years of service). But McGee's successor, Speaker George Keverian, immediately rescinded any pension adjustment to Craven, and the public humiliation for his unsuccessful maneuver forever eliminated any chance of an electoral comeback.

·   ·   ·

Politics is the way we decide who gets what, when, where, how, and why. Tom Loftus got the office of sixth-grade class president at St. Luke's grammar school in 1964 by taking advantage of a debate opportunity to offer something to his fellow students that separated him from me and the other contenders. I got the office of state representative in the Twelfth Suffolk District in 1984 by organizing a smart and effective campaign that offered voters a clear alternative, by taking advantage of a weakened incumbent whose traditional base was eroding and who was unable to reach out to the new populations, and by taking full advantage of some lucky breaks.

Both campaigns were politics, nothing more and nothing less— exciting passions, organizing people, generating support—all for a purpose, to get something. The distance between the sixth grade and the Twelfth Suffolk seemed quite far to me in 1984. But sixteen years after the latter campaign, the connections between these two events seem immediate and close. Both required making the decision to run, planning the effort, and doing what needed to be done to ensure victory. Both had winners and losers. Both evoked passions and surprises that could never have been predicted at the outset. Both provided lessons that I carry to this day. Each, in its own way, was a "baptism of fire" for the political episodes that follow in this book.

Both provided me with one other important lesson. Politics, at its core, is about relationships. (The negative way of saying this is that politics is about "who you know.") In both campaigns, the individual who was able to establish the more secure bond with the voters was victorious. There are many ways to establish relationships, and many steps and obstacles along the way. But one should never forget that at the heart of the process rests the ability to make people believe a candidate and, in the process, believe more in themselves. Once the bond is set, it becomes hard to break and forms the basis for everything that follows, including the rest of this book.

CHAPTER TWO

The Stories We Tell
and the X-Men

I am always at a loss to know how much to believe of my
own stories.

Washington Irving

The two months between election and swearing-in day are frenetic for
any new rep, less an interregnum and more a new and exciting phase of
the perpetual campaign. This is the time to file one's first package of proposed legislation, to meet veteran and fellow first-year legislators, to swap
experiences and war stories, and to share interests and ideas. I recall a
revealing conversation over coffee in December 1984 with another rep-
elect from a suburban community south of Boston. We were both young,
idealistic, progressive reformers who saw ourselves as elected to help clean
up the House of Representatives. There were few others with whom I
considered myself so simpatico. Knowing that my friend had a special
interest in transportation issues, I related a story about my district's proud
and heroic transportation milestone.

Back in the late 1940s, the state's urban designers developed a master plan for highway construction across Massachusetts. The plan included building a monster eight-lane expressway—with mostly federal
dollars—through the heart of the Boston neighborhoods of the South
End, Roxbury, Jamaica Plain, Roslindale, and Hyde Park. In the 1960s,
the state began using its eminent domain powers to seize homes along
the route and tear them down to make way for the road. Around this
time, people from these neighborhoods, helped by skilled community organizers, assembled a Herculean and seemingly futile effort to stop the
highway, which was to be the final connection of Interstate Route I-95
from downtown Boston to southern suburban communities. In 1970, Re-

publican Governor Frank Sargent stunned the political community, especially powerful highway construction interests, by canceling the I-95 project. Several years later, for the first time, the U.S. Congress voted to permit highway funds to be redirected toward construction of a new mass transit line, which was finally completed in 1987. In my neighborhoods, this victory was our liberation, a titanic achievement over interests thought unbeatable. Indeed, a plaque at the Roxbury Crossing station on the Orange Line commemorates the many ordinary citizens who were the veterans of this campaign, not unlike war memorials that dot the nation's landscape.

"It's too bad," the rep-elect commented quite sincerely to me, "that the state caved into the selfish political demands of those small groups. Because of that stupid decision, it takes forever for my constituents to drive to downtown Boston."

This conversation with a friend left me wondering even at that early point in my career: Is everything in politics relative? Does where I stand depend solely on where I sit? Is there such a thing as right versus wrong, or is it all just where one is coming from? Over thirteen years in the Massachusetts legislature, I went back and forth on those questions, at times seeing everything as self-interest, at other times seeing right versus wrong, and other times seeing an incoherent mix.

In my later years, I saw a third way of understanding that was more helpful. That perspective, sometimes called discourse theory, shows how the ways we talk and the ways we tell our stories shape others' understanding and ideas. In this chapter, I describe the discourse approach to understanding political language, using the writings of Deborah Stone.[1] I then illustrate the value of the approach by telling a story about a Hispanic street gang, the X-Men, that had an intense impact on a tough part of my legislative district called Egleston Square.

DISCOURSE THEORY:
HOW WE TALK WITH EACH OTHER

Most people approach politics with one of two powerful frameworks embedded in their minds. Many approach political conflict with a strong sense of right and wrong. I entered the Massachusetts House of Representatives in January 1985 with my own sense of good versus bad. I had fought very hard to win my first election in 1984 so that I could wage battles for right and justice and join my ideological soul mates in the legislature in numerous struggles for the greater good. My priorities were varied—

housing, health care, tax fairness, public safety, urban development—but generally occupied the political left of center. Political scientists call this framework a *normative* outlook in the sense that I held to—or at least thought I held to—a clear set of *norms* about how the world *should* work.[2]

Others enter the political arena with a sharply different outlook. In this view, it's all about self-interest: mine, yours, interest groups', citizens', both enlightened and unenlightened. I want to get mine, my colleagues want to get theirs, my constituents and supporters want to get their share, and the challenge is to figure out how we can all get the most of what we need and/or want. It was in my interest to do my best job representing the people of my district so that they would continue to re-elect me to pursue my self-interest, whether that involved moving up in the House hierarchy, running for higher office, or moving to some other job. We're all just looking after our own hides, doing the best we can (in economic terms, trying to "maximize our own utility curves"), and it just so happens that the better we do for our constituents, the better we do for ourselves. If I got carried away doing favors for special interests and ignoring my district's needs, some young wanna-be would come along and defeat me, just as I did to my predecessor, Jimmy Craven. Political scientists refer to this perspective as *rationalist:* we all pursue self-interest in a form that appears rational to ourselves.

I explore the interplay between self-interest and public interest in more detail in chapter 4. In this section, I describe a different way of understanding political behavior and ideas by focusing on the way we use—and misuse—language, stories, metaphors, symbols, numbers, and other devices to create—or fake—shared meaning. This is an application of discourse theory, and the best place to begin is with our stories.

STORIES

In life, as in politics, we communicate with each other most of the time by telling stories, stories that are necessarily selective and incomplete. We arrive home after work and tell our loved ones interesting stories from our day. We meet friends and share stories telling how are lives have gone since our last connection. In my classes, I frequently ask an unsuspecting student to tell the rest of us the story of his or her day thus far. The tale ordinarily is mundane: early-morning preparations, time at work, lunch, studying, rushing to class, sprinkled with other details and events. I then ask the other students to think about details the narrator may have omitted, deliberately or not. This second request always produces a flood of information the narrator left out. (What did you have for lunch? Where? With whom? What did you wear? How did you get to work? What happened on the trip? Did you talk with anyone on the telephone? What did you do at work?) Out of this develops a sense of how necessarily selective we are in telling the stories of our lives. There is no lying or misrepresentation, just the normal mental process of picking out details and incidents that have some personal meaning and that help to communicate the message behind our stories.

A similar process occurs in journalism. A newspaper or television news program is not composed of random facts or incidents. Each consists of stories (assigned by an editor) written by a reporter who takes facts, incidents, quotes, and other data and constructs a narrative about a particular event or phenomenon. By necessity, even the most thorough reporters and the most prestigious newspapers are selective in the construction and presentation of their stories. Reporters and editors choose what they believe to be the most important and interesting elements to include in a story and discard those elements that, in their judgments, are not as important or don't fit into the allotted space. Lots of times, the journalists are right in their judgments of what is most important and what is not, and lots of times they are wrong. Often, they know ahead of time what story they want to tell and then look for facts, data, and quotations fitting their predetermined premises. Above all, they always try to tell us a good story within their own time and space limitations.

In psychotherapy, one school of practice, called *narrative therapy*, takes the idea of the story one step further. This approach focuses on understanding and analyzing a client's story—how it's constructed, what meanings it holds, and how seeing the story from a different perspective can be helpful. For example, two sets of parents, each with a severely disabled child, can construct extraordinarily different stories of their new lives: one set is strengthened while the other is crushed by the enormous responsibility. Narrative therapy can help them to imagine different stories or ways of dealing with their challenges. In a similar way, individuals and groups seeking a political solution to a problem can construct vastly different stories about their challenges that can either liberate or thwart them. Imagining can't guarantee success in itself but can be a useful first step.

In the political world, the process of storytelling is also an essential element of daily life. Just as in other parts of our lives, people communicate politically with each other by means of telling selective stories, with one crucial difference. In politics, the stories are told in order to *get* something. Stories in politics are constructed to convince others of the legitimacy or illegitimacy of some individual or group claim.

One of my favorite examples of political storytelling involves the perennial legislative war between optometrists and ophthalmologists that occurs in nearly every state. Ophthalmologists are medical doctors with a broad scope of practice to diagnose and treat eye ailments. Optometrists have a much more limited scope of practice and constantly seek approval from state legislatures to expand the boundaries of what they are permitted to do. As a legislator, and especially during my time as the Health Care Committee chairman, I would listen regularly to the stories told by representatives of both sides to make their respective cases. First, the optometrists:

> Thank you very much for seeing us today. We want you to support our bill so we can diagnose and treat common and simple eye ailments in our patients. We know their problems. We can treat them very simply, and save them the cost and inconvenience of having to go to an ophthalmologist. If you let us do these things, it will lower the cost of care, increase accessibility, and improve overall quality because lots of these people can't go to the ophthalmologists. Oh, and by the way, when the ophthalmologists come to see you, please understand that they are greedy bastards who are just out to preserve their shrinking base of income.

"Thank you very much," I say. "That was most informative and helpful." As they leave through one door, in through the other come the ophthalmologists:

> Thank you very much for seeing us today. What you need to understand most of all is that we are *physicians*. We are trained for many years in diagnosing and treating illness. These other people, these *glass dispensers,* can't be held responsible for what they say because they are not properly trained and they don't know any better. But if you let them do these procedures, there will be more serious eye ailments because of their inadequate training, and we will still have to see these patients. It will end up raising the cost of care because necessary treatment will be delayed, and the overall quality of care will drop. By the way, we are only concerned with the quality of medical care provided to patients. These other people are greedy bastards only interested in lining their pockets.

"Thank you very much for your input," I say. "That was most helpful and informative." These groups are telling me their stories as they see them, including facts and arguments that they consider important, and leaving out lots of details that others might consider relevant. Just as it is impossible in real-life conversation to include everything that could be said about a particular topic, so also there is a necessary selecting and editing process in political discourse. The critical difference in political discourse is that the selecting and editing are done for a political purpose: to get something or to stop someone else from getting something.

But wait a minute, some will object. Who is right and who is wrong in the interplay between the optometrists and the ophthalmologists? Where is the truth? The best answer to this question was written by the legendary community activist Saul Alinsky:

> This grasp of the duality of all phenomena is vital in our understanding of politics. It frees one from the myth that one approach is positive and another negative. There is no such thing in life. One man's positive is another man's negative. The description of any procedure as "positive" or "negative" is the mark of a political illiterate."[3]

Princeton health economist Uwe Reinhardt reminds his readers and audiences that health care cost containment is so difficult because one person's cost is nearly always someone else's revenue. In much of politics, searching for absolute truths is mirage chasing. There is no end to the arguments and data that either side can produce to bolster their own arguments. There is no point at which one side surrenders to the other. There is only the convincing of third parties that one side's arguments are more in keeping with the outside groups' values. Story construction is one of the key techniques in that process. The side that does the better job, and that persists, has the advantage.

Whether fiction or nonfiction, whether politics, business, sports, love, school, or just about anything else, we communicate most effectively with each other by telling stories. To be effective in politics, it is helpful to be ever conscious of the narrative, of the techniques we all use, consciously or not, in constructing our stories, in making them interesting and convincing, in picking various rhetorical techniques and tools to win over our listeners or readers. We all use these techniques and tools every day to enhance our stories, in politics and everywhere else. Three techniques are especially useful in political discourse: metaphor, numbers, and synecdoche. They are each presented in turn.

METAPHORS

Metaphors are figures of speech that suggest a comparison between two objects or concepts that are not literally related. We become so accus-

tomed to the use of metaphors in speech and writing that we often di-
gest them without notice. "It was hot as hell today." "I worked like a
dog yesterday." "You look like a princess in that dress." "I slept like a
log." When I first began to notice the extent of metaphoric usage in everyday speech—especially my own!—it was disarming. We use metaphors
so frequently because they perform a service: speakers adept at the creative use of metaphors enjoy an advantage over more pedestrian speakers in capturing and holding our attention.

In political discourse, metaphors are universal. George Lakoff and
Mark Johnson wrote in 1980: "In all aspects of life, not just in politics
or in love, we define our reality in terms of metaphors and then proceed
to act on the basis of the metaphors."[4] When we confront a new situation or phenomenon, our instinctive reaction is to ask what this matter
is most like. When we decide what it is most like, we then hold a road
map (metaphorically speaking) to figure out how to regard it and how
to deal with it. In late 1996, I listened to a radio debate on the issue of
federal budget entitlements, chiefly Social Security and Medicare. One
of the discussants, former U.S. Secretary of Commerce Peter Peterson, a
critic of entitlement spending, began by declaring that the problem of
entitlement spending within the federal budget was "metastasizing." His
implication was clear: spending on these items was growing like a cancer in the human body. What do we do when confronted with cancer?
We drop everything else we possibly can to battle the dread disease, putting our bodies through intense medical regimens that cause sickness
and severe reactions to rid ourselves of the menace. Yale's Mark
Schlesinger, the other discussant, began not by arguing facts or numbers but rather by challenging Peterson's choice of metaphor. It is invalid, he countered, to suggest that controlling entitlements requires the
massive and radical intervention the metaphor suggests. The problem
is not so great or severe.

The essential difference in the use of metaphor in politics versus
everyday life is that in the former, it is used with a political purpose in
mind, to convince someone of a likeness—as opposed to another potential
likeness—in order to get something or to prevent someone from getting
something. It is may be valid or invalid reasoning, but it is almost never
innocent. Metaphor is, in Stone's words, "strategic portrayal for persuasion's sake, and ultimately for policy's sake."[5] It is used to craft more compelling stories to convince others to support the user's political agenda.
It is not inherently good or bad—it can be either. For those seeking to advance a political cause, it is valuable to use metaphor creatively and skill-

fully. For those on the receiving end of a political message, it is essential to be intelligent and skeptical consumers of others' metaphors.

George Annas of the Boston University School of Public Health wrote a powerful article in 1995 on the need for a new metaphor for our health system.[6] Between the end of World War II and the early 1970s, he argued, the organizing metaphor for our system was *military*. We waged "war" on cancer and "battled" heart disease, in a system designed by those whose outlooks were shaped by war. The implication of the metaphor was important: in war, the imperative is to throw everything possible into the fight to vanquish the enemy regardless of budgets or other limitations. Applied to health care, this metaphor helps to explain our desire to develop technological weapons to conquer disease without regard to cost. The war metaphor continues today most prominently in our approach to drug abuse, the war on drugs. In health care, though, this metaphor was replaced in the 1970s and 1980s by a new metaphor, the health system as a *market*. Hence, we observed the corporatization of the system, the emergence of for-profit, shareholder-driven medicine, and the transformation of the patient into the consumer-customer, all driven by the failure of the previous metaphor in a new epoch of exploding health care costs. Annas concludes by proposing a new organizing metaphor, *ecology*, to reshape the system into one focused on addressing problems upstream, maintaining balance, recycling resources, and more.

We often assume that logic, facts, and data rule the day. In fact, the winners in political dialogue—and thus in politics—are often those most skillful in crafting compelling stories and using metaphor creatively.

NUMBERS

Often, when speaking before groups or classes, I write the following on a board in large figures:

$$1/9$$

and then ask if anyone knows what the number means. Nearly always, a large number of women in the room answer that the number refers to the lifetime risk of a woman's developing breast cancer. These days the number is between 1/8 and 1/9, but that's beside the point. Next I ask if anyone knows the lifetime risk of a woman's developing heart disease. Mostly silence. The answer is between 1/3 and 1/4. Why are people aware of the first number but not the second, which is far worse?

The answer is that in the former case, a well-organized political group decided that creating broad public awareness around a number, 1/9, would help to advance its agenda to obtain more financial support for breast cancer education, treatment, and research, while those concerned with cardiovascular disease have made no such effort. I have no problem with this use of a number to attract support (though most Americans are unaware that a woman's risk of dying from heart disease is far greater than her risk of dying from breast cancer; polls show most Americans believe breast cancer is the leading cause of female mortality). My point is that in political discourse, numbers are most often simply another form of rhetoric. They do not carry the same level of authenticity they carry in scientific arenas (how numbers may be abused in other fields is beyond my purpose here). They are frequently presented without context or in self-serving ones. Just as we selectively construct stories and metaphors for political purposes, so also political actors use numbers to help get something or to prevent someone else from getting something. Behind any number, there usually are multiple hidden stories that cast the original number in a different light, as with the breast cancer/heart disease numbers. Numbers present only a partial view of reality—Stone suggests they are simply another form of metaphor—and always must be consumed in the political arena with great caution and care.

In chapter 7, I show how I created and used public awareness of two numbers—700,000, the number of uninsured persons in Massachusetts, and 160,000, the number of uninsured children—in building momentum to win passage of health care access legislation in 1996. No one suggested that the numbers were false; they were as accurate and scientifically grounded as possible. We strengthened our argument by adding an additional number, 50 percent, the size of the increase in the uninsured population since 1989. Governor William Weld and his allies tried to minimize the impact of these numbers by showing that the state's proportion of uninsured citizens was still lower than the national average, also a true assertion but one that didn't harm our efforts. Part of the reason they were unsuccessful was our generation of still other useful numbers, especially polling numbers showing that nearly 80 percent of the state's population agreed with our plan. Judy Meredith, a lobbyist and friend, notes that in politics, unlike other arenas, *opinion counts as fact*. Legislators deciding how to vote on my bill had to confront the *fact* that nearly four out of five voters supported it. In this political fight, as in most others, we used numbers as weapons to get what we wanted.

Just as it is important to be a careful user and consumer of stories and metaphors, so is it also crucial to be a skeptical and cautious recipient of numbers. There is always more to a number than appears on the surface, especially in politics!

SYNECDOCHE

There are many interesting and challenging facets to discourse theory as described by Stone. I mention one more to illustrate the use and manipulation of symbols for political advantage. *Synecdoche* is a rhetorical device whereby a small part of a larger phenomenon or population is used—fairly or not—to represent the whole. This is a harder concept to explain than to illustrate.

In 1988, a criminal named Willie Horton was used in the U.S. presidential race to represent the Massachusetts prison population and the criminal justice policies of Democratic presidential candidate Michael Dukakis. The Massachusetts corrections system, prior to 1988, permitted some prison inmates to have so-called furloughs or releases from prison for brief periods. Horton, a convicted rapist who was released on furlough, fled the state and reached Maryland, where he raped a woman in her home. Supporters of Republican presidential candidate George Bush ran national television ads featuring Horton's black face and showing a revolving door into a prisonlike structure. Horton became a household name during the campaign. His public exposure was attacked by some as an indicator of racism within the Bush campaign. But the message behind the image—that Dukakis was untrustworthy on crime—was conveyed effectively. The Massachusetts prison population, and especially those let out on furlough, was substantially more diverse than Horton's image suggested. Fairly or not, Horton was made a synecdoche for that population in order to harm Dukakis politically.

In the 1980s, a young Florida boy named Ryan White, who had contracted the AIDS virus from a blood transfusion, became a pariah in his small community where he and his family were viciously harassed. When AIDS advocacy organizations and their supporters in Congress lobbied hard to win passage of national legislation to support education, research, and treatment for AIDS, they used Ryan White as the synecdoche for their cause. Of course, the part of the U.S. population suffering from AIDS is substantially more diverse than young white boys with hemophilia and includes parts of the population that generate far less sympathy. The final legislation became known as the Ryan White Law because the groups and legislators supporting it decided that the boy would be a helpful symbol of that population and would help in future reauthorization fights.

Synecdoche doesn't refer only to individuals. Consider the universal symbol for people with disabilities, a stick drawing of an individual in a wheelchair. The population of people with disabilities is substantially more diverse than people confined to wheelchairs, yet that symbol—easy to recognize and more sympathetic than, for example, people disabled because of addiction to drugs or alcohol—helps to evoke greater feelings of support among the public. A partial representation of a diverse group is effectively used to characterize the whole.

In these three examples, the individual or symbol chosen was genuinely a member of the stated group. In none of the cases did the individual or symbol accurately represent the entire group. The attempt to turn each into a representative of the larger group is strategic and political, done for a specific purpose—to get something or to stop someone else from getting something—which wins praise from some and enmity from others. It is not accidental or random. The choice of symbols in these and many other cases is deliberate—recall President Ronald Reagan's evocation of the Chicago welfare queen (who turned out to be mythical). At each presidential State of the Union address since the Reagan era, one can observe the strategic placement of sympathetic individuals in the visitors' gallery seated near the first lady. Synecdoche is a compelling example of the manipulation of symbols for political ends. Those seeking to advance an agenda or cause should consider its use. The rest of us should accept all such symbols with caution.

WRAPPING UP

In a powerfully important insight, Stone suggests most of politics is debates about values masquerading as debates about facts, numbers, and data. The search for political "truth" will always be constrained by differences in values. In the process, she raises challenging and troubling questions: In politics, is there right versus wrong? Is there truth versus falsehood? Or is everything strategic, manipulative, and contextual? My answer is: yes, yes, and no—with reservations at each step.

Discourse theory relates to a larger ethic known as *postmodernism,* which minimally suggests that all knowledge must be evaluated from the context in which it emerges and maximally that all knowledge is only a social construct of one's environment and culture. Postmodernism is a reaction to "metanarratives"—whether Christianity, Islam, modernism, socialism, capitalism, or others—that purport to represent universal truths for all humanity for all time. At the extreme, postmodernism's most ardent adherents claim all knowledge, in all spheres, is relative. But there are facts, data, events, and other phenomena that are indisputably real: Lincoln *was* assassinated; humans *can* build machines that enable us to fly; abortion, within certain restrictions, *is* legal in the United States; all U.S. citizens sixty-five and over can get certain health services paid for through the federal Medicare program; the U.S. Constitution *does* contain particular words that we can all read and cite; and so on. While we must be especially careful of what we define as fact, we can agree on lots of them.

When we move from facts to interpretation of them, we enter truly contested terrain. What was the meaning of Lincoln's assassination? How has human flight changed our society and lives? What is the impact of legalized abortion in the United States? What value does the Medicare program provide for American society? What do the Constitution's words concerning, for example, impeachment or the right to bear arms, mean? In the struggle to define the meaning of events and phenomena, particularly in politics, we should always engage with humility and a sense of the limitations of our own points of view. Any two persons can take the same facts—agreeing on them completely—and devise radically divergent meanings and lessons from them. So much of our sense of the words *right* and *wrong* is, in fact, socially constructed and contextual. It is in deriving meaning from facts that our values intrude and guide us. In our own minds, our values, more than facts, shape our understanding.

Does this suggest, then, that we can never condemn another's behavior because he or she just has another value system or cultural background? I don't think so. We just have to proceed with caution and respect and be sure to consider how our own cultural background and biases may distort our perspective. In some parts of the world, for example, female genital mutilation has been an accepted practice in certain cultures for many centuries. An extreme postmodern approach suggests it is no one's business but their own. But as human beings we have rights and responsibilities to act in behalf of others, regardless of cultural and other divides. We can't presume to know the correct and moral answer to every problem and situation, but just as surely, we must not ignore those situations where right versus wrong is so abundantly evident.

In the next section, I tell the story of a street gang that created intense controversy, conflict, and crime in a disadvantaged part of my legislative district known as Egleston Square, straddling the neighborhoods of Roxbury and Jamaica Plain. Metaphors, numbers, synecdoche, and the story all play parts in this tale. A metaphor, peeling the onion, became a plan of action. A number, the number of bullets fired into a gang member, symbolized the divide in a badly fractured community. A synecdoche, one gang member, was used to help reunite neighbors and to win new resources. Finally, I show how seeing a particular situation through a variety of eyes and working to "change the story" can help to achieve political objectives.

THE X-MEN

Looking around the hot, tightly packed room filled with about 250 angry, mostly Hispanic residents of the Egleston Square community, I suddenly realized that it would be awfully hard for me, Boston Police Commissioner Mickey Roache, and the other few city officials present to escape from the building if things got out of hand. It was a cold Monday night, November 26, 1990. We were all on the second floor of a vacant, two-story office building that had been abandoned recently by a sign manufacturing company because of instability in the community. I was standing in the front of a room behind Roache, who was seated on a metal chair with his hands folded on a flimsy table, when I noticed that I was standing directly in front of a closed, gray metal door.

Speaker after speaker came to the front of the room to express their hostility and emotions—many in a loud and rapid Spanish that I could not understand—to Roache and the rest of us about suspected policy brutality in the Saturday night shooting death of Hector Morales. Because all the attention was focused on Roache and whoever was speaking, I discreetly moved my hand up behind my back and placed it on the silver doorknob, just to check whether it would turn or not, in case it might be helpful to know. I grabbed the doorknob and gave it a slight turn. Locked.

Oh, well. I knew that Pablo Calderon, a longtime friend, community leader, and translator for the evening, had been checking people for weapons before they came into the empty office building. Only about 200 feet from the building was the spot where two Boston police officers had shot Morales two nights before after he opened fire on them with a sawed-off shotgun. A large portion of the local Hispanic community firmly believed and stated publicly that the officers had kept shooting bullets into Morales after he had fallen critically wounded, thus unnecessarily causing his death hours later and continuing a trend they saw of excessive police force.

Meanwhile, another large segment of the community was meeting a quarter of a mile down the street at the local police station, outraged at the past year's coddling of Morales's notorious street gang, the X-Men, by me, mayoral aide David Cortiella, and the local Catholic parish pastor, Father Jack Roussin. All I had wanted to do was to get the gang off the street so economic development in Egleston Square could move forward and the crime problem plaguing the Square could be minimized. I regularly heard complaints from other parts of my district that I spent too much time in Egleston to the neglect of other neighborhoods. Now, six years of intense work to rebuild the Square was coming unhinged in a matter of days. How could things have got so terribly out of hand? Did it even matter anymore? Was all progress a lost cause now? None of us in the room even knew whether we would get out of this building tonight in one piece. My mind raced over the events of the past tumultuous year. . . .

JANUARY 1990: TONY MOLINA'S HOUSE

There are many metaphors that can be used to describe the work of an urban state representative: legislator, social worker, preacher, negotiator, salesman/saleswoman, coach, street worker, to name a few. I especially liked one metaphor, plumber: I fixed problems and tried to improve systems using my special box of tools. In Egleston Square, though, my key role until 1990 had been urban planner, of sorts. Egleston Square stood at the crossroads of two Boston neighborhoods, Jamaica Plain and Roxbury, both disadvantaged and struggling to move forward. Jamaica Plain had a vibrant mix of old Irish, white affluent yuppies, African Americans, Hispanics, Asians, and others, mixing incomes, ideologies, and cultures. Roxbury was one of Boston's poorest neighborhoods, occupied mostly by African Americans, with a growing Hispanic presence.

For about eighty years, Egleston Square was known primarily as the name of a station stop on the Washington Street elevated rail line that led from Forest Hills in Jamaica Plain to the downtown Boston subway. The train made an intolerable racket passing overhead, and the "el" (for "elevated") cast a permanent shadow on the motley collection of businesses and homes along its line. The 1987 opening of the new Orange Line rapid transit train a few hundred yards away from Egleston meant the end of the noisy, ugly railway that shaded and defined the neighborhood for generations. It took nearly two years to dismantle the old line, and expectations were high during the economic boom years of the mid-

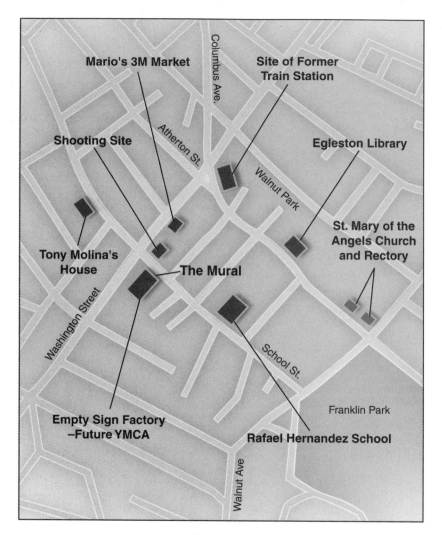

Egleston Square

1980s that sunshine spilling onto the street would lead to renewal and opportunity for the mixed but overwhelmingly poor community.

Unfortunately, by the time Egleston Square was ready to catch up in 1989, the economy had already begun to deliver the worst recession since the 1930s. New housing and commercial development ground to a halt; jobs disappeared; storefronts became abandoned and boarded up; apartments that had been snapped up in hours now went empty and unwanted; and kids and young adults with nothing to do found escape from boredom and opportunity on the streets dealing cocaine and marijuana. Across the city, street gangs had become a growing and dangerous feature of the urban environment. Graffiti was only the most visible manifestation, and in Egleston Square, the most common and omnipresent tag was, simply, "X-Men."

Beginning in the late 1980s, increasing numbers of neighbors began telling me that they were afraid to walk through the Square, daytime or evening, because of the young toughs with the rosary beads around their necks hanging out in front of the stores and at both key street corners: Washington Street and School Street, and Washington Street and Columbus Avenue. Frequently, I would call the area police superintendent, Gerry McHale, and urge him to get his officers into the Square to get rid of these kids or young adults, whoever they were. Gerry had an aggressive and effective can-do style and was always eager to respond to requests or complaints from elected officials. He had run unsuccessfully for a seat on the Boston City Council in 1981 and understood how much elected officials needed the police. His officers would repeatedly and unsuccessfully try to broom the X-Men away from the Square. But the more the officers pushed, the harder the gang pushed back, and the louder community leaders complained, as the tensions and hostility mounted.

My responsibility, I felt, was to keep the feet of the police to the fire, making sure that they, in turn, kept pressure on the gang and eventually convinced them to leave. I plowed ahead with neighborhood activists and city officials to develop an Egleston Square Economic Development Master Plan, a project that we had begun during my first year in office in 1985. The centerpiece of the plan was a strategy to redevelop the old Egleston Square train station into a commercial plaza that would attract other business development. The residents who had the patience to put up with endless planning meetings made clear that they wanted a bank and a pharmacy on the site, two things that Egleston Square had lacked for more than a generation. The master plan was a good-times document that had little relevance to the real economic plight facing the community in 1990. We plowed on, hoping to be ready to catch the next favorable economic wave.

Trying to overcome considerable community apathy to the planning process, I began organizing a series of house meetings to bring neighbors together in their homes to learn about the plan. One freezing Saturday morning in January 1990 brought me to the living room of Tony Molina, a respected community leader in his fifties, a voice for the Puerto Rican community, owner of his own radio station, and a political mover and shaker. At my request, Tony had brought together about ten community leaders and residents, including Mario Melendez, longtime owner of the 3M Market, and Pablo Calderon, an old friend and president of the Egleston Square Neighborhood Association, which he and I had started together in the mid-1980s. To my surprise, Tony also invited Boston Mayor Ray Flynn's policy adviser, David Cortiella, the highest-ranking Hispanic in City Hall. I knew David slightly from various events but had never worked closely with him.

As I started the session by presenting the rationale and background behind the draft plan, Tony interrupted me, somewhat impatiently. "How can we be talking about building up the Square economically when most people are afraid to even walk through there? We had a near riot in the Square just two weeks ago and one of these gang members actually tossed a Molotov cocktail from a roof at the corner of School and Washington onto a police cruiser. It seems to me that that's what our priority should be. But what are we doing about that?"

"I know that's a big problem," I said. "We've been working with the police to try and get these guys to stop hanging out and intimidating people. The police have been putting a lot of pressure on them that I hope will pay off soon."

"These kids who are hanging out there are not strangers," Tony replied. "We've watched them grow up. They act tough now, calling themselves the X-Men and all that nonsense. But we're kidding ourselves if we think we can just chase them away, because they live here. This is their home. We've got to find a different way to reach them."

"Well, what would you suggest?" I asked.

There was no easy answer. Throughout the city, relations between the police and minority youth on the street had never been more tense. While police responded to frantic public calls to address growing gang violence, drug dealing, and illegal weapons, youths and some community leaders responded angrily to aggressive police tactics such as "stop and search," whereby police required kids to drop their pants while leaning spread-eagled against the wall. The January Molotov cocktail incident in Egleston Square was a signal to city leaders that tensions were mounting and that other interventions might be needed. Cortiella had argued to Mayor Flynn that different tactics were needed to deal with the violence and that police pressure would backfire if used alone. After Flynn gave him the OK in January to do some work in Egleston Square, David contacted his friend Tony Molina, who invited him to come to my planning meeting.

David suggested that we needed to address the reality on the street before we could turn the Square around economically. I could hardly disagree. We decided to call a meeting with the X-Men. We would hold it at the Egleston Square Library. Mario Melendez, owner of the 3M Market, knew nearly all the members of the gang because the front of his store was one of their favorite hangout spots. He was fearful of them but also was able to maintain a rapport. They actually stopped someone from robbing his store once, he said. He volunteered to let them know that a group of city and state officials, along with some neighborhood leaders, wanted a meeting. Would they come? None of us knew, but nobody had a better idea. We picked a date, Monday evening, February 5, and a time, 7:30.

For the time being, the Egleston Square Master Plan was on the shelf.

FEBRUARY: THE EGLESTON SQUARE LIBRARY

In 1983, a librarian at the Egleston Square Library was assaulted leaving the building one night. The city promptly closed the facility saying that none of the staff would agree to work there anymore. One of my earliest victories as a new representative, working with the newly formed Egleston Square Neighborhood Association, was convincing the city in 1985 to reopen the library. Thus I always had a soft spot in my heart for the facility, joining with neighbors to remove graffiti and fix other occasional acts of vandalism. It seemed an appropriate place to meet the X-Men, whose activities were undermining our efforts to build up and improve the Square. If any of these guys wanted to give me a hard time and ask what I had done for Egleston Square, I would just point my finger at the fluorescent lights.

The "adults" arrived early: David Cortiella, Mario Melendez, Father Jack Roussin, pastor of the local Catholic church, St. Mary of the Angels, and I. "Father Jack," as he was universally called, was unlike any Catholic priest I had ever met—earthy, irreverent, independent, at ease on the streets, and wickedly funny. He took over a parish in the 1970s that was headed for dissolution and made it financially independent with a United Nations congregation of Anglos, African Americans, Puerto Ricans, Dominicans, Cambodians, Laotians, and others. He knew nearly every kid who lived around Egleston, their siblings, their parents, and their grandparents.

I had told Father Jack about the meeting and was relieved he wanted to come. He told me he first realized something funny was going on in the Square when young Hispanic men started showing up at his rectory door asking if he had any rosary beads he could spare. He was happy initially to oblige, thinking some grassroots prayer and religious revival might be brewing. Only later did he learn that the X-Men, in their early days, identified their membership status by wearing the beads around their necks.

Most people I told of that night's meeting said I was seriously crazy to go into a situation like that without police protection. Following the Molotov cocktail incident and another widely publicized altercation with police in the adjacent city of Chelsea, the X-Men already had developed a citywide reputation as one of the toughest gangs of outlaws in a city now full of them. Some police estimated their membership numbers at as high as five hundred and suggested that this gang was tightly organized and disciplined, military-style.

At 7:30, on time, about twenty-five Hispanic teens and young adults arrived, dressed uniformly in dark trousers, sneakers, and dark jackets, many with wool caps—the street uniform that was by now so familiar. We didn't ask the numerous cigarette smokers to put out their butts. Maybe I was naïve, I thought, but my first impression was that they didn't appear to be particularly tough or intimidating. Some sat in chairs across from us, while others stood around, near the chairs or closer to the door. For an awkward few minutes, we just stared at each other, sizing up our opposites.

David broke the ice and did most of the talking for our side that evening.

"We wanted to meet with you because what's going on is creating real problems for the community and the city. We know that you guys have your own complaints and problems, and we're here to listen to them. We want to work with you so that you get some things that you need, and we get some things that we need."

Celio (pronounced see-low) did most of the talking for the group. He was tall, in his midtwenties, with a loud voice, broken teeth, and an easy, goofy grin. He would most often stand up to speak, walking with heavy steps and waving his arms in the open space among the chairs.

"You don't understand us at all. We are the guardians and defenders of the Square. When the gangs from other parts of the city wanted to claim Egleston for their own turf, we had to stand up and chase them out. We had no other choice. We won't let any of the crack or the heroin in. We don't allow guns on the street. If people come in and try to make trouble, we push them out. We stopped a robbery at Mario's store—I bet you didn't know that? And for all that, the cops come by and harass us, push us around, insult us, pull down our pants on the street in front of everyone. They try to humiliate us. To us, the cops are just another gang with better weapons, and we defend our streets from them just like from everyone else."

On it went for about an hour. David appealed to their Hispanic pride, digging at them for putting their "X-Men" graffiti all over the Square and especially on the Rafael Hernandez Public Elementary School across Columbus Avenue from the library. No one could answer when he asked if they even knew who Rafael Hernandez, the famous Puerto Rican composer, historian, and educator, was. He talked about his own growing up in Brooklyn, being part of a gang that hung out at Second and Fifth Avenues. He told them about his own struggle to escape, about staying in school and eventually becoming a lawyer and, now, a respected and influential city official.

Hector Morales was sitting there, next to Celio, generally quiet, but among the most vocal and bitter about the behavior of the police. Toward the end, several of the guys stated what they wanted: jobs, a place to play basketball, and fair treatment from the cops. David told them that as long as they peddled drugs of any sort, they could expect trouble from the cops and no support from us; but if they were harassed unfairly, we would stand up for them. He offered to try to get the Rafael Hernandez School gym opened on Saturday mornings for their use to play basketball, with one condition: that they agree to become the protectors of the school and make sure that all graffiti tagging on the building would stop. David asked if we had a deal.

Celio put on his broadest grin: "Well, we all know who does that, and we think we can hold him back." All X-Men eyes turned to one quiet younger member of the gang, who said nothing and shrunk low in his seat.

We made a tentative agreement, each side doubtful that the other would hold up its end of the bargain but pleased to sense something coming out of the session. At the end of the meeting, Hector walked up to David to offer some personal advice: "Next time, don't come here wearing your wingtip shoes."

After the meeting, many of us—gang members and adults—hung around to talk for a while. I approached one of the group whom the others called "Sinbad," a nickname given to him in recognition of his loose resemblance to the movie character played by Douglas Fairbanks Jr. He introduced himself as Eddie Ortega. He was decidedly different from the others, well spoken and groomed, easygoing with none of the machismo swagger of his fellow X-Men. He shied away when I called him by the name Sinbad. He was dismissive of the evening's discussion and the promises made by us.

"What about if we get the gym in the school across the street opened for basketball," I asked.

"That doesn't matter to me. I don't like to sweat," he said. I immediately felt a special bond with him.

"What would make a difference to you, then?"

Eddie was in his early twenties and wanted to get some GED instruction to obtain his high school equivalency degree, but he was too old to enroll in the instructional program at the Ecumenical Social Action Committee, a social services agency in the Square. I knew the director well and asked Eddie if he would like me to help. "Sure," he said suspiciously, and gave me a phone number to reach him.

It was about 9:30 when the X-Men left us at the library. We stayed to compare notes. "We're off to a good start," said David, who then offered the metaphor that defined our work for the next ten months. "What we're trying to do now is to 'peel the onion,' one piece at a time. We'll help the ones who are looking for a way out, with jobs or school or recreation or whatever, and that will leave the hardcore dealers and troublemakers exposed."

Father Jack, much to my surprise, knew just about every one of them—not just the gang members but their entire families. "What you have to realize," he told me, "is that some of these guys use the money off the street to support their incredibly messed-up families. In a lot of cases, believe it or not, they are actually the least screwed-up members of their households."

APRIL: A FRIDAY NIGHT IN THE SQUARE

David, Father Jack, and I began meeting every week with the X-Men at the rectory of St. Mary of the Angels Church, though their numbers dropped precipitously after the first few weeks. Increasing numbers, though, began to show up on Saturday mornings at the Rafael Hernandez School. David and I convinced the principal, Margarita Muniz, that we could keep things under control and keep the school graffiti-free in the bargain. About fifteen members of the Hispanic Patrolmen's Association, with equipment and financial support from the Police Athletic League, made playing and working with the X-Men one of their own special projects. And so for the rest of the winter into the spring, I would watch cops and gang members who had often been at each other's throats playing basketball in the school gym. At the first Saturday basketball session, Police Commissioner Mickey Roache showed up to offer support. More and more of the younger kids in the neighborhood started coming to watch the X-Men play the cops.

The graffiti came off the building and stayed off, as X-Men members kept their word by keeping the school building graffiti-free. While I landed a few jobs for some of them along with other things such as a GED slot for Eddie, David used his well-placed network at Boston City Hall to steer full-time and seasonal jobs to members of the X-Men who were looking for a way out. David also steered funding to Father Jack, who hired and supervised X-Men willing to do community work. The three of us never spoke of "peeling the onion" to anyone but each other, but it became our common reference point.

A lengthy April article in the Jamaica Plain community newspaper lauded the work being done to redirect the energies of the X-Men, adding momentum and legitimacy to our drive. The gang members even volunteered to participate in the annual spring cleanup, offering to form the bulk of the Egleston cleanup crew. One X Man, Ariel Ruiz, told the paper, "Lately, I've been reevaluating things—looking at the situation I've put myself into. I've decided I want to make a difference in this neighborhood."

David became especially close to another young X-Man, Jose Ojeda, a seventeen-year-old who dropped out of school in the ninth grade, and got him a job working in the city's Retirement Board at $375 a week. In February, David and Jose signed a written contract with each other, David promising a full-time job through the summer, with part-time work after September, while Jose agreed to sign up for school beginning in the fall. "For a while, Jose was the happiest person in the world," David remembers. "He was giving all his pay to his mother. He worked on the Mayor's Youth Campaign as a volunteer, calling up kids to sign up for summer jobs. He proposed that we create a billboard against violence, showing twelve mothers crying, with the caption "Is that what you want to leave for your mother?"

One Thursday evening in late April in the Square, Jose's sister got involved in a bad fight with her boyfriend that led to shoving, pushing, and punching among a group of friends. The police showed up to stop the fight and began pulling people away from each other. Jose lost his cool, threw a punch at one of the more aggressive cops, and was arrested. He expected he was going to get rough treatment in return for his swing and got it on the ride to the station. David arrived with Father Jack and referred to himself as Jose's attorney, demanding to see him. When he reached the cell, he saw bruises and black-and-blue marks on Jose's face. David told Jose to strip down to his underwear and point out all the marks on his body so that David would know if any new ones were added during the night after he had left. The night commander at the station was furious at him.

Back on the street, the X-Men knew immediately what had happened and heard Jose had been roughed up on the way to the station. "Look what happened," Celio said to David, Father Jack, and me. "The cops continue to do whatever they want and get away with anything. You got no juice."

In an increasingly familiar pattern for all of us, David took grief from both sides. He soon faced a fierce confrontation in the Mayor's office with Gerry McHale, the local police commander. "You're coddling these gang members; you're covering up for criminals," Gerry yelled. "And you're undermining our ability to do our jobs by making it look like we don't control the streets." David brought in Jose, who apologized for his behavior, but he also convinced the police commissioner to remove from Egleston Square duty one police officer who had been particularly aggressive against the X-Men.

Concerned that reaction to the events would undermine our relationship with the X-Men, David, Father Jack, and I spent that Friday evening from about 6 to midnight standing on Washington Street in the Square near Mario's 3M Market. Our purpose was just to "be there" to talk with anyone who wanted us and to show that we were going to stay involved. It was a mild spring evening, and Father Jack, who rarely wore his priestly clothes outside of church services, wore his Cuban "guayavera" shirt and chain-smoked Marlboros despite our constant harassment. Many people walking by or driving their cars recognized one or more of us in this highly unusual spot—three adult men standing in a place most recognized as a gang hangout. "What the heck am I doing here?" I thought to myself repeatedly. The X-Men moved their base of operations a little further down the block that night, periodically coming near us in groups of two or three. They were steamed and accusatory about what they heard had happened to Jose. David asked them to draw a different lesson from the experience: "Look, you're right that this kind of thing happens. But the difference this time is that the cop who was out of line got transferred away from the Square. That happened only because you guys have become participants in the political process. You got something out of this, not nothing. And if you stay involved, you can make other changes happen as well."

It was an evening full of heated talk, unusual characters, and strange looks. Sometime around 10, I mentioned to my two companions that it seemed to be awfully peaceful for a Friday night. Shortly after I made that statement, a fast-driving car screeched to a halt on the other side of the street from us. One man jumped out of his car and ran to someone standing across the street from us. The driver was quickly joined by several others who began to punch the other man severely. Almost instantly, as if from nowhere, there were more than a hundred people out on the street watching this fight, some getting into the fray. The three of us stood about thirty feet from the altercation, frozen in disbelief, uncertain what to do or which way to go. I heard a bottle smash on the street amidst the yells. Then, just as quickly as it had begun, it was over. Within two more minutes, the street was as empty as it had been minutes before the fight. A few minutes later, a police squad car arrived, but there was nothing left to find. And the "three amigos," standing puzzled and dazed on the sidewalk, could only shrug when asked what happened by the police officer. "Beats us." Their looks told us their reaction: "Yeah, sure!"

Our presence in the Square that evening had not gone unnoticed by the X-Men or the police. It was an indication we were willing to play with the balance of power in the Square in order to achieve our larger objectives. As we headed out of the Square that evening, David remarked that "we scored a lot of points tonight." I couldn't help wondering what game I was really playing.

The next morning, we were back in the Square, doing the annual cleanup, with about half of the workers members of the X-Men. The events of Thursday and Friday got no attention, while the Saturday cleanup was fully covered and photographed. We successfully created one image for the community, but I was more aware than ever how complex the real image was.

SUMMER: AROUND THE SQUARE

Throughout the spring and into the summer, David, Father Jack, and I continued to meet, getting together less occasionally with the X-Men. But we kept peeling the onion, pulling individuals out, one at a time, whenever they asked, getting jobs, help, and whatever else we could. David arranged for Father Jack to get a large pot of money from the city for summer jobs for kids in the Square, and he picked out a number of X-Men to help organize the work crews. It may have been that I was just getting more familiar with them, but somehow they seemed to lose their edge, their fearsomeness, their threat to progress in the Square. I had a routine of driving through the Square after my nightly community meetings to see what was going on. It struck me as strange when the X-Men on the street recognized me and waved as I passed.

David and I both were getting distracted by our other work priorities. David had been named executive director of the city's Fair Housing Commission, a position that gave him less time to spend in the Square. I was absorbed by a number of State House concerns, not the least of which was an endlessly growing state fiscal crisis which had forced us into severe budget cutting and a major tax increase in 1989 and an additional round of both in 1990—running right into the November statewide elections.

A goal I started to pursue was establishing a permanent youth center in Egleston Square, something that gang and nongang members agreed was a priority. Pablo Calderon, the head of the Egleston Square Neighborhood Association, and I spent time over the summer visiting the heads of various social service organizations to identify an interested party. We received a lot of smiles and best wishes but little action, until Pablo bumped into the executive director of the Greater Boston YMCA, Peter Post, who had a gym locker next to his. Pablo, Mossik Hacobian, the entrepreneurial director of a local community development corporation called Urban Edge, and I arranged a walking tour of the Square for Peter and some of his senior staff, giving them history and identifying a number of potential sites. They were more interested than any of our other prospects but were not able to make a clear commitment.

While the X-Men lost much of their dangerous image to me, others were communicating a different picture. The weekly newspaper the *Boston Phoenix* ran a series of articles on gangs in Boston, highlighting the X-Men as the baddest and most threatening of them all. The articles enraged me because they encouraged hard-core members of the gang who wanted to stay out on the street to see it as worthwhile. "The total package of the 90's Boston gangs," said the *Phoenix* of the X-Men. "'We are ready to fight the power if it comes to that,' says Cee. 'And,' says J., 'we ain't scared to die either.'"

While David, Father Jack, and I pursued our strategy of "peeling the onion" and carefully breaking up the group, some other neighborhood leaders began to encourage the remainder of the X-Men to express themselves more proudly. They obtained an arts grant to hire an artist to work with the gang members to paint a huge mural on the wall of a vacant School Street building across from one of their favorite hangouts.

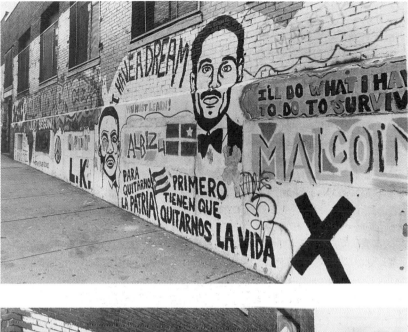

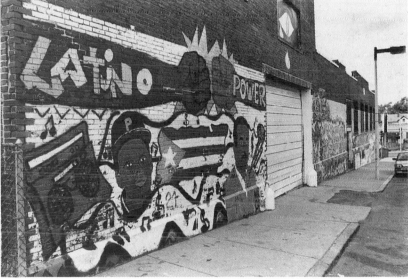

Throughout the summer, they worked on the wall: a broad painting full of provocative images of civil rights leaders Malcolm X and Martin Luther King, baseball player Roberto Clemente, and renowned Puerto Rican signer Willie Colon. They emblazoned the mural with the slogans "We are all in the same gang," "Latino power," and more. Toward the end of the project, Willie Colon, in Boston for a concert, visited the site and signed his name on the work.

The X-Men and their friends were hugely proud of this new and tangible symbol of their influence. Some community leaders felt that it would move gang members away from illegal and destructive activities. But a larger number of longtime community leaders were appalled and outraged. They were aghast that a community with a healthy mixture of whites, blacks, and Hispanics was symbolized by a mural that they saw as celebrating Latino toughs. They thought it was pretty ugly to boot. Mostly, they felt it legitimized and glamorized a group they felt to be threatening, a group engaged in illegal activities, a group that was holding back community progress. Father Jack challenged X-Men members about these concerns expressed by many solid community leaders and lost their respect and friendship as a result. As usual, I had mixed feelings about the episode. Mostly it said to me that bringing the community together and ending the fear and divisions caused by the emergence of the X-Men were going to be much harder and longer-term challenges than I had believed or bargained for.

LATE NOVEMBER

On Saturday evening, November 24, around 9:20, two undercover Boston police officers, Darrin Greeley, age twenty-four, and Thomas Gomperts, age thirty-three, stopped their unmarked car in front of the doorway to 87 School Street, one of the most favored hangout spots for the X-Men, a group of whom were standing in and around the open door. Gomperts followed one suspicious-looking member into the hallway. Greeley, standing outside, saw Hector Morales, who appeared to be holding something inside his coat. "Hey, what's up, Hector," asked Greeley. "This is what's up, motherfucker," yelled Hector, who pulled out a sawed-off shotgun and began shooting it at the officers.

Luckily for Greeley and Gomperts, Hector's gun was loaded only with birdshot, which could not penetrate their bullet-proof vests. Hector got off about half a dozen shots, wounding Gomperts in the forehead and cheek and Greeley on his right hand. The officers fired back, striking

Morales four times in the stomach and chest. He was fatally wounded and died shortly after midnight at Boston City Hospital. The two officers were taken to Brigham and Women's Hospital to be treated for their wounds.

I was at home when I heard the television news report about the shooting, and I arrived at the scene around 10 P.M. While the crime scene was cordoned off with police tape, lots of police and residents were standing around and already were making their feelings known, feelings that would explode during the coming days. The police officers and some community members were angry that a gang that carried such dangerous weapons had been permitted such free rein in the neighborhood. Other residents were already decrying what in their minds was another example of excessive force and brutality by the police. "They shot him one or two times, and he was down," one resident told the *Boston Globe*. "Why did they have to shoot him until he was dead?" One of the X-Men, identified in the paper only as Frankie, gave his own account: "He dropped his gun, he had his hands up and he was saying, 'Don't shoot any more. For my mother, don't shoot no more' . . . I yelled out the window, 'you're going to kill him,' and the cop shot him four more times." On the street that night, residents were spreading the word that Hector had been murdered by the cops.

Hector Morales was a most unlikely candidate for martyrdom. Three times that year, he had been arrested: in March for possession of marijuana, in June for possession of stolen property, and in early November for driving a stolen car. Shortly before the November 24 shooting, Hector had told Eddie Ortega, "If I'm ever caught with a gun, I'm not going to let them take me." Eddie had once told me, "You had to be afraid of the guys who were really quiet, and Hector was really quiet." What little he had said at the February meeting at the Egleston Library was characteristically with an angry intensity aimed at the police. He was nineteen, small, influenced by hard leftist ideas, drawn to Malcolm X, revolution, a group that would show up occasionally in the Square called the Revolutionary Community Party, and "fighting the power." David remembered his being heavily influenced by the Spike Lee movie *Do the Right Thing*.

Numbers took on a great degree of importance for all concerned in the shooting aftermath. How many times had Hector been shot? Those charging police brutality and claiming to be eyewitnesses suggested that he took as many as a dozen bullets. How many were too many? That was difficult to say, but it was all academic until an autopsy was performed, and the results of the report would not be available for several days. Ultimately, the report showed that Hector had been shot four times, a number that quickly diminished suggestions of police overreaction or brutality in the face of his own precipitating action. But that news didn't come out until well after the most heated action was over.

David, Father Jack, Pablo, and I shared one common goal, working to make sure that there would be no further incidents or reprisals by the X-Men. I kept wondering to myself if the Square would ever be able to recover from this incident, but those thoughts seemed distinctly remote at that point. Throughout Sunday and Monday, tensions in the Square were high. Police maintained a strong presence, but the X-Men made clear that they wanted revenge with blood. We heard all kinds of stories about weapons the gang had in hiding, including three Uzi machine guns. All the goodwill that had developed during the Saturday morning basketball games in February quickly vanished. To the X-Men, the police were once again the enemy, the biggest, baddest gang of them all—some of the police even had T-shirts with the slogan "Boston's Bad Boys"— with the most weapons. To many of the police, the feelings were mutual. On Sunday afternoon, some police forced a group of X-Men to lean against the wall with their legs spread. "Cops one, X-Men zero," one of them crowed.

Sunday evening, David, Father Jack, and I brought a group of the gang members to meet at City Hall with Mayor Ray Flynn and Police Commissioner Mickey Roache. We got a commitment from the X-Men for no retaliation through Hector's wake on Tuesday, but we didn't put much weight in their ability to control their wilder members. We needed some way for community residents to blow off steam and let out their anger, legitimate or not. One large portion of the community was outraged at excessive police force that killed one of their own; the other large portion was outraged that police and officials (such as I) had been coddling a violent gang that was not afraid to shoot at the police. We decided to have two meetings. One would take place right across from the shooting site at 87 School Street in an old office building (the site of the mural) that had housed a sign factory until about a year before and was now largely empty; this meeting would be for the residents angry at the police. The other would be held three blocks away at the local police station for the part of the community outraged at the gang and their coddlers. My purpose was the same as it had been since that Saturday morning in January at Tony Molina's house: to stabilize the Square so that we could move ahead on economic development and to hold onto the progress we had made—a prospect that now seemed pretty remote.

The scene at the old sign factory was outrageous. Hundreds of residents and youth gathered at the intersection of School and Washington Streets, where the shooting had occurred, and X-Men placed a black wreath for Hector on the street sign. TV news reporters looked for anyone willing to make outrageous statements, until the reporters themselves became too intimidated to stick around. They were deliberately excluded from the community meetings. Pablo took it upon himself to check everyone who walked into the building for weapons. He took five guns and thirteen knives, promising to return them to the owners after the meeting. But Pablo also served as the meeting's MC and translator and wasn't able to search people who came in once the meeting had started. In the middle of the meeting, one person shouted that someone in the room had a hand grenade, but after a brief moment of panic, nothing further came of that. Everyone stood except for two people. The police commissioner sat on a metal chair, his hands clasped together on a folding table, with Pablo, the translator, standing in front of him, partially as a form of protection. David, Father Jack, several police officials, and I stood behind him. In front of the table, seated in a chair, was Hector's mother, Clara Hernandez, silently crying. For about two hours, one community resident after another spoke up to express their outrage at the actions of the police. Some claimed that Hector had been shot more than a dozen times, again and again, after he was lying on the ground unconscious. Commissioner Roache responded calmly that no conclusions could be reached until the conclusion of the autopsy. Near the end, Clara Hernandez stood, bringing silence to the room. She fell to her knees, facing the commissioner, with outstretched arms, speaking in Spanish. I leaned over and asked Father Jack for a quick translation. "She's talking about the need to stop the violence and to bring the community together," he said. "Now she's saying, 'My poor little lamb has been unjustly taken to the slaughter.' The poor little lamb," he added parenthetically, "who had a police record as long as your arm."

Ms. Hernandez's statement provided a convenient point to end the meeting, which could have gone on endlessly. On the way out of the building, word spread that the X-Men intended to seal the exits and to hold all of us hostage. It was part of the lunacy of the evening that the threat seemed entirely plausible. Every raising of voices seemed to indicate a further unraveling of control. People wandered out and stood around the site where everything had come unglued just two nights before. David stayed with the street scene, which culminated later in the evening with more than a hundred police surrounding a large cadre of X-Men and other gang members up the street in Franklin Park. Other gangs from across the city had come to Egleston to show their support for the X-Men. The police responded by bringing to the neighborhood the riot squad, ready for whatever trouble might emerge. David and Pablo walked into the park where the gang members were gathered to cool them down and prevent further trouble. The night ended with only a couple of arrests.

Down the street, at the district police station, about a hundred community leaders met to express their own outrage and anger. I did not find them out of line or unfair, even those with the harshest words. Many wanted to know why I and others were not publicly critical of the outrageous conduct of the X-Men, why we were so silent. Others wanted to know what we intended to do to prevent other episodes and to eliminate this gang. I felt more torn and emotional than at any other time in my years as a representative.

"We had one priority over the past couple of days," I said, "and that was to prevent any more violence. Heavy statements expressing our anger and outrage would have limited our ability to work with them to keep a lid on things. It may have been right or wrong, but that's what we were doing. The important work for us now is to make sure that we don't allow this to stop our efforts to revitalize the Square. This can be the event that destroys all of our hard work leaving us with nothing, or it can be one incident that challenges us to work even harder to make things better. I want it to be the latter."

AFTERMATH

Hector Morales fired at two police officers and was killed by their return gunfire. That was an event, a fact about which everyone and anyone who cared agreed. But what was the *meaning* of that event for the future of Egleston Square, or more appropriately, what should the meaning of that event be? On that point, there was no agreement. To some, it meant that the police should crack down even harder to eliminate the gang menace and stop any pretense of coddling or working with gangsters and criminals. To others, the shooting meant the police were out of control, and members of the community were justified in seeing them as the enemy, as simply another gang with better weapons and the power of the state behind them. To still others, myself included, the shooting meant we had to work even harder in multiple directions if we were to create conditions from which Egleston Square could emerge and thrive. One more thing was certain to me: nothing was written, nothing was destined, nothing *had* to happen—it was up to the community and its leaders, me and others, to work together to create and to fashion the story we wanted to see happen.

On at least one count, we were able to use the crisis that gripped Egleston Square during that week in November to good effect. The group of community leaders who had been working to open up a youth center in Egleston Square found significantly more support for our efforts in the wake of the well-publicized violence. Doors suddenly were opened for funding and other kinds of support much more readily than had been the case prior to the shooting. After the shooting incident, YMCA officials were eager to make a firm commitment to locate a center in the Square. Mossik Hacobian, the tenacious director of Urban Edge, negotiated to buy the old sign factory building across the street from the shooting site and began working with YMCA officials to finance and construct their new center at that location.

In December 1991, a little more than one year after the Morales shooting, in the same space that held that tense, packed, and angry community meeting, neighbors and community leaders once again crowded in tightly and without chairs, but this time to celebrate the opening of a new YMCA for the Egleston community. It was an emotional and important event for those of us who had been involved in the work to hold the community together during those difficult days of 1990 and 1991. It represented our unwillingness to permit the events surrounding the Morales shooting to defeat us and our collective commitment to transform the horrible story into a good one. The most symbolic and dynamic element of the new YMCA program was the appointment of its first site director, Eddie Ortega, once known on the streets as Sinbad, a member of the X-Men.

Eddie had been working in a grocery store and restaurant near Egleston in 1987 when his brother-in-law, Frankie, invited him to participate in the growing and lucrative drug trade developing around the Boylston Street section of the Square. Eddie and Frankie referred to themselves as a "Batman and Robin" team, with Eddie providing the business skills and Frankie the muscle, selling marijuana and cocaine. As the business grew with more guys joining in, and pressure from the police developed, the group of between fifty and a hundred claimed its own identity as the X-Men, named after the Marvel comic book characters. The money was the major intoxicant for Eddie, who got used to fast cars and fancy restaurants and was able to fool the police because of his suave manner and wallet full of credit cards. But Eddie had something else that was different from the other guys joining the trade: two hardworking parents who let him know how they felt about his activities. "They didn't talk to me for quite a while," he said. "That hurt me a lot. It took a long time for them to trust me again. . . . The other guys didn't have that."

By the time we organized the February 1990 meeting at the Egleston Library, Eddie had already been thinking about how to get out of the action. He recoiled that night when I addressed him as "Sinbad," calling himself Eddie instead. He grabbed at the chance I gave him to get into the GED program at a social service agency in the Square. He pushed David and me to help him get a job as a street worker for the Boston Housing Authority in the South End in the spring of 1990 and worked at it hard to start a different track record for himself. When the YMCA was looking for someone to manage their new program and deal with the unique dynamic of the players in Egleston Square, David, Father Jack, and I all pushed to give Eddie the chance.

"I used you guys more than you thought," Eddie told me years later. "But I kept my end of the bargain." We all used him, too. As the director of the Egleston YMCA, Eddie became our synecdoche for what gang members could become with the right attention and support. He became a spokesperson around the country on issues of gang violence, talking about what really goes on and what is realistic to expect. I would refer to him in my own speeches in the House of Representatives and elsewhere for why we had to invest in services and support for disadvantaged communities, and not just in more police. Eddie had a difficult time managing the new YMCA branch at first. His former X-Men compatriots all expected the site to be their own private clubhouse, and Eddie had to struggle to establish rules and expectations so that the center would be open and comfortable for youth throughout the community. But he did it. Eddie's successor in that position is also worthy of note. In 1998, Willie Morales, Hector's older brother, became director of the Egleston Y. Willie had been serving time in prison at the time of Hector's shooting, an incident that made him resolve to find another direction in life. After his release, he became a respected community organizer in the neighborhood until his appointment to the YMCA job.

If Eddie and Willie seemed to represent one side of the coin, Jose Ojeda represented the other. He was David Cortiella's protégé and kept faithful to the contract they had signed with each other in the spring of 1990, though his older brother stayed on the dangerous side of the street. One night in 1991, the pair of brothers were in the Square together at the intersection of Washington and Atherton Streets when two men approached them in the dark. Mistaking Jose for his older brother, the two aimed their weapons at him. Their first bullet hit his spine, paralyzing him from the neck down for life. In his days in a wheelchair, he became bitter about his former gang friends and girlfriend who never bothered to visit him in the hospital. He became a regular speaker at youth events to warn others about the realities of violence, but he was unable to overcome the depression that accompanied his loss of mobility. "It turns out it wasn't real," he told a *Boston Globe* reporter in 1994, speaking of his relationships with the other gang members.[7] He died in 1996.

The X-Men as an identifiable group vanished. Some went on to finish their education, get jobs, and go straight. Others ended up with long stretches in prison, paralyzed, or dead. A few others were still out on the street years later, though their numbers were considerably diminished, and their methods more discreet.

Economic development in the Square picked up in the early 1990s. By 1996, the residents of the Square finally had both the bank branch and the pharmacy they had desired for such a long time, along with a host of other new businesses and services. By then, Egleston Square had become a celebrated citywide symbol of rebirth and redevelopment, a dramatic turnaround from its image only a few years earlier.

In 1992, David Cortiella began a term of several years as the executive director of the Boston Housing Authority. He presently runs a Latino housing and community development program in Boston's South End. Pablo Calderon still lives in the Square, and works in Massachusetts state government.

Father Jack Roussin fulfilled a lifelong ambition in 1992 by becoming pastor of a Catholic parish in Lima, Peru. His departure from St. Mary of the Angels was marked by overwhelming expressions of gratitude and sadness at his departure. When St. Mary of the Angels Church was first built decades before, construction on the small church at the intersection of Columbus and Walnut Avenues had been interrupted halfway because of a lack of funds. From its beginning, the church had always been on the edge financially, the center of a community perpetually on the edge, and the missing roof was an appropriate symbol. Jack rebuilt the church financially, socially, theologically, and physically, eventually raising the funds to construct the roof that had always been missing from his church.

Father Jack returned for visits to the Boston area periodically to visit his family, to drop in on the Egleston community, and to seek financial support for his desperately needy parish in Peru. He was thrilled and amazed with the challenge. In 1995, he contracted tuberculosis and was forced to return quickly to the United States for emergency hospitalization. It was too late, however, and he died within one month. In the spring of 1995, the Egleston community had its second round of mourning for the loss of Father Jack Roussin.

I was getting ready to attend one of the numerous memorial services for Father Jack on the Friday afternoon shortly after his death. I had been thinking about him all day long as I went through my routines at work, straightened up my house, and washed my car. I had a little extra time before the service to work off some energy, and decided to take a quick run in the Arnold Arboretum near my home. Near the end of the run, I was passing through my favorite section, one with tall, majestic pines, spruces, and firs that reach far into the sky, sending out a strong and pleasing fragrance. Ever since about the age of sixteen and a half, when I first got my driver's license and could ride out to Walden Pond in Concord instead of going to Catholic Mass, I have considered myself agnostic. I choose "to let the mystery be," as the Iris DeMent song suggests, focusing on the work of this planet. But at that moment, heavily sweaty, out of breath, and full of thoughts of my many times with Father Jack, I veered in the belief direction and began talking to him as I walked alone along the path in the woods.

"Jack," I said, "I have no idea if you can hear anything I'm saying right now. But I just wanted to let you know that we all miss you very much, and we're all thinking about you. And, even though I'm not very religious, well, if you would like to give me some kind of sign, signal, or message to let me know that you're OK, well, I just want to let you know that—I wouldn't at all mind, and would really appreciate it."

Having let the words out of my mouth, I shut up. Nothing happened. I looked around, checked my pulse, wiped some more sweat, did a few stretches, and headed out the back gate of the Arboretum to my car a few hundreds yards away, already forgetting about my impudent request.

Back at my freshly washed car, on the roof right above the driver's side, was the largest pile of bird shit I had ever seen in my life. I could not say, of course, that there was a connection between my request and this particular gift. All I can say, most definitively, is that if there *was* a connection, it was entirely consistent with the character of Father Jack.

PART TWO

Themes

Whatever the controversy in political life, certain themes repeat that slice into issues in both familiar and unexpected ways.

- Why do politicians fight with each other so much instead of just sitting down and working things out?
- Is everything in politics just about self-interest? Is there room for ideas and the public interest, or is that just a convenient cover for self-interest?
- How do political leaders reconcile their responsibilities to their respective constituencies with their own consciences, preferences, and ideas?
- What is the role of relationships in political life: do they matter too much or too little?

No effort is made in this collection to be comprehensive. Many other themes could have been explored in addition to these. The themes in this section, though, resonate universally in politics. Indeed, while each chapter's theme is paired with one or two case stories, it should be immediately apparent that all of them connect in one way or another with all the stories in this book.

CHAPTER THREE

Landlords, Tenants, and Conflict

Conflict is the essential core of a free and open society.

If one were to project the democratic way of life in the form of a musical score, its major theme would be the harmony of dissonance.

Saul Alinsky

My 1984 election to the House of Representatives also brought membership in a special subgroup called the "Boston Delegation," a collection of approximately twenty legislators whose districts encompass portions of the capital city. Because of the delegation's size and distinctive personalities, its members were presumed to possess a degree of political savvy and insider knowledge that was the envy of the institution. Non-Boston legislators assumed a level of cooperation and conniving among Boston's senators, representatives, city councillors, and mayor that assured only crumbs and leftovers for the rest. The moniker "a Boston pol" carried the scent of legends such as Governor James Michael Curley, Mayor John (Honey Fitz) Fitzgerald, the grandfather of John F. Kennedy, and the archetypal ward boss Martin (Mahatma) Lomasney, remembered for his quiet advice: "Never write when you can talk, never talk when you can nod."

On the basis of such billing, I expected to find an advanced degree of cooperation and scheming within the delegation. Instead, I found a cast of characters who fought mostly with each other—behind the scenes and in full view of the public. In 1991, largely because no one else wanted the position, I was chosen as chairman of the delegation. I spoke to many of my city colleagues of my desire to minimize conflict among the members. Typical was the response I received from then Mayor Ray Flynn, who lustily enjoyed the rough-and-tumble of political confrontation: "I don't see anything wrong with us fighting with each other—that's the normal way things get done politically around here."

I came to see that people assume one of two roles in a given political fight: those looking for conflict who most frequently set it off or quickly dive in, and those who seek to avoid or settle it. Over time, I came to appreciate conflict as more than a necessary evil or inconvenience: it was an essential and vital core of politics. I also learned how various dimensions of conflict can be recognized and manipulated to enhance one's opportunities for political success.

In this chapter, I identify key dimensions of political conflict, drawing on a range of diverse sources and ideas. I then relate two case stories (out of many) concerning perpetual conflict between landlords and tenants that occurred during my years in the State House. Both stories illustrate different key dimensions of conflict.

CONFLICT: SCOPE, SITE, AND INTENSITY

As a society, we seem to be of two minds about conflict. In many respects, we celebrate and idolize conflict and aggressive competition—in sports, elections, the business world, and academia. We constantly devise ways to pick winners and losers and to measure and score each other.

At the same time, many of us are taught from our earliest years that conflict is bad, something to be avoided, repressed, and discouraged at all costs. While many children are taught to put up their dukes and slug it out with a bully, many more are counseled to walk away. Many citizens wonder why political leaders—whether in campaign or governing mode—must be so relentlessly conflictual and negative. Why can't they just resolve their differences maturely and without rancor? Doesn't all the relentless negativism undermine public confidence and demean the public process? Wouldn't it be much better if we could all, in the words of Los Angeles police beating victim Rodney King, "just get along"?

To understand why we just can't, it is helpful to visit the early sixteenth century to examine the writings of one of history's first political scientists, the much-disparaged Niccolò Machiavelli. Machiavelli is best known for his volume *The Prince,* which has been mistranslated and misinterpreted to suggest that "the end justifies the means" and caricatured as a handbook for would-be tyrants and despots. The key contention, properly translated, holds that "in the actions of all men, and especially princes, where there is no impartial arbiter, one must consider the final result."[1] While it has attained the status of a universal guide for political connivance, *The Prince* was actually written in haste responding to a specific contemporary crisis in Italian politics. Machiavelli wrote a second, longer, and neglected volume, *The Discourses,* which lays out in a calmer and more deliberate fashion his essential ideas. These ideas represent a framework for understanding conflict that has relevance for us today.

Machiavelli starts with twin assumptions of insatiable human appetites for more and inevitable limits on our ability to obtain all we desire:

> [H]uman desires are insatiable, for we are endowed by Nature with the power and the wish to desire everything and by Fortune with the ability to obtain little of what we desire. The result is an unending discontent in the minds of men and a weariness with what they possess; this makes men curse the present, praise the past, and hope in the future, even though they do this with no reasonable motive.[2]

The more humans possess, the more they want. This is certainly not true in the case of every individual (from Mother Teresa to my own mother) but easily confirmable collectively by examining human societies from the least to the most advanced throughout human history. While technological and economic progress continually expand the boundaries of potential consumption, our aspirations always have outstripped the wealth of the planet and always will do so. Even if humans were able to reach a point of balance between resources and desires, it could not last long because we would quickly demand more.

A critical task for human societies, then, is to figure out how to distribute limited resources in a context of insatiable human desires—the ultimate and essential application of *who gets what.* As described in chapter 1, humans have two ways at their disposal to reach this determination. The first way is by physical force, the use or threat of violence that enables the most powerful to set the terms of distribution. The second way is by law, the use of civil government (often backed up by the threat of force) that enables citizens to establish nonviolent rules and procedures to determine who gets what. A vital challenge is therefore to organize society in such a way that its members can reasonably pursue their interests and desires without resorting to violence.

Here Machiavelli offered insights that were unique in his time. Instead of advocating government suppression of conflict to enforce a false stability, he suggested that the strongest societies were those organized to encourage a healthy dose of political conflict and social friction, that allowing properly channeled conflict would enhance rather than undermine social stability. His model society in this regard was ancient

Rome, which he contrasted with his contemporary and politically ane-
mic Florence:

> [T]hose who criticize the conflicts between the nobles and the plebeians con-
> demn those very things which were the primary cause of Roman liberty.
> . . . [E]very city must have a means by which the people can express their am-
> bition, and especially those cities that wish to make use of the people in im-
> portant affairs. . . . [N]othing makes a republic so stable and strong as or-
> ganizing it in such a way that the agitation of the hatreds which excite it has
> a means of expressing itself provided for by the laws. . . .[F]or experience
> shows that cities have never enlarged their dominion nor increased their wealth
> except while they have existed in freedom.[3]

A healthy society, according to Machiavelli, exists not in spite of persistent and vigorous conflict among different classes but because of it.
(Interestingly, recent international research studies have demonstrated
that democratic societies have *never*, without exception, initiated war
against one another.[4])

The designers of the United States Constitution did not share Machiavelli's affection for conflict. The nation for which they designed a new
government in 1787 was riddled by "the violence of faction . . . this dangerous vice," according to James Madison.

> Complaints are everywhere heard . . . that our governments are too unstable,
> that the public good is disregarded in the conflicts of rival parties, and that
> measures are too often decided, not according to the rules of justice and the
> rights of the minor party, but by the superiour force of an interested and over-
> bearing majority.[5]

At the same time, they recognized the importance of legitimizing conflict
in order to ensure a stable and free society:

> Liberty is to faction what air is to fire, an aliment without which it instantly
> expires. But it could not be a less folly to abolish liberty, which is essential to
> political life, because it nourishes faction than it would be to wish the anni-
> hilation of air, which is essential to animal life, because it imparts to fire its
> destructive energy.[6]

As had Machiavelli, the designers of the new Constitution understood
that at the heart of conflict and faction were issues related to control and
distribution of society's resources and wealth:

> But the most common and durable source of factions has been the various
> and unequal distribution of property. Those who hold and those who are with-
> out property have ever formed distinct interests in society. . . . [T]he regula-
> tion of these various and interfering interests forms the principal task of mod-

ern legislation and involves the spirit of party and faction in the necessary and ordinary operations of government.[7]

As we shall see in this chapter's case stories involving relations between landlords and tenants, a core dynamic connects then and now.

The U.S. Constitution is a document deliberately designed to permit the open expression of factional conflict by citizens, while it structures a government that restricts the ability of the majority to overrun the rights of minorities. This goal is accomplished through several means. One is by establishing a nation so large and with so many competing factions that no single interest is likely to be able to assert its will over the entire polity for any length of time. A second is by establishing a governance structure through which power must be shared by equally influential branches, each chosen according to differing methods and timetables, each jealously guarding its own prerogatives and privileges.

> It may be a reflection on human nature that such devices should be necessary to control the abuses of government. But what is government itself but the greatest of all reflections on human nature? If men were angels, no government would be necessary. If angels were to govern men, neither external nor internal controls on government would be necessary.[8]

Modern political scientists have advanced, not rejected, the ideas of Machiavelli, Madison, and others who recognized the purpose and necessity of controlled conflict in democratic societies. One of the most intriguing is E. E. Schattschneider, who defined politics as "the socialization of conflict." Not all conflicts, in his view, are political, but become so only "when an attempt is made to involve the wider public."[9]

A commonly used metaphor for political conflict is sports. Frequently, politicians, media figures, and others will invoke sports metaphors to explain political rivalries. Political parties are treated as "teams" that "play offense or defense" in a particular dispute. A successful "player" hits "a home run" with a particular initiative. One side in a conflict "moves the ball down the field" by advancing a bill in the legislative process. An injured party cries "foul" at an unsavory campaign tactic. One active group "controls the ball." Another group that can't achieve its full objective settles "for a field goal." Every season, there are rookies and veterans on the field together. On and on. In order to better understand Schattschneider's ideas, it is helpful to consider some ways that political conflict is *not* similar to sporting contests.

Consider the most common of sports metaphors—those related to football. In a football game, two teams of eleven players each occupy set positions on the field, for fixed periods of time, watched by their fans in the stands and sometimes at home. In political conflict, there is no requirement that the opposing teams be of equal size. Moreover, there is no reason why the field of conflict is limited to only two teams. Three, ten, and literally hundreds of teams can claim a spot if the conflict draws sufficient attention. Players can change teams at will in the middle of the game. Spectators are by no means confined to the stands during the game and can jump down and assist any or several sides whenever they desire. Even the fans watching the game at home can join the fray. Though a legislative session may conclude, the game is not necessarily over at the final bell and can resume without missing a beat at the start of the next round. Finally (though we could go on), there is no reason why the conflict needs to be confined to the particular playing field where it began: it can easily spread into the stands, out to the parking lot, over to another field, or onto the stadium access road.

Schattschneider understood political conflict as a form of controlled chaos. He disparaged theories popular during his time that the outcome of a conflict was predetermined (and could be predicted) at the outset by knowing the relative powers of those who start a dispute:

> Can we really assume that we know all that is to be known about a conflict if we understand its *origins?* Everything we know about politics suggests that a conflict is likely to change profoundly as it becomes political. It is a rare individual who can confront his antagonists without changing his opinions to some degree. Everything changes once a conflict gets into the political arena— *who* is involved, *what* the conflict is about, the resources available, etc. It is extremely difficult to predict the outcome of a fight by watching its beginning because we do not even know who else is going to get into the conflict. The logical consequence of the exclusive emphasis on the determinism of the private origins of conflict is to assign zero value to the political process.[10]

Schattschneider was disdainful of another school of thought during the 1950s and 1960s, the pluralist school, which held that no single group or set of groups held sway and that the dominance of any one interest would inevitably create an effective counter-organizing effort among interests adversely affected by the former's growing influence. "The flaw in the pluralist heaven," he writes, "is that the heavenly chorus sings with a strong upper class accent." Political mobilization is an activity heavily concentrated among wealthier interests. While there was less grassroots citizen mobilization in the 1950s than in the 1990s, it is still true today that serious political mobilization is more often the province of the affluent and professionals. "If everybody got into the act, the unique advantages of this form of organization would be destroyed, for it is possible that if all interests could be mobilized, the result would be a stalemate," Schattschneider observes. "Pressure politics is essentially the politics of small groups."[11]

Schattschneider was much less interested in the activities of individuals and much more alert to groups as the key to understanding political conflict. He powerfully characterized *organization* as "a mobilization of *bias* in preparation for action."[12] We may react negatively to the word *bias* but still see its fit. The National Rifle Association is an organization biased toward preserving the rights of Americans to own guns. The AFL-CIO is an organization biased toward defending and advancing the rights of workers to engage in collective bargaining with employers. The American Cancer Society is an organization biased in favor of treating and preventing cancer. Local neighborhood crime watches are organizations biased toward eliminating criminal activity from their streets. New organizations are formed every day by individuals and groups seeking to advance their particular biases in new ways.

Inevitably, biased organizations confront other groups biased in different directions, leading to conflict. Here, Schattschneider introduces the first important variable in analyzing conflict, its *scope*. Who usually starts a fight? Some one or group that wants to get something someone else has or someone else can give. A fight can start with a simple verbal or written demand, a petition, a lawsuit, legislation, or the like. Generally, an organization that already has what it wants will seek to minimize conflict, try to make it go away, and even pay a price to do so if not too high. But if the price demanded by the challenging group is too high, the latter group will seek to politicize the conflict by dragging it into public view. This, to Schattschneider, is the key moment:

> Private conflicts are taken into the public arena precisely because someone wants to make certain that the power ratio among the private interests most immediately involved shall not prevail. . . . This is so true that it might indeed be said that the only way to preserve private power ratios is to keep conflicts out of the public arena.[13]

This observation helps to explain why there can almost never be harmony—or the absence of conflict—in a partisan legislative body such as the U.S. Congress. By definition, a minority party will always want to create conflict and to bring more parties into the fray—*broadening the scope of conflict*—to make its case to become the majority party. It will seek issues and positions to unite its members, to win the support and attention of outside groups, and to place the majority party at a disadvantage. The majority party usually seeks to minimize conflict to demonstrate its ability to maintain control. (The activities of the congressional Republicans in 1995 seem to violate this last prediction, though that caucus was consciously creating conflict then to get something it wanted in 1996, the White House.)

Lawyers in a legal dispute follow this pattern as well. The attorney who is winning a case will seek to narrow the argument to those terms most likely to produce a favorable outcome. The attorney on the losing side will seek to broaden the list of issues under consideration, hoping to find at least one that will unbalance the opposition. "Throw everything on the wall to see what sticks" is the common expression.

I observed this dynamic in an amusing way at a 1998 conference on proposed federal regulation of managed care. The broad though not unanimous consensus at the session was that some degree of new regulation to protect the rights of HMO members was appropriate. Karen Ignani, president of the American Association of Health Plans, the leading HMO trade organization, was brought up to speak. She began: "The problem with this debate over managed care regulation is that we are looking at it in terms that are too narrow. We need to broaden the issues under consideration. For example, we need to talk about 'values.' What do we really want from our health care system. . . ." In this case, Ignani's industry preferred the status quo to proposed changes which would restrict the ability of HMOs to operate as they saw fit. But it was not just consumers seeking redress; there was also a panoply of health industry providers chafing at the restrictions imposed on them by managed care. Schattschneider must have had a crystal ball when he wrote:

> It is the losers in intrabusiness conflict who seek redress from public authority. The dominant business interests resist appeals to the government. The role of government as the patron of the defeated private interest sheds light on its function as the critic of private power relations. . . . It is the weak, not the strong, who appeal to public authority for relief. It is the weak who want to socialize conflict until the balance of forces is changed. In the schoolyard it is not the bully but the defenseless smaller boys who "tell the teacher." . . . It is the function of public authority to *modify private power relations by enlarging the scope of conflict.*[14]

We can readily observe this dynamic in the first of the two case stories that follow, involving landlord-tenant conflict over the regulation of the conversion of rental apartments to condominiums. The outcome of this conflict, four years in duration, was determined by dramatic changes in its scope.

The second critical element in understanding the dynamics of conflict is the *site*. It is common sense that physical combatants will seek to wage a fight on terrain they believe gives them an advantage. This is also true in political conflict. Parties to a conflict who are losing—or who lose in one particular setting—often seek to change the site of a conflict in hopes that a different locale might produce a more favorable outcome.

(Van Horn, Baumer, and Gormley identify six sites—or "rooms"— where the bulk of political conflict is played out in American politics and policy. Each site typifies a distinct form of political activity:[15])

—> 1.   *Boardroom Politics:* This site involves decision making by business elites and professionals that has substantive public consequences. Here, decision making is highly centralized and is principally focused on one goal, the maximization of corporate profits. The issues addressed typically tend to be highly complex and have low degrees of salience or appeal to the general public.

—> 2.   *Bureaucratic Politics:* This site involves rule making, adjudication, and implementation responsibilities carried out by agency bureaucrats with input from organized clients and professionals. At this level, issues are defined to be as compatible as possible with standard agency methods of operation. The standards for decision making are usually quite explicit, though subject to quick and dramatic change by outsiders. As is true with boardroom politics, the issues tend to be complex and to have low-to-moderate degrees of salience with the public.

—> 3.   *Cloakroom Politics:* This site involves policymaking by legislators, whether in the U.S. Congress, state houses, county boards, or city/town councils. Legislative bodies react to a wide array of issues but tend to be slow in making decisions. Decision making is most often decentralized, subject to numerous influences, especially by well-financed and well-organized interests. Issues tend to have a high degree of public salience and to generate higher levels of conflict than at the two previous levels.

—> 4.   *Chief Executive Politics:* Presidents, governors, mayors, county executives, and their advisers dominate this part of the process. Chief executives generally address highly visible issues and dominate public and media perceptions about government. Their actual policy influence is most often quite different from the image they project. For chief executives, leadership involves the ability to persuade other policymakers, especially legislators, to adopt his or her priorities and to turn them into policy or legislation. Issues at this level normally have high salience, as well as a high degree of conflict.

—> 5.   *Courtroom Politics:* This site issues court orders in response to claims made by aggrieved groups and individuals. This level of politics generally addresses a more restricted range of issues but is capable of decisive policy actions that may have huge effects. Some chafe at the mingling of courts and politics, believing this level to be outside of politics. But large portions of the nation live with a state and county judiciary that runs for office. Even appointed members of the bench reach their perches via nominations by elected officials. Courts generally interpret statutes and regulations that have been crafted by elected politicians or political appointees. Also, courtroom decisions often have dramatic impacts on politics (e.g., decisions on voting rights and voting districts) and policy. The courtroom is a frequent stop for interest groups seeking their most favorable venue.

—> 6.   *The Living Room:* This site represents public opinion, expressed in the voting booth for candidates and ballot initiatives, through public opinion surveys, and through the media. An aggrieved party that loses in the other five sites can always turn to the living room by opposing an official's reelection or by proposing a ballot initiative (permissible in twenty-four states). The public, when effectively mobilized, can have a profound impact on public policy yet can be more subject to manipulation by other government officials and the media than the other sites of conflict.

In the second case story in this chapter, we will see how one determined group of small-property owners that kept losing in site after site kept moving to other venues until they found a room in which they could win.

In addition to the scope and site of conflict, a third key variable to recognize is *intensity.* Though one participant in a conflict may be mammoth in size and huge in perceived influence, a much smaller group can beat it depending upon the respective intensities of interest in a given dispute.

For example, in 1986, with the support of gay-lesbian and AIDS advocacy organizations, I succeeded in winning passage of legislation to protect the confidentiality of HIV tests that detect the presence of the AIDS virus, requiring that no one in Massachusetts could be tested without his or her written, informed consent. During the course of this debate, the Massachusetts Medical Society, representing the interests of physicians, was consumed with other priority issues at the State House. When the law was passed, an influential group of their members who were unaware of the legislation during passage erupted with anger that a physician would no longer be permitted to tell a spouse, or a significant other, of an individual's HIV status without the infected individual's permission. They angrily demanded that their lobbyists file legislation to exempt physicians from the new law.

Over the course of the next five years, Medical Society lobbyists regularly filed legislation, sponsored by an influential state senator, to change the law to permit broad disclosure of HIV status by physicians without the infected individual's consent. Each year, they fought me and the same loose coalition of AIDS and gay-lesbian advocacy groups who sponsored the original law and who were fiercely opposed to the Medical Society's proposal. On paper, the Medical Society's wealth, influence, and clout overwhelmed its opponents'. Yet each year, it failed to amend the law. Why?

In 1993, after it had given up, a Medical Society lobbyist agreed to speak before my public health class to discuss its role and strategy in this dispute. He was kind enough to tell my class what he never told me when we were engaged in the fight: "The truth is that we always had a number of other issues that were of higher priority, and we were never able to invest sufficient resources and attention into winning this bill." When publicly asked, the Medical Society lobbyists always asserted that winning passage of their bill was a top priority; but their actions told a different story. The intensity brought to this conflict by the AIDS and gay-lesbian advocacy groups easily outmatched the superior resources and clout of the Medical Society.

The following two case stories illustrate two key aspects of political conflict, first the scope and second the site.

CONDOMINIUM CONVERSIONS
AND THE SCOPE OF CONFLICT

In December 1979 hundreds of middle-class and elderly tenants at the Towne Estates apartment complex in the Brighton section of Boston got an unwelcome Christmas present, notices from their landlord that their apartments were being converted into condominiums and that they had sixty days to buy their apartments or else move out. Immediately, the phenomenon of condominium conversions hit newspapers and evening news-casts as an important story. Tenants, especially the elderly who had lived in their apartments for decades, felt abused and angry and looked to their elected officials and to the organized tenants' movement for support.

Tenants as an organized political force in Massachusetts had a spotty history. Tenants' rights were a recurring theme during the social and economic upheaval of the 1960s. *Condominium* was largely an un-known word, but large rent hikes were real. Tenants successfully or-ganized in some larger cities during this period to establish rent control but found that the Massachusetts constitution—specifically the "home rule" provision—prevented any city or town from adopting laws such as rent control without the express approval of the state legislature and governor. Turning their sights to the State Capitol, tenant groups in 1970 won approval of "enabling" legislation allowing any city or town with more than 50,000 residents to adopt controls by vote of the local city council or town meeting. One important hitch was that the law contained a "sunset" clause making it—and all local laws enacted pursuant to it—expire at the end of 1975 if not renewed by the legislature. Local ten-ants' groups formed all over the state and won the adoption of rent con-trols in Boston, its neighboring communities of Brookline and Cambridge, and the western Massachusetts college town of Amherst, which adopted a weaker "rent review" system.

In 1975, real estate interests mobilized to block renewal of the state rent control enabling law. Tenants' group leaders, many of whom saw themselves as part of a larger "antiestablishment" movement, under-mined their own influence with ideological bickering that included the unfurling of communist flags in legislative hearings and intense ideologi-cal infighting over events such as the 1975 revolution in Portugal. The legislature failed to renew the state rent control enabling law, but the four communities with rent control at that time were permitted to continue their systems through four separate enabling laws specific to each of those locales. With the demise of the statewide statute, the cohesion of a statewide network quickly evaporated and activist tenants focused in-stead on their local community conflicts.

But the condominium conversion wave that kicked off in an aggres-sive form in 1979 provided a shock to activist and inactive tenants across the state. Activist tenants saw in the conversion wave an erosion of af-fordable rental units threatening the political base that maintained local rent controls. Inactive tenants were stunned by the bullying tactics of the "condo converters," particularly toward elderly and vulnerable tenants.

Triggered by the Towne Estates conversion, a number of local tenants' groups came together to form the Condo Conversion Task Force (CCTF), which packed a state legislative hearing room in April 1980 in support of a bill to ban all conversions. Instead, the legislature's Committee on Housing and Urban Development reported favorably a bill which provided only minimal notification to tenants before they could face eviction. The CCTF members raised enough of a political ruckus to keep that bill from moving further in the legislative process, but they recognized the need for a stronger statewide organization if they were to win legislation to meet the threat.

At the end of 1980, the CCTF filed a bill for consideration by the legislature in its 1981 session to ban conversions in any community with a rental housing vacancy rate below 8 percent, effectively a statewide ban. But the CCTF quickly folded into a new statewide group, which held its inaugural meeting in January 1981. The Massachusetts Tenants Organization (MTO) began as a coalition of about twenty tenants' rights groups from across the state and—in contrast to previous statewide efforts— would focus exclusively on issues of concern to tenants, mobilizing them into a political force modeled after the successful New Jersey Tenants Organization (NJTO), which had won rent controls in more than a hundred local communities and was courted and feared by the state's political leaders.

The two initial MTO staff members—working unpaid for the first six months—were Lew Finfer, a Harvard-educated, mild-mannered yet intense, community-organizing phenomenon, and I, most recently of the Amalgamated Clothing and Textile Workers Union (ACTWU), assigned to work on its national consumer boycott of J. P. Stevens sheets and towels because of that company's staunch antiunion activities. ACTWU and Stevens reached an agreement in November 1980 that left me looking for new organizing opportunities. A friend and Tufts sociology professor, Peter Dreier, had been pushing for the creation of a statewide tenants' group modeled on the NJTO and urged me to help start it. Lew was made executive director and focused on building the organization and new local affiliates; I became associate director and was given responsibility for state legislative activities.

MTO had plenty of bravado in our early days. Another friend, the late Kirk Scharfenberg, ran the *Boston Globe*'s editorial page and wrote a column about us in our early days titled "The Giant Is Waking." We won—for our size—a major funding grant from the social action funding arm of the Roman Catholic Church, the Campaign for Human Development, giving us the financial resources needed to build MTO's foundation. We established state and local political action committees to mobilize tenants to support our friends and punish our enemies. We obtained the professional lobbying services of "poor people's lobbyist" Judy Meredith and her able assistant, MaryAnn Walsh, via support from Greater Boston Legal Services. We thought that the political creatures making up the Massachusetts House and Senate would shudder at the reality of tenant power and submit to our demands, first and foremost being the passage of legislation to ban condominium conversions. After that, we would resurrect the battle for rent control. There would be no stopping us.

We began our State House campaign with an influential ally, State Senator Joseph Timilty, who cochaired the legislature's Joint Committee on Housing and Urban Development that would be the starting point for our legislation. Timilty had run unsuccessfully for mayor of Boston three times, losing in 1971, 1975, and 1979 to incumbent Mayor Kevin White. Though he had close ties to real estate industry interests (and later became a developer), he felt loyalty to Judy Meredith and me because we had worked hard for him in 1979. We had strong support from several dozen other representatives and senators, but none with a leadership position as well placed as Timilty's.

Our new, revived tenants' movement had a debut in a March 1981 legislative hearing before Timilty's committee, pushing the bill initiated by the CCTF to ban conversions in all communities with rental housing vacancy rates below 8 percent. At the same time, a growing number of cities and towns were passing their own local laws to regulate conversions and filing so-called home rule petitions with the legislature seeking the needed state authority to implement them. Despite Timilty's support, we lacked the votes on the committee to report favorably our bill as written. Instead, the committee reported favorably a compromise bill to ban conversions in communities with more than 150,000 persons (only Boston, Worcester, and Springfield) and to grant all other 348 cities and towns "home rule authority" to pass and implement any protections they chose without having to obtain enactment of home rule petitions beforehand. Though disappointed, we felt that we would use the law to win protections in the big three cities and come back for broader authority in 1982. Because of Timilty's support, we successfully urged that the bill be sent first to the Senate, where we could gather momentum and begin building for the expected confrontation in the House, where we lacked any leadership support.

Naïvely expecting that the bill would move quickly through the Senate, we cooled our heels from May through September, waiting for Timilty to use his influence to pry it loose from the Senate Committee on Ways and Means. Finally, in late September, the bill reached the floor of the Senate, and we were ready. The two public galleries in the elegant, blue-toned Senate are located so that—from each—one can see only the opposite half of the chamber and half of the forty members. Knowing the location of each senator's seat, we directed our supporters—many of whom took the day off from work—to sit in the section of the public gallery that enabled them to eyeball their own senators. We successfully packed both sides, assuming that our show of force would compel their support. Our bill, "An Act to Regulate Condominium Conversions," was printed on the official Senate calendar. It was show time.

After hours of waiting, the clerk of the Senate read the bill's title. Timilty took the floor, explained the bill, and addressed some of the criticisms that had been raised. After he had finished, a Republican senator was recognized: "Mr. President, I move that this matter be laid upon the table."

Senate President William Bulger, whose reputation as a harsh authoritarian leader did not jibe with the day-to-day reality in his chamber, calmly replied: "The Senator from . . . moves that the matter before the Senate be laid upon the table. Under the rules, the matter is held over until the next formal sitting." He then moved on to the next bill on the calendar.

Our supporters looked at each other puzzled. "What happened?" they asked. I didn't know but soon found out that a Senate rule permits any member to move that any bill—or an amendment to any bill—be "laid upon the table," whereupon all debate and action that day stops and the matter is put off until the next formal session of the Senate. At that time, the first matter of business relative to the bill is the senator's motion to lay the matter on the table. Because the Senate meets only once or twice a week in formal sessions, moving to lay a bill on the table was an effective device to eat up valuable legislative time.

At the next formal session, we again gathered our forces, though our numbers were somewhat diminished by members who could not forgo a second day of work. We again filled the gallery. When the condo conversion bill was reached on the calendar, the senator who moved to lay the matter on the table allowed his motion to be defeated on a voice vote. Again, debate began, with Timilty leading off. We thought we were flying. After another fifteen minutes of talk, another senator sought recognition. "Mr. President, I move that the matter be laid upon the table."

"The Senator from . . . has moved that the matter be laid upon the table. Under the rules, the matter is laid aside until the next formal sitting. . . ."

For nearly three months, the State Senate toyed with our bill, delaying and amending in ways that made it unrecognizable. A senator from Worcester—one of the three communities in which conversions would be banned—threatened to hold the bill up indefinitely unless his city was removed from the trio; we agreed to that change, uncertain of its impact on the bill's legality. The chamber's sole African American senator, Bill Owens, took the floor regularly to castigate us as "racist" because the legislation would impede minority developers who were "starting to get a piece of the action" and to charge that we were determined to "keep black people on our knees!" By the time the Senate gave its final vote of approval in mid-December, the bill had been altered to make it meaningless. The legislative session was scheduled to conclude at the end of the month, and we had no ability to move the matter in the House. The new aggressive statewide tenants' movement had entered the State House and hit a brick wall. We refiled for 1982.

In January 1982, battered by the Senate's watering down of the provisions that would have banned conversions in the three largest cities, and emboldened by a growing number of outlying communities that were enacting strong local measures and seeking State House approval for them, I convinced the MTO board to abandon the push for state-mandated bans and move instead for a simple home rule bill to allow all 351 cities and towns to adopt whatever condo conversion protections they chose. Because this portion of our bill had been noncontroversial in 1981, we assumed that it would sail through, and we could use the new law to bolster our growing local organizing efforts.

But as we moved to a more moderate position, Senator Timilty— feeling his IOUs to Judy Meredith and me were paid—moved to the side of the real estate industry and formed his own study group to develop an industry-friendly bill. Through our local organizing efforts, we had developed a strong base of support in his Housing and Urban Development Committee and were able to garner enough votes in April to have our bill reported favorably by a 2-to-1 margin over the negative votes of *both* committee chairmen, Timilty and the House chairman, realtor Jack Cusack from Arlington. We had had our fill of the Senate and used our strength among committee members to have the bill referred to the House of Representatives.

On the face of it, the House was not a hospitable locale for us. Speaker of the House Tommy McGee was a gruff, World War II Marine veteran, a cigar-chomping authoritarian whose methods were already generating a rules reform backlash among his members. He held near-total control over the flow of legislation and, like most of his key leaders, was friendly with the real estate industry and its lobbyists. For two months, he held our condo conversion bill in the clerk's office, refusing to permit it to come to the floor of the House for a vote. In response, we circulated a petition among legislators and brought our burgeoning network of local tenant leaders back to the State House to track down their own legislators and ask them to sign. We got 105 of 160 reps to sign, leading McGee to bring the bill to the floor of the House in mid-June. After more than two hours of debate and several unsuccessful attempts to block us ("laying a bill on the table" is a motion rarely used in the House because it does not lead to automatic postponement until the subsequent sitting), the bill was "ordered to a third reading" by a vote of 131 to 15.

The point at which the House or Senate "orders a bill to a third reading" is also known as the "second reading of the bill." Every bill requires three separate readings in each chamber, with the first being pro forma; after the second, the bill is referred to the Committee on Bills in Third Reading, where House legal counsel review the legislation to ensure that it is properly drafted and ready for the third and final reading. But the committee also serves as a legislative graveyard from which hundreds of bills each session fail to emerge. Bills are only released from that committee when the Speaker gives his OK. Given our lopsidedly favorable vote in the House, we had hoped for a quick release. Instead, June, July, August, September, October, and November passed (the session was scheduled to end at the end of December), and the bill remained stuck. We organized press conferences, rallies, letter campaigns, phone call drives, and more, all to no avail. Finally, after we had held a late-November press conference in front of McGee's office, the Speaker told a reporter that he would release the bill, adding: "Oh, why didn't they ask for it?"

When the bill emerged in early December, it received final approval on a voice vote and was sent to the Senate. We already understood the game that had been set in motion, but there was nothing we could do except play along. The final day of the 1982 legislative session would not occur until January 3, 1983, after which all bills not yet signed into law would die. The governor, Edward J. King, had been defeated in the September 14 Democratic gubernatorial primary by his archnemesis, former Governor Michael Dukakis, whom King had beaten four years earlier, in 1978. King was a staunchly conservative, pro-business leader who switched his party allegiance to Republican shortly after his departure and was known nationally as "Ronald Reagan's favorite Democratic governor." King had no interest in tenants, supported efforts to undermine our bill, and left our new "Mass. Tenants Political Action Committee" no choice but to endorse and work hard for Dukakis. We knew that whenever the legislature sent King our bill, it would be payback time. If the bill was not sent to him quickly, he could run out the clock so that there would be no opportunity for a veto override in the House and Senate.

The State Senate gave our legislation initial approval, by voice vote, without debate, in mid-December, and final approval in the same manner on December 20. Timilty sat quietly during the proceeding.

"What a change from last year," I said to our lobbyist, Judy Meredith, as we climbed the stairs from the third-floor Senate entrance to the fourth-floor gallery. "I guess they must have already dug the grave for us."

"Don't say that!" she slapped me hard on the head. "We keep this thing moving as hard as we can and as long as we can!"

When our bill reached Governor King's desk on December 20, he had ten working days to decide among four choices: (1) sign the bill (inconceivable); (2) veto the bill (unlikely, because we had sufficient votes to override a veto in both chambers); (3) let the bill become law without his signature (inconceivable); or (4) send the bill back to the legislature with an amendment, an option the state constitution permits the governor to exercise once per bill that had the added advantage of running down the clock. On December 29, he chose option 4, sending the bill back, substituting for it the legislation favored by the real estate industry. On January 2, the full House rejected his proposed changes, and on January 3, the final day of the session, the Senate did likewise in the early afternoon, returning the bill to his desk once more. Option 4 was now gone. Option 3 had now changed: because the legislative session would be over at the end of the day, failure to sign or veto would become a "pocket veto" and the bill would die. Except . . . on the next day, January 4, Michael Dukakis would be sworn in as governor, and King wanted to take no chance that Dukakis would sign the bill.

At 11:52 P.M., eight minutes before the constitutional end of the session, King returned our bill to the House with a veto, leaving no time for an override vote. Dead again! Back to square one.

Departing Massachusetts governors engage in a unique ceremony upon leaving office. The center doors to the State House (only opened for the visits of U.S. presidents and foreign dignitaries) are swung open, and the new ex-governor walks alone down the front steps of the famous structure, with friends and well-wishers standing on either side. I had been given tickets to attend the Dukakis inauguration but gave them away and went to watch King take his lonely leave instead. I wanted to make damn sure he left!

In early December 1982, we refiled our home rule legislation for consideration during the 1983 session, knowing full well that much could go wrong. In February, new Governor Dukakis surprised us by agreeing to speak at MTO's first statewide tenants' convention, held on a Saturday at Boston University. He delivered an encouraging speech, promising to sign our condo conversion bill if it reached his desk and giving MTO terrific media coverage the next day. But in the House and Senate, all was not well. In addition to a new governor, 1983 brought a new sitting of the House and Senate, meaning that the membership of all standing committees would be reconstituted. Committee assignments were made at the respective and total discretion of the House Speaker and the Senate President. On the key Housing and Urban Development Committee, every one of our strong supporters was removed by Speaker McGee. Meanwhile, the Massachusetts Association of Realtors and the Greater Boston Real Estate Board, our two principal opponents who were upset at the lopsided 1982 votes in our favor, hired a new lobbyist, a savvy, chain-smoking former state cop named Billy Delaney, who specialized in nurturing friendships and favors with rank-and-file legislators, something their previous lobbyist, the austere J. Kinney O'Rourke, eschewed.

The Housing and Urban Development Committee began its hearing season in March with two key bills relative to condo conversions, the MTO home rule bill and the weak landlord bill. After a fierce April committee battle—including a last-minute appointment of an MTO foe by Speaker McGee—we lost, 8 to 7. For the first time since 1980, the landlord's favored bill would be the committee's bill, with our legislation receiving a negative committee report. The bill was sent first to the Senate under Timilty's tight control.

In early May, Timilty called me into his office, saying he wanted to negotiate. The MTO board authorized me to meet with him to explore a deal. I felt in a completely weak position: after three years of excruciating work, we had *nothing* to show. Our member groups were weary and frustrated. We had lost the key committee vote. The legislature would soon be wrapped up in writing the state budget, with little time for other matters. I already saw the clock ticking away toward December. In our discussions, Timilty refused to budge from the landlords' hard-line position, offering to allow cities and towns to adopt only minimal protections that gave tenants a little more time before facing eviction and prohibiting local governments from doing anything more. He agreed to none of the items my members told me were key.

"Our bill will pass this year," he told me straight. "This is your last chance to be on the winning side." Reluctantly, I concluded he was right. In early June, I brought his offer back to my board.

The MTO board, made up of the most committed tenant activists in Massachusetts, had followed my advice since 1981; this time, they strongly rebuked me. We've come too far, they said, to settle for this. One of the most fiercely pro-tenant members of the legislature, Representative John Businger of Brookline, was equally appalled at my proposed capitulation and approached his fellow Brookline resident, Governor Michael Dukakis, for assistance. Dukakis had pleased us by attending our February convention but never indicated any particular interest in helping our lobbying efforts. His chief housing adviser expressed no desire to help us, as she was absorbed in other priorities. The governor asked to meet with us.

This was a pleasant switch, being *invited* into the governor's office. Dukakis told my board members, Lew Finfer, and me that it was much too early to throw in the towel, that he wanted to help, and that he would make our bill one of his top priorities. We happily agreed and began preparing for a July showdown in the Senate: Dukakis and the tenants versus Timilty and the landlords sounded good to us. The governor began calling senators, bringing them into his office one at a time, finding ways to convince them to commit to voting for the MTO bill over the Timilty-landlord bill. He ordered his key aides and lobbyists to work aggressively on our bill, including his chief secretary, John Sasso, a legendary political strategist and hardballer. I became a daily visitor to Sasso's office. The Senate President agreed to the governor's personal request to schedule the matter for a showdown debate and vote on the last day of July before the summer recess. Hours before the debate, Timilty called Dukakis and asked for a delay to negotiate. We had counted enough votes to win and smelled a stalling tactic. But Dukakis said, "Let's talk if they want to." July ended, the legislature went home for the summer, and we were still nowhere.

In August, Dukakis and representatives of the real estate industry met in his office. Some of them were simply owners of rental properties, but a number of them were also developers who knew Dukakis was committed to investing large amounts of public money in the construction of affordable housing. Knowing the governor would be around for at least four years, and maybe eight, they said to him, "We don't want to fight with you." Dukakis replied, "I don't want to fight with you." After further discussion, they reached an agreement in principle: cities and towns would have home rule authority to do whatever they wanted to regulate conversions, except that any new regulations would require a two-thirds instead of a majority vote in the local city council or town meeting; in exchange for this concession, all tenants in the state would receive basic legal protections regardless of their community—at least one year's notice for all tenants and two to four years' notice for elderly and disabled tenants. Everyone left smiling, Sasso told me.

Agreements in principle have a tendency to break down over details, and this deal was no different. Numerous minor issues divided the two sides, and many landlords not attending the meeting balked when they heard the outline of the deal. Timilty balked. But the governor plowed ahead as though he had an agreement signed in blood. In September, a bill reflecting the agreement was brought to the floor. We won a few technical amendments that were important to us, and the landlords won none of their requested changes. After the Senate passed the bill on September 21 by a 33-to-0 vote and sent it on to the House of Representatives, the landlords held a press conference near the House chamber in front of brightly painted Civil War and Spanish-American War images. They insisted that any "deal" was off and that they would oppose passage of the legislation in the House.

While we still had overwhelming support among rank-and-file representatives, we had no support from any House leader. Stony silence greeted our requests for meetings. Speaker McGee refused to answer legislators' questions concerning his intentions for our bill. Governor Dukakis pressed him, but without the success he enjoyed with the Senate leaders. The House leaders were listening to the landlords, and we began to foresee another empty Christmas box as our fate, even with Dukakis's strong and committed support.

Then something happened.

Since 1975, Tommy McGee had ruled the House with an iron fist, rewarding his allies and punishing all who did not follow his orders. His majority leader, George Keverian from working-class Everett, had waited patiently for McGee to retire and had a promise from the Speaker that he would not run for reelection in 1984, clearing the path for Keverian's ascension in January 1985 to the Speaker's office. But in 1983, McGee started making broad hints that he might change his mind and instead run for reelection as representative and as Speaker. With the strong backing of Representative Charlie Flaherty of Cambridge, the ambitious chairman of the Taxation Committee, Keverian announced on October 18, 1983, that he was soliciting support from members for election as Speaker in January 1985. On October 20, Keverian and McGee met on the cold, windswept Revere Beach Parkway for a private, face-to-face showdown. Unbeknownst to them, they were followed by a photographer from the *Boston Globe,* which ran a series of three front-page photographs on October 21 showing the two of them arguing. Neither would back down, and a showdown had begun.

Civil warfare erupted immediately in the House. On October 25, McGee unilaterally removed Keverian and Flaherty as majority leader and taxation chair, respectively, and faced a nearly unprecedented motion on the floor to "vacate the Speaker's chair." He survived that motion without difficulty but knew that Keverian already claimed a sizable portion of the House Democratic caucus that would choose the next Speaker. Every issue from that moment forward became fodder for the leadership struggle—including, prominently, our condo conversion legislation.

Prior to the schism, neither side in the leadership struggle had been helpful to our cause. Suddenly, neither side in the McGee-Keverian conflict wanted to be publicly identified with the landlords. Both camps openly embraced our bill. With a final strong push from Dukakis, the Speaker promised to move our bill to the House floor in mid-November. At the last minute, his Committee on Ways and Means released a completely rewritten bill that reflected the landlords' position. MTO leaders, Dukakis, and our legislative allies screamed bloody murder, the bill was hastily withdrawn within hours, and our preferred version was approved in the House in sixty-eight seconds on November 15.

On November 30, Michael Dukakis signed the condominium conversion legislation into law in front of an apartment building scheduled for conversion in the South End of Boston. The governor's reputation was as a mediator and consensus builder, but this victory gave him his best chance in the first year of this second term to show his fighting instinct and his willingness to play power politics. He relished the win.

Schattschneider's essential points about the scope of conflict are amply in evidence in this story. One can rarely predict the outcome of a fight at the beginning, because it is nearly always impossible to know ahead of time who will enter the fray once it gets under way and how their entry will change the dispute. Neither tenant nor real estate leaders could have predicted the twists and turns over the four years of this fight, and especially could never have foreseen the shifting cast of players. Michael Dukakis was the critical new element in 1983 that altered the scope of conflict by shifting the power and weight of the governor's office from the landlord to the tenant side. But this was not enough. The other vital change was the McGee-Keverian Speakership fight that erupted in October 1983, shifting alliances in fateful ways.

Many politicized environments are full of "wise guys" and "smart players" who claim marvelous predictive powers for themselves. From my experience, the smartest players are those with the greatest amount of humility regarding their predictive powers. The smart ones know that no one can really predict the outcome of a fight and constantly look to manage the scope of conflict for their own advantage.

RENT CONTROL AND THE SITE OF CONFLICT

The *iron triangle* was a durable and accepted concept in political science for many years. The notion was that a tripartite alliance—a politically active industry lobby, an executive branch department, and the Senate-House oversight committees—would link arms, dictate policy, and freeze out intervention by forces not part of the triangle. The most familiar examples were in agriculture (the farm lobby, the U.S. Department of Agriculture, and the House and Senate Agriculture Committees) and in national defense (the arms industry, the U.S. Department of Defense, and the House and Senate Armed Services Committees). But political scientists who closely examined these areas found the triangles far less impenetrable than predicted and have since discarded the rigid construct of the iron triangle in favor of more pliable *policy networks*.[16]

Apparently, these later researchers never examined rent control in Cambridge, Massachusetts. Known as one of the most durably liberal communities in America, Cambridge boasted healthy mixes of Harvard and MIT university students, working-class families, professionals, poor, and elderly—Irish, Italian, African American, Portuguese, Hispanic, and others. In 1970, the city adopted one of the most pro-tenant rent control systems in the nation in an era when protesting racial and sexual discrimination, the war in Vietnam, economic injustice, and unfair rent hikes was all part of the "movement," the seamless progressive fabric of the times.

To foster and protect this key city program, supporters developed a local version of the iron triangle. The first corner—the bureaucracy—was found at the Cambridge Rent Control Board, the city agency charged with enforcing the law, determining allowable rent increases, and eventually regulating condominium conversions as well. The five-member and staunchly pro-tenant board, appointed by the city manager, determined policy while the staff enforced the law on the ground. The second corner—the legislative branch—was found in the Cambridge City Council, where at least five of the nine members throughout the twenty-five-year history of the rent control program had always pledged to support continuation of the strongest possible controls. The third corner—the outside lobby—consisted of a strong, active network of local tenant groups that closely monitored the board and the council on housing issues and worked feverishly every two years to elect a pro–rent control majority. Tenant forces were also a core part of the Cambridge Civic Association (CCA), the successful coalition of liberal-progressive groups that endorsed a slate of candidates during each council election. No candidate could win CCA backing without first unconditionally backing the vigorous continuation of rent control. Thus, the tenants elected the councillors who sustained rent control and appointed the city manager who made all appointments to the Rent Control Board that ruled on all proposed rent increases, evictions, and condominium conversions.

Under Cambridge rent control, landlords could only raise rents according to allowable annual adjustments based on increases in the consumer price index. Adjustments could also be requested for physical improvements to property, though owners had to go through a hearing process to do so and could only recoup their investments over many years. New apartments constructed after 1970 were exempted from rent regulation in order not to discourage new construction. Over time, the disparities in rents between controlled and uncontrolled apartments grew dramatically, and many owners jumped at the opportunity presented by the emerging market of the late 1970s for apartments converted to condominiums. But the City Council—using a broad interpretation of its rent control authority granted by the Massachusetts state government (an interpretation upheld by the state's highest court)—directed the board to strictly regulate and discourage these conversions. During the early days of the hot condominium market, many units were purchased by individuals ignorant of or indifferent to the new city regulations. The city responded by legally prohibiting these owners from living in the units they had purchased and forcing them to rent their units at the low regulated rents.

This structure was created and maintained in the name of preserving affordable housing, particularly for elders, the disabled, and low-income residents and families. The system also provided equal protection to disputed numbers of affluent tenants as well as high-powered Harvard and MIT students making an educational pit stop on the road to comfortable incomes. Seething at these strictures were landlords—owners of several units to many—as well as condominium owners unable to occupy their own homes (owner-occupied two- and three-unit structures were specifically exempted from the system). Over time, various groups of owners joined together, formally and informally, to challenge the system without success. In 1987, a group of owners, most owning only one or several units and many aggrieved by actions of local rent control officials that prevented them from residing in their own properties, formed the Small Property Owners Association (SPOA).[17] Among these was a soft-spoken, determined woman named Denise Jillson, who became an anti–rent control activist when the Rent Control Board subjected her and her family to a lengthy delay in moving into a four-family house they had purchased in North Cambridge; by 1992, she was a cochair and driving force. Over the course of eight years, the SPOA provided a powerful example of Schattschneider's thesis that losers in political conflict—those who don't give up—will seek to change the *site* of conflict until finding a locale that enables them to win.

Between 1987 and 1994, the SPOA visited all of the "rooms" (most on multiple occasions) that Van Horn, Baumer, and Gormley identified as the various sites for political conflict.[18] First, they—as other property owners had tried before—approached the *bureaucracy,* the Rent Control Board, for changes; but most SPOA members had been to that room before with results they found unsatisfactory. Second, the SPOA approached the *cloakrooms* of the Cambridge City Council and the Massachusetts legislature. The council held numerous sessions to consider various changes but always rejected their proposals for system changes. The state legislature—heeding the opposition of the Cambridge legislative delegation—refused to intervene in a local home rule matter. Third, the leaders reached out to *boardrooms,* specifically, the statewide realtor associations, but found those leaders unwilling to raise a rent control ruckus that could reverberate in other communities; confining rent regulations to Cambridge, Brookline, and Boston (the latter two moving through a gradual deregulation process because of the adoption of vacancy decontrol) was fine for them. Fourth, the SPOA sought help from *chief executive offices,* specifically the Cambridge city manager and the governor, and received expressions of sympathy but the same cold shoulder given by local and state legislators. Fifth, the SPOA tried the *living room,* placing a referendum on the Cambridge municipal ballot to appeal to Cambridge voters directly for help; on this count, they again lost soundly in the 1989 municipal elections. Finally, the SPOA entered the *courtroom,* many times, seeking judicial relief and were also rebuffed, with a dismissal of their claims by the State Supreme Judicial Court and, most recently, by a Superior Court judge in March 1993.

From the perspective of the tenants' movement, the landlords always had an important tactical advantage in that the tenants had to win in every room, every time, or else face the elimination or watering down of rent protections. The landlords could keep going until they were able to achieve a victory in any one room that could lead to the eventual demise of controls.

Nonetheless, it seemed to be a clean sweep: a defeat in every venue until 1993, when a new SPOA member, an attorney named Jon Maddox, suggested appealing to a much larger *living room,* the statewide electorate, through a ballot initiative to be placed before all Massachusetts voters in the November 1994 general election. The Commonwealth had granted Cambridge the authority to regulate rents and condo conversions, and thus there should be a way for the voters of the Commonwealth to take that same right away. But devising a legally appropriate ballot question would not be simple. The rules to obtain ballot access were onerous and intricate, loaded with booby traps that had thwarted many determined groups of all persuasions. Since the 1975 expiration of the statewide law permitting communities to adopt rent controls, Cambridge, Boston, Brookline, and Amherst each maintained their systems through individual enabling laws specific only to those communities. To win the required approval from the attorney general, ballot initiatives had to affect more than several municipalities. Thus, the version Maddox devised, with SPOA's endorsement, titled "The Massachusetts Rent Control Prohibition Act," authorized all 351 cities and towns to adopt rent controls but only under three conditions: (1) six months after adoption, compliance by owners had to be voluntary; (2) exempted were all units with fair market rents over $400 per month and all owners with fewer than ten units; and (3) any municipality with such regulation had to compensate property owners for the difference between the controlled rents and the fair market rents. All other local laws would be nullified. The title, in short, was apt.

To win a position on the 1994 statewide ballot would not be easy.

SPOA, with financial backing from state realtor groups and assistance from paid signature gatherers, needed to obtain signatures from 70,286 registered voters between early September and the first Wednesday in December 1993, with no more than one-fourth coming from any single county in Massachusetts. SPOA established a political committee, the Massachusetts Homeowners Coalition (MHC), to receive donations and to run the campaign, with Jillson as chairman. Before filing their signatures with the secretary of state on December 1, 1993, however, MHC first had to file its collected signatures in each city or town from which the petitions were obtained for certification by local officials that the signatures represented true registered voters in each respective community. By December 1, organizers had filed 73,769 signatures; however, that total exceeded the county maximum in Middlesex and Suffolk Counties by 3,843, leaving MHC with only 69,926 signatures, 360 fewer than needed. On December 7, Jillson was notified by the secretary of state's office of the shortfall.

With advice from Barbara Anderson, the state's premiere ballot question initiator and tax cut activist, MHC filed suit in Superior Court against the secretary of state alleging that enough signatures in local communities had been wrongfully denied by local election officials to overcome the shortfall. Two days later, eleven rent control supporters from Boston, Brookline, and Cambridge filed a motion to intervene in opposition to MHC. At the end of an eight-week trial that included exhaustive testimony from competing handwriting experts, Judge Martha Sosman ruled on April 22, 1994, that MHC had collected 34 more signatures than necessary to win ballot certification. Meanwhile, on March 8, the city of Cambridge and six registered voters filed suit in the Supreme Judicial Court arguing that the attorney general erred in certifying the MHC petition as conforming to the requirements of the Massachusetts constitution for ballot initiatives. It was not until July 14 that the court voted to uphold the legality of the attorney general's certification. By then, MHC had collected the final round of 11,714 signatures needed. The MHC initiative would appear on the November ballot as Question 9.

The year 1994 proved to be one with an unusually large number of ballot questions: adopting a graduated income tax, establishing term limits for officeholders, regulating corporate spending on ballot questions, repealing the state's seat belt law, allowing retail stores to open on Sunday mornings, regulating college student fees, and more. The Massachusetts constitution's provisions on ballot initiatives require that a "fair, concise summary . . . of . . . each law submitted to the people, shall be printed on the ballot." This requirement was never a problem for communities that used paper ballots and had never been a problem in cities and towns using voting machines—until 1994. There simply was not enough physical space on the voting machines to print appropriate summaries of all the questions. As a result, in the voting machine communities, the initiative section looked this way:

Question 1	Question 2	Question 3	Question 4	...	Question 9
Yes No	Yes No	Yes No	Yes No	...	Yes No

with no indication as to the subject matter of each question. Under a requirement recommended by the secretary of state and approved by the legislature (I was involved at the time as House chairman of the Committee on Election Laws), each voter on approaching the machine was to be handed a sheet of paper by a local election official that included the summaries of each question. Unclear was whether this modification violated the provisions of the Constitution, provisions that had been strictly interpreted by the Supreme Judicial Court in prior cases.

Despite this controversy, the campaigns for and against each ballot question moved forward, including MHC's. Its motto, blazoned on bumper stickers and house signs distributed by realtors and small property owners across the state, was a shouted "Get Gov't Out." Its literature, however, took a different approach, relating stories of vulnerable property owners who had been victimized by rent control. One example, the MHC campaign's own synecdoche, was Barbara Pilgrim, an elderly African American woman in Cambridge with an invalid husband, who was not permitted by local authorities to collect rents to cover her mortgage, "even though," the handout noted, "one of her tenants can afford to winter in Florida and summer on the Cape."[19] The MHC had resources totaling over $1 million, including donations of $75,000 in the campaign's final days from the National Association of Realtors and the Institute of Real Estate Management, both located in Chicago. Though its campaign was identified as an effort by small property owners, more than half of MHC's money came from trade organizations and large property owners and managers in donations of $4,000 or more. In comparison, Question 9 opponents spent less than $200,000. Unlike the proponents, the Question 9 opponents had no substantial statewide network to employ, and they concentrated their efforts in the three communities with rent controls.

On November 8, Question 9 received 1,034,594 "yes" votes (51 percent) and 980,723 "no" votes (49 percent). It was defeated in Cambridge, 58 to 42 percent, and in Boston and Brookline by narrower margins. The MHC-SPOA had narrowly won its first and major victory by shifting the site of conflict to the statewide living room. But the conflict was by no means over, as rent control supporters immediately shifted the site of conflict back to the cloakroom and the courtroom, two previously friendly venues.

On the legislative front, political leaders in Boston, Brookline, and Cambridge all moved within days to begin the process to win local approval for new laws that would be submitted as soon as possible to the legislature as proposed home rule petitions. Each community took a different tactic. Boston filed a bill that would simply have restored its broad legal authority to write a new rent control ordinance. Mayor Thomas Menino publicly promised that any new system would target only vulnerable groups, and he was backed by a unanimous City Council endorsement, something that had never occurred in the long history of Boston rent control. Brookline, through its town meeting, voted to seek authority to reinstate its system that had been in existence prior to the November ballot. Leaders in both communities felt the controversy surrounding Question 9 had primarily involved the Cambridge regulations, and because their local voters did not support Question 9 and because both communities had implemented vacancy decontrol, endorsement by the legislature of their proposals would not be difficult or controversial. The Cambridge City Council, recognizing the controversies connected with its system, and having been told by its key local legislator, House Speaker Charles Flaherty, that any new system would have to be limited and temporary, voted to end all controls except for lower-income families and elderly and disabled tenants. By Thanksgiving, all three communities had filed petitions with the legislature.

As chairman of the Boston Legislative Delegation and as a known former tenant activist, I became the point person and lead sponsor in the House on behalf of the Boston petition. As a member of Flaherty's leadership team, I became his point person on the broader rent control issue and consulted with him regularly on all strategic questions. For the legislature, the issue presented a sharp policy conflict between respecting the rights of voters to establish state policy through the ballot initiative process and respecting the rights of local communities, through the home rule process, to determine their own fates. Because any legislator may need the House and Senate's approval of his or her own home rule bill at some time, respect for local community prerogatives is a key cultural theme within the walls of the State House. We sought to play that orientation to the hilt.

On November 28, the legislature's Joint Committee on Local Affairs, the first stop in the legislative process for most home rule petitions, held a packed, daylong hearing on the three petitions in Gardner Auditorium, the largest hearing room of the State House. Mayor Menino and I sat together as the leadoff witnesses, with the mayor stressing the human costs of complete decontrol: "You have to think about the human factor, especially for seniors," he told the committee. "It's the anxiety." I stressed the home rule factor, as well as the special role played by Boston as a haven for people in need: "We have always opened our doors to those in need. We have more shelters and homeless than the rest of the state combined, as well as more public housing, and we accept that responsibility. We ask those communities that do not open their doors to please allow us to continue to meet that human need." We knew ahead of time that we had the votes to win committee approval: both the House and Senate cochairs were on our side, and most other members did not want to vote against legislation personally important to the House Speaker.

The next day, November 29, the House of Representatives passed first the Boston petition, 89 to 56, then the Brookline petition, 84 to 60, and finally the Cambridge petition, 105 to 35. Importantly, the Cambridge bill passed with more than two-thirds of the vote, more than enough to override a potential veto from Governor William Weld, while the other two bills fell far short of that mark. Those of us from Boston and Brookline who had been working this issue found it ironic that the bill from the community that created this mess was the only one that received more than two-thirds support. But we knew that the extra votes for the Cambridge bill were cast in courtesy to the Speaker and also that this drama had many more rounds to play. We held our tongues.

Meanwhile, another front opened up on that same day, as rent control supporters joined forces with other groups on the losing side of ballot questions to challenge the legality of the entire voting procedure, asking the courts to declare the votes on all 1994 ballot questions null and void. Their claims were twofold: first, that handing voters a separate sheet of paper with summaries of the ballot questions violated the stringent provisions of the Massachusetts Constitution; and second, that many local officials did not follow even these procedures, leaving many voters illegally confused. Superior Court Judge Hiller Zobel (later to achieve notice as the presiding judge in the 1997 Louise Woodward "nanny" case) immediately issued a temporary restraining order barring the secretary of state from certifying the results on five of the nine ballot questions—including rent control—and stating that he was "troubled" by the plaintiffs' claims. The key legal question was: What exactly is a ballot? Is it the printed material physically attached to the voting machine, or is it the totality of official literature distributed by voting officials? While the issue was semantic, the implications of the answer for thousands of citizens were quite real.

Both sides in this controversy—landlords and tenants—were now engaged in a massive game of bluff and chance. MHC leaders were in a quandary. They had begun to recognize in the early fall that Question 9 was deficient in not providing any transition rules to protect the most vulnerable tenants. They feared that some landlords would impose huge rent increases on vulnerable tenants, triggering a public outcry that would legitimize the call for new and strong regulations in spite of the November 9 vote. They also worried that the legislative process—in the guise of transitional rules—would produce new controls that would eliminate their hard-won gains. They anguished over the unpredictable potential actions of the courts. Finally, and importantly, they knew that if the legislature produced an acceptable transitional law, the new statute would supersede the law approved by the voters on November 9 and thus end all the judicial uncertainty.

For tenants and their advocates, the stakes and uncertainties were of equal magnitude. Judge Zobel's decision emboldened many of them to hope that the courts would nullify the entire initiative balloting, restoring all controls, and that agreeing to any compromise would trade away this potentially critical card. But they also understood that failure to adopt new legislation combined with an adverse judicial ruling would leave all tenants—even the most vulnerable—with no protections. They were heartened by the support in the legislature for the three replacement bills but also knew the prospects for generating the two-thirds vote needed to override a likely gubernatorial veto already looked not encouraging.

Governor William Weld, a libertarian Republican opposed to much government regulation, moved on November 30 to eliminate any uncertainty about his intended action, announcing that all three petitions approved by the House the day before would be vetoed, thus strengthening the bargaining position of the real estate industry. But on that same day, state Appeals Court Judge Christopher Armstrong refused to lift the earlier injunction blocking the rent control ballot question from taking effect and repeated Judge Zobel's stated concerns that the entire election procedure may have been invalid, thus strengthening the tenant advocates who wanted to forgo the cloakroom in favor of the courtroom. One riddle we asked ourselves was: if the courts did throw out the entire balloting process, what could they require as a remedy? A new, special election would draw a very low turnout, and there would still not be space on the voting machines to print question summaries. Not permitting any new ballot at all would harm all of those who had endured the onerous process of obtaining ballot question access. These questions made me doubt the judgment of those relying strongly on the courtroom option.

It soon became clear that we had major reasons to doubt the viability of a legislative approach as well. On December 6, the State Senate took up the three petitions and dealt surprises on all three. The Senate approved the Cambridge legislation intact, but only by a 19-to-17 vote, far short of the two-thirds needed to override a veto. The Senate rebuffed Mayor Menino and amended the broadly structured Boston petition to continue benefits only to low-income tenants and to require a phaseout of all controls within five years, approving that by only a 19-to-16 vote. Senate Minority Leader Brian Lees called the Boston bill "a crappy piece of legislation."[20] Finally, the Senate voted down the Brookline petition, 22 to 13, a vote interpreted as an institutional slap in the face to liberal Brookline State Senator Lois Pines, who had angered many senators by siding with Governor Weld at a critical point in the debate over welfare reform legislation. Before Pines could move reconsideration, a Christmas tree in Senate President William Bulger's office burst into flames, requiring the hasty adjournment of the Senate.

In public comment, Governor Weld said that five years was too long and vowed again to veto all three bills. Several days later, he kept his word by vetoing the Cambridge petition. His veto message stated, "Although I appreciate that Cambridge has attempted in good faith to fashion a balanced conclusion to rent control, it is not one which is appropriately consonant with the results of the referendum." The MHC's Jillson was delighted: "Now we just have to make sure we sustain the veto and wait for the outcome of the court case." Boston Mayor Menino said, "It's sad, but the courts are the only hope we have."[21]

The Cambridge and Brookline bills were dead. The Boston petition was back in the House, but substantially and unacceptably changed by the Senate and yet still veto bait. The state's Supreme Judicial Court scheduled a hearing on the ballot questions for December 22, though no one could predict when it would act. And the local newspapers began to fill with stories of vulnerable tenants receiving exorbitant rent increases:

> CAMBRIDGE—Bill Marcotte, whose partner and roommate is dying of AIDS, received a notice the day after Thanksgiving: The rent for their one-bedroom rent-controlled apartment would be going up to $800 from $576 a month. Across the Charles River, in the South End [of Boston], Judy Desmarais, who has lived in her rent-controlled apartment for 19 years, faces a rent increase of $500 a month.[22]

Just before Christmas, I spoke with Speaker Flaherty about our gloomy predicament. He brushed aside my suggestion that he probe Governor Weld for a possible compromise. "He has no interest in talking about it," he said. We agreed that I would approach the governor's chief policy adviser, Mary Lee King, to see if a deal was possible. King was the most popular member of the governor's staff in the legislature. She had served there for a dozen years before joining Weld and his lieutenant governor, Paul Cellucci, for whom she had worked for many years. Senator Stan Rosenberg and I had worked directly with King earlier that year in sensitive negotiations on the campaign finance reform law. I thought maybe we could resume our good relations. She agreed to meet me the day after Christmas in the governor's outer chamber, a very public spot surrounded by large portraits of recent former governors.

I made King an offer that key local officials from Boston, Cambridge, and Brookline, as well as tenant advocates, told me they could accept: two years of extended rent controls for elderly, disabled, and low-income tenants. This would end the controversy over the ballot question, prevent the issue from exploding with the increasing number of horror stories, and allow local officials time to prepare other plans for the worst-off tenants. I gave her a draft and asked her to get back. Her message later in the day indicated that the proposed plan was acceptable. I was delighted and started putting the legislative pieces together.

Tuesday, December 27, was a turbulent day for both sides. First, the Supreme Judicial Court released a decision upholding the legality of all ballot questions except Question 9, the rent control issue. The court stayed implementation of Question 9 pending a lower court trial on whether the balloting process was implemented correctly. They ordered the lower court hearing for the next day. Meanwhile, the full House of Representatives voted to amend the Boston home rule petition with my redraft, providing two years of protections for elderly, disabled, and low-income tenants in all three communities. A legislative deal seemed to be coming together.

The *Boston Globe* reported: "Weld signaled support for the latest rent control plan, provided it was backed by landlords and real estate interests who pushed Question 9. Weld said, 'If this is something they think is a good idea, I'm certainly not going to stand in the way.'"[23]

But the next day, the real estate groups—increasingly tense and divided among themselves—announced that the bill approved by the House was not acceptable and left too much room for abuse by tenants and local governments. The deal we thought had been set with the governor was off as he repeated his intention to veto any bill unacceptable to the landlords. "If they are satisfied, I am satisfied. I am almost a spectator here."[24]

On Thursday, December 29, Superior Court Justice Wilkins extended the injunction preventing the implementation of Question 9 until after the official end of the 1994 legislative session on January 3, 1995, and explicitly expressed hope that the legislature would devise a resolution to take the matter off his lap. Failing that, he would hold a trial:

> It was granted by all that some irreparable harm would result if the law . . . were allowed to come into effect and thereafter it were determined that the vote on Question 9 was invalid. . . . In my view, the plaintiffs [the rent control supporters] have a difficult but not impossible task of demonstrating that departures from proscribed procedures were reasonably likely to have affected the result on Question 9.

The message to Question 9 backers was that a long implementation delay was possible.

Though Weld apparently had rejected the agreement, the Senate moved ahead on Thursday and approved the same legislation sent over from the House. The margin was close, 19 to 15, and insufficient to override a veto that, once again, appeared certain. In case there was any doubt, the MHC's Jillson stated, "No way, no way. Nope. It is not acceptable."[25] A friend and the State House reporter for the *Boston Herald* asked me why I had not included a means test for seniors in the new legislation:

> McDonough (D–Jamaica Plain) bristled when asked why he did not include the means test, explaining that Weld's chief policy adviser, Mary Lee King, had "passed" on the bill before he submitted it, McDonough said. "We're talking about the elderly. We're talking about people who've lived in their apartments for at least 20 years," McDonough said. "We're not talking about a 'means' test here. We're talking about a 'mean' test."[26]

The next day, King steamed at me: "I *never* have my name mentioned to the papers. *Do you understand?*" I did then. In a moment of frustration,

I had unknowingly broken a cardinal senior staff rule. Our brief era of collaboration was over.

The legislation reached the governor on Monday, January 2, 1995, and sat with him until the next day, the final day of the 1994 session, Tuesday, January 3. The real estate industry, fearful of a trial and of the public relations consequences of no transition legislation, wanted legislation, and so did Weld. Both the House and Senate were meeting that last day in "informal session," meaning that bills could move until midnight as long as no member in either chamber objected—everything that moved did so by unanimous consent. In midafternoon, Weld sent back the legislation with an amendment, something the constitution permits him to do once on any legislation sent to his desk (and as Governor Edward King had done to the condo conversion legislation in December 1982). If the House and Senate concurred, the bill would go back to his desk for his signature. If they disagreed and sent it back to him in its original form, he could veto it or fail to sign it. The new version he sent back was written by the Massachusetts Association of Realtors, only covered low-income tenants, only for one or two years depending on the number of units in each building, and contained numerous loopholes that permitted many thousands of apartments—many of which included bona fide low-income tenants—to lose any protections at all. The local officials from Boston, Cambridge, and Brookline, along with tenant advocates, were dismayed. This was a fig leaf that would permit real estate interests and the governor to pretend that problems for needy tenants had been solved.

Around 6 on Tuesday evening, we held the first and only meeting between both sides. I was the point person for the tenant and local communities position; Jillson of the MHC and Bob Nash of the Massachusetts Association of Realtors led for the realtors. This was my first and only face-to-face with Jillson. Nash and I had dealt with each other many times before during condominium conversion fights of the early 1980s, lead poisoning debates of the 1980s and 1990s, and lots more. Both Nash and I wanted to strike a deal. I had a list of changes that would add protections for low-income tenants in units that were not included in the realtors' draft and that would allow each side to claim resolution. Jillson was reserved and steely. One after another, the answers were all "no." There was no accommodation to be reached. We adjourned the meeting after about thirty minutes.

I spoke with Speaker Flaherty at around 8 P.M., and suggested that he make one more approach to the governor on some key points. He said it was over, the governor would not move, we had lost, and we needed to approve the governor's proposed redraft in order to protect as many people as possible. We had carried the fight as far and as hard as we could, and now it was time to take what we could get. I was out of options and energy and couldn't disagree. I had a splitting headache. I went to my office in the basement of the State House and sat in the dark, thinking about what I could have done to obtain a better outcome and to avert this dismal failure. No answers were obvious.

At two minutes before midnight, the measure written by the landlords and filed by Governor Weld was sent to his desk, the last bill approved by the House and Senate in the 1994 session. I decided to be as upbeat as I could. "We're not talking about restoring rent control," I told the reporters outside of the House chamber, "but rent control's death with dignity." The rent control iron triangle in Cambridge—after many tries—had been defeated.

·   ·   ·

Filing a bill, starting a court suit, filing a complaint with an agency, or initiating a ballot petition that requires some group or set of individuals to give up something without their prior consent is a polite way of picking a fight, a civil form of setting off conflict. It is nearly always the group or individual that wants to get something it doesn't have that sets off the action. It is normally the group or individual that is losing that seeks a broader base of allies and supporters (why create unnecessary IOUs that will have to be repaid at some point?). It is the group or individual that is struggling and losing that typically will appeal to the government for relief. Though not always, we have a tendency in society to root for the underdogs, the Don Quixotes who take on fights against seemingly unwinnable odds.

We can detest what a group or individual is trying to get. We can abhor the way they may try to get it. Organization is, as Schattschneider suggests, "the mobilization of bias," and many times those biases are not pretty. But the base right of groups and individuals in a society to organize to use the civil mechanisms in society to press their demands is one of our most fundamental freedoms.

CHAPTER FOUR

Interests
and a Fiscal Crisis

I don't believe in princerple,
But O, I du in interest.
      James Russell Lowell

In the fall of 1995, a giant Massachusetts-based defense contractor, Raytheon, asked for a giant tax break from the legislature. Company leaders made it clear that their taxes in Massachusetts were demonstrably higher than in other states such as Tennessee where they also had plants, and that they were being offered tempting financial incentives to move to competing states. Rather than using executives in suits, the company convinced thousands of their anxious employees to do the lobbying in the halls of the State House. To the workers, keeping Raytheon in Massachusetts was all that mattered, whatever the cost or precedent. To many legislators, myself included, it also mattered that this was corporate blackmail. Nonetheless, the company had done its work, lining up a comfortable House majority to approve the legislation enacting the deal. On the afternoon of the vote, I pushed the red "no" button on my desk. Within a minute, the House majority whip, Joan Menard, came over to me and said in her cheery, soft-spoken manner: "John, the Speaker wants a green from you on this."

I answered back plaintively, "But he has more than enough votes to win this. Why does he need me?"

"He just does," she replied.

I looked up to the Speaker's rostrum where Charlie Flaherty stood serenely, directly eyeing me. He must have been about two hundred feet from me, but I could feel the weight of his stare as though he were two feet away. I walked over to my desk and pushed the green "yes" button.

As I thought about my switch, I first knew that my vote in either direction would have no substantive impact on the outcome. I held mixed feelings on the issue and could have gone either way, originally voting red as a symbolic protest. Had the vote been close, I might have voted green on my own. I had received no calls or letters from my constituents at all, so that was not a factor. But more importantly, I knew that within the next nine months, I would be bringing to the floor my own controversial legislation on health care access expansion, and I fervently hoped that when my turn came, the Speaker would deliver the votes of recalcitrant members as he was now delivering me. Was my switch an example of naked, opportunistic self-interest or of a hard trade-off necessary to achieve a higher good? Anyone can characterize my action either way. The most honest answer is that both perspectives contain some degree of truth.

Attaining a true understanding of the real and personal interests of participants in a political conflict is always a critical step in analyzing what happened and in planning future steps. This process is important in understanding the moves of players inside government as well as the actions of interests that try to influence what goes on from the outside. Many observers and participants believe that all parties always act out of self-interested motives, while others hold onto a sense of public good and public interest as a motivator of political behavior. Over time, this dispute has tipped back and forth from one side to another, most often reflecting the ethic of the age when the question is posed.

In this chapter, we first explore the ongoing debate between self-interest and public interest as motivators of political behavior, examining what is known about the actions of public officials and interest groups as they pursue their objectives. The case story describes the Massachusetts economic and fiscal crisis of 1989 and 1990 and shows individuals, myself included, acting from self- *and* public-interested motives, most often intertwining the two in ways that can never fully be teased apart.

INTERESTS: SELF- AND OTHERWISE

In my thirteen years as a member and chairman in the House, no individual or organization ever asked me to do anything that was contrary to his or her perceived self-interest. Over the course of thousands of bills, regulations, issues, and disputes, I just *never* saw it. Period. Trying to convince an interest group to support a bill or policy change that served my sense of the public interest but violated its own, I came to learn, was most often a waste of time. The trick was to massage a proposal to make it supportive at best or neutral at worst. Public officials, as well, seemed overwhelmingly motivated by the impact of any action on their own concerns and priorities. As the state's economy hovered near collapse in the late 1980s, I saw any sense of the public good drown in a sea of self-interest. Around 1990, I came across a book that, for the first time, seemed to make sense of it all to me. *The Politics of Health Legislation,*[1] by health economist Paul Feldstein, caricatured the legislative arena as a "Chicago Board of Trade" where—instead of pork bellies and soybeans—the tradable commodity was the publicly bestowed benefit via statute, regulation, or appropriation:

> [I]ndividuals act according to self-interest, not necessarily the public interest . . . legislators (and regulators) are assumed to act so as to maximize the political support they receive. Legislators require political support to be reelected. Organized groups that are able to provide greater political support are expected to have greater political influence than other groups or than voters who are not organized. Organized groups seek to achieve through legislation what they cannot achieve through the marketplace.[2]

Feldstein's analysis hit home with me. Organized lobbies, he wrote, tend to have a *concentrated* interest in legislative outcomes that can have immensely positive or negative impacts on their bottom lines. To them, the substantial cost of investing in heavy lobbying, sizable campaign donations, and up-to-the-minute monitoring of public processes is dwarfed by the potential financial impact of success or failure. Citizens and consumers, on the other hand, have a *diffuse* interest in the fate of most legislative battles, and the price they pay for others' legislative deals normally will have only a marginal impact on their personal budgets and will be weighed against hundreds of other daily distractions, public and private.[3]

The politics of auto insurance presents an example of this dynamic. Insurance companies, trial attorneys, chiropractors, and other well-heeled groups invest huge sums to monitor and influence legislators and regulators to advance their respective positions and to check their opponents. When I chaired hearings of the legislature's Insurance Committee, executives—notified by their cell-phoned lobbyists—would phone messages to my office about a statement I made at a public hearing, even before the session had concluded. They pay good money to know what is going on, at times on a minute-by-minute basis. Even though legislative decisions affect all drivers in the state, consumer voices are overwhelmingly silent, with the few public interest lobbies far outweighed by their industry counterparts.

Everywhere I looked, I found confirmation for the dominance of self-interest. I hated the notion that public good was merely a mask for the pursuit of private agendas, but it made more sense than anything else I had found. I discovered that Feldstein's analysis was but a piece of a much broader school of thinking most commonly referred to as *rational choice theory,* closely related to *public choice theory, social choice theory, game theory,* and more. The word *rational* does not imply that choices are inherently good or logical but simply suggests that individuals weigh choices as best they can and select on the basis of their own perceived self-interest.

I discovered that self-interest, as a concept and a motivator of political behavior, has a long history in political thought, tracing back to the Sophists in fifth-century B.C. Athens, who argued that humans came together for the self-interested purpose of mutual defense and that all laws were based on self-interest. Thomas Hobbes in seventeenth-century England saw self-preservation and mutual defense as the self-interested rationale for subjects to submit to the will of a sovereign. Some seventeenth- and eighteenth-century thinkers contended that a government based upon self-interest would result in a far healthier society for individuals than one based upon the available alternatives. John Locke, for example, concluded that a passion for self-interest as a governmental organizing principle would be far less damaging than passions for honor, glory, and conquest that frequently led nations to destructive wars.[4]

Many other thinkers throughout history, though, recognized *dual motivations* of self-interest and public spirit in the structure and conduct of public affairs. Saint Augustine's *The City of God* divides all humankind into two cities: "That which animates secular society (*civitas terrena,* the earthly city) is the love of self to the point of contempt for God; that which animates divine society (*civitas caelestis,* the heavenly city) is the love of God to the point of contempt for self."[5] Adam Smith saw numerous motivations in humans, with benevolence and self-interest being only the most prominent. James Madison and his contemporaries relied on a mix of self-interest and virtue to balance the needs of the new American nation, suggesting in *The Federalist Papers* in 1787 that the proposed U.S. Constitution could mitigate the "causes of faction" that thwart "the true interest of the country." Even during the American Revolutionary War, George Washington saw a role for both dynamics:

> I do not mean to exclude altogether the Idea of Patriotism. I know it exists, and I know it has done much in the present Contest. But I will venture to asert [*sic*], that a great and lasting War can never be supported on this principle alone. It must be aided by a prospect of Interest or some reward. For a

time, it may, of itself push Men to Action; to bear much, to encounter difficulties; but it will not endure unassisted by Interest.[6]

But in the maelstrom of depression and world war in the 1930s and 1940s, political theory based on normative assumptions of the existence of a common good fell into disfavor. The popular ethic of *utilitarianism*—the greatest good for the greatest number, or majority rule—that traced back to Jeremy Bentham in the nineteenth century was fatally discredited by fascism's capacity to obliterate one minority after another. In 1942 Joseph Schumpeter published an influential book discarding notions of dual motivation in politics or a common good, advocating instead theory based on self-interest alone. "Adversary democracy," in his view, had no place for public interest or common good: voters follow their self-interest, making demands on the political system to satisfy their own needs. Elected officials, in turn, adopt policies to win votes and elections, seeking to satisfy as many and alienate as few as possible. The sum of people's preferences, combined with the self-interested moves of their elected brokers, is all there is.[7] Schumpeter's work signaled a sharp turn in political science away from normative studies seeking to identify the common good and toward a more value-free discipline concerned with the study of interest groups, pluralism, behaviorism, and self-interest.

The growing curiosity of political scientists about self-interest led to collaboration with economics. In 1951, economist Kenneth Arrow demonstrated that majority rule—especially when applied to three or more options—was subject to manipulation and distortion depending upon, for example, the ordering of choices.[8] Thus, majority rule could no longer assume the majority as "right" but only conscious of their interests and alternatives. Anthony Downs pushed the union of political science and economics further in 1957 in creating his "economic theory of democracy." Democratic governments, he suggested, favor producers over consumers because the former are more likely to reward actions favorable to their interests. Calling his theory "political rationality from an economic point of view," and naming self-interest "the cornerstone of our analysis," he asserted that "parties formulate policies in order to win elections rather than win elections in order to formulate policy."[9] In 1962 James Buchanan and Gordon Tullock extended the analysis to the behavior of voters: "Voters and customers are essentially the same people. Mr. Smith buys and votes; he is the same man in the supermarket and in the voting booth."[10]

An explosion of rational-public-social choice–based research followed during the 1960s and 1970s. In political science, new works appeared on the U.S. Congress finding evidence to suggest that members were solely motivated by the desire for reelection.[11] The rational choice approach was extended by George Stigler to the field of governmental regulation—in the theory of economic regulation—to assert that "as a rule, regulation is acquired by the industry and is designed and operated primarily for its benefit. . . . Political intermediaries—parties, legislators, administrators—are not believed to be devoid of influence, but in the main, they act as agents for the primary players in the construction and administration of public policy."[12] In the Cold War–Vietnam era of "realpolitik," James Bond, and "destroying the village in order to save it," a "value-free" study of politics and economics based solely on self-interest was in sync with important themes of the times. Many heralded the new intellectual supremacy of rational choice:

> As Gordon Tullock put it, triumphantly, in 1979, "the traditional view of government has always been that it sought something called *the public interest,*" but "with public choice, all of this has changed." In the profession of political science, "the public interest point of view" is now obsolete, although it "still informs many statements by public figures and the more old-fashioned students of politics."[13]

There is a tendency in the social sciences for the exuberant adherents of valid and helpful theories to claim more explanatory power than is justified, to go overboard in their enthusiasm for a particular construct. Today, some proponents of postmodern theories, for example, take helpful and compelling perspectives to extremes by asserting the relativity of all knowledge. In this same way, rational choice theorists set themselves up for attack by claiming more power for their theories than could be proved. As rational choice theory rose in prominence during the 1960s and 1970s, other researchers made findings that went beyond narrowly framed self-interest as an all-purpose behavioral explanation. For example, Richard Fenno, in *Congressmen in Committees,* found that many members sought seats on particular committees to make good public policy, not to bolster their reelection prospects.[14] In the arena of government regulation, Martha Derthick and Paul Quirk concluded in *The Politics of Deregulation* that the power of an idea—in this case the ability of markets to do a better job than government in controlling industries—was far more influential in moving a deregulation agenda in communications, airline, trucking, and other industries than the positions and lobbying of the affected corporate interests.[15]

The straw that broke the back of all-powerful claims for the predictive power of self-interest-based models—or in the words of Morris Fiorina, "the paradox that ate rational choice theory"[16]—was voting. According to a pure rational choice–self-interest model, the only rational reason to vote is if one genuinely believes an election result would be different because of the absence of that *one* vote. Absent that belief, there is no rational explanation for an individual to make the effort to learn about choices and to make the extra effort to show up at the polling station on election day. Over the better part of a decade, rational choice theorists tried without success to construct a rational choice explanation for voting. In the end, an individual's belief in the importance of voting (or "civic duty") was found to have a far greater effect on his or her voting behavior than any rational choice explanation. There is more to life, and to explaining one's political behavior, than narrow, economic self-interest.

During the 1980s and 1990s, the intellectual challenge has shifted more to understanding the appropriate role of self-interest and rational choice and less to proving its theoretical hegemony. One important reason is that many of its strands, including the theory of economic regulation, for example, have been "devastated by the empirical literature."[17] Most assaults have not tried to dismiss the importance of self-interest in understanding politics, just its place as the dominant motivator of human behavior. Stephen Kelman writes: "Self interest does a great job explaining the location of a new federal building in Missoula. It fails with regard to the major policy upheavals in the United States of the past decades."[18] Similarly, Donald Green and Ian Shapiro suggest a more productive role for rational choice models: "The question would change from 'Whether or not rational choice theory?' to something more fruitful: 'How does rationality interact with other facets of human nature and organization to produce the politics that we seek to understand?'"[19] At the same time, the objective for those who oppose an all-inclusive rational choice approach has been less to prove the existence of "public interest" or "public good" and more to demonstrate the "power of ideas" as an important motivator of political behavior and policy choices.[20]

Rational choice has an important contribution to make in understanding political behavior. But it is illogical to ignore the panoply of other motivations that also explain human behavior: love, envy, sexual drive, patriotism, prejudice, fear, competitiveness, ego, charity, religious belief, hatred, compassion, addiction, and so much more. It is impossible to watch the competing partisans on the sidewalk outside a women's health clinic that performs abortions, or the young men and women who volunteer for military service during times of war, or the many who volunteer time at homeless shelters and other services for the indigent, and conclude that individuals act solely out of concern for their personal pocketbooks.

Over time, even the most exuberant advocates of self-interest and rational choice moderated their claims. The same year that he won a Nobel Prize in economic science for his work in rational choice modeling, James Buchanan wrote that "both images (self and public interest) are partial. Each image pulls out, isolates, and accentuates a highly particularized element that is universal in all human behavior. . . . Each political actor, regardless of his role, combines both of these elements in his behavior pattern, along with many other elements not noted here."[21] Gary Becker won the 1992 Nobel Prize for his efforts to incorporate a much wider class of attitudes, preferences, and calculations in rational choice modeling beyond economic self-interest, including forces such as racism, propensity for violence, and affection.[22]

In the past decade, we have not returned to earlier ideas of "dual motivation" but instead have moved toward beliefs that "multiple motivations" explain human behavior, models that are based not just on economics or political science but also on our rapidly expanding understanding of psychology, the human mind, genetics, and other sources of human motivation. Behavioral psychologists, for example, have demonstrated that empathy is not exclusively learned behavior but also biologically programmed. We have also learned that though we can construct systems that encourage and direct individuals to act only in accordance with self-interest, we can develop structures that help to engender other more "communitarian" forms of behavior as well.

Even politicians, we have come to recognize, are not solely motivated by narrow self-interest. Certainly, the vast majority of successful political figures follow the advice of the late U.S. Senator Everett Dirksen: "The first law of politics is to get elected. The second is to be re-elected."[23] Nonetheless, empirical studies have shown that members' beliefs about how to improve society will often be a stronger explainer of voting behavior than the economic interests of constituents or campaign contributors; still others have identified "ideological shirking" as an important political phenomenon in certain political contexts.[24]

The sources of influence on an elected official's votes and work priorities are multiple, and change from official to official, issue to issue, and year to year. These sources include personal beliefs and interests, colleagues, party leaders, constituents, campaign contributors (time and money), newspapers and magazines, TV shows, radio talk shows and other programs, friends, relatives, professional background and training, interest groups, lobbyists, books, religious leaders, and many, many more. Any seasoned elected official is always aware, to the extent possible, of his or her self-interest in any particular issue, though self-interest most often can be interpreted in multiple ways. It is one of the most important factors in understanding political behavior. It is always vital to recognize and to consider. Failure to do so can easily and often be fatal. But it is only one factor of many.

Most elected officials—though not all—cast votes or take positions at times that represent calculated risks contrary to their perceived self-interest. Individuals unable to do that, from my observation, quickly lose the respect and trust of their colleagues. As we would tell each other in the House, "that's what we get paid the big bucks for." Most rare, though, are those instances when an elected official knowingly takes a position that places his or her future in certain jeopardy. We have a name for those instances. In 1958, U.S. President-to-be John F. Kennedy received a Pulitzer Prize for his book *Profiles in Courage* that presented examples of U.S. senators who placed their careers at serious risk for principle. We call them profiles in courage because they are so rare—not nonexistent, just rare.

The following case story chronicles two years in the life of the Massachusetts legislature when the state's economy and budget approached collapse. The account describes what happened and how my colleagues and I, in our own ways, tried to deal with it. Interests and self-interest abounded; public interest and principle were more scarce.

THE MASSACHUSETTS FISCAL CRISIS: 1989–90

These are some personal images and memories from a state fiscal collapse:

As I was standing in a long line at a local quickie-mart on Centre Street in Jamaica Plain holding a half gallon of milk, a man I had never met angrily walked over to me and began shouting: "You are a cockroach! How dare you vote to raise my taxes. You are a disgrace! You should be ashamed! We're going to run you out of there fast!" Before I could say anything, he stormed out the door.

Walking home from the Forest Hills public transit station along Washington Street and Hyde Park Avenue, I had the habit of reading books

and magazines along the way. At least a dozen times, my attention would
be broken by a beeping horn. I would look up and see the driver or a
passenger giving me the finger and yelling something I usually could not
quite make out.

Sitting on a crowded Orange Line train, again reading a book, I noticed a strange middle-aged woman standing over me, talking at me.
"Please Mr. Representative," she pleaded. "We can't take any more of
these taxes." She got down on her knees, every eye on the train now staring at us. I looked both ways, giving a perplexed shrug. "We just can't
take any more," she insisted. "You have to stop it!"

•   •   •

JANUARY 1989

Conventional wisdom holds that Governor Michael Dukakis's huge popularity ended with his sound shellacking in the November 1988 U.S. presidential election against Vice President George Bush. But two events this
month were the more reliable cause for the rapid drop—to the low–20
percent range—in his favorability ratings among the electorate. On January 4, he announced that he would not be a candidate for reelection in
the November 1990 gubernatorial election, ending twelve years as chief
executive. On January 13, he announced his intention to seek legislative
approval for $604 million in new taxes to balance his proposed fiscal
year 1990 state budget, which he would submit for legislative consideration by the end of the month.

The tax proposal was an abrupt and harsh signal that the years of the
"Massachusetts Miracle" during the mid-1980s when the state's economy wildly outperformed the rest of the nation were over. The Miracle
was based on phenomenal growth in computers, real estate, banking, construction, and defense—all key parts of the state economy that Dukakis
used to legitimize his bid for the nation's highest office. The Miracle
bought sizable budget increases for human services and other programs
at the same time as major tax cuts. But the signs of a weakening economy and fewer dollars became increasingly evident over the course of
the 1988 campaign, and the administration and legislature found it
difficult to slow spending as revenue growth began to taper off. By the
time Dukakis announced his tax proposal, his political enemies had already prepared the public to believe that the state fiscal crisis was all about
paying bills for his failed presidential campaign, bills that could have been
avoided but for his national ambitions. Now, it looked to many as though

he was sticking everyone with the tab and getting out at the same time. The fiscal crisis and the demonization of Dukakis were fully under way.

.   .   .

One of Dukakis's fiercest critics was Jerry Williams, an aging, aggressive radio talk show host credited with killing the governor's mandatory seat belt law in a 1986 ballot referendum through his determined radio opposition. In mid-January, I was invited to be a panelist on his Channel 25 TV talk show to discuss state issues. Jerry was jovial and pleasant, joking and chatting with us, until his producer said, "30 seconds, Jerry." Suddenly, he became serious and leaned forward staring hard at us: ("Look, I want you all to argue with each other, interrupt, get mad, disagree, and be as outrageous as you can—because the second you get all nice and congenial my viewers [he extravagantly flicked his right hand] switch the channel." Show time.). .

.   .   .

FEBRUARY 1989

Richard Voke was the mercurial, flamboyant chairman of the House Committee on Ways and Means, the key budget-writing committee in the House of Representatives. A keenly bright, sharp-tongued, and successful attorney representing the poor, working-class city of Chelsea, he was a reluctant endorser of the spending increases of the 1980s and an open skeptic of key Dukakis initiatives including the Universal Health Care Law passed in the waning days of the Miracle in April 1988. With Dukakis's departure from the 1990 governor's race, Voke saw himself as a potential contender for that office or for another statewide post such as state treasurer. In late January, Dukakis's proposed budget, new taxes and all, came to his committee. Opportunity knocked, and Voke welcomed it.

Believing that the state budget had expanded far more than was sustainable and that the groundwork had not been laid to justify new taxes, Voke directed his budget staff to ready the House Ways and Means version of the fiscal 1990 budget (Massachusetts fiscal years run from July 1 to June 30) by late February, far earlier than the normal April/May release. On February 22, he unveiled a no-new-taxes budget plan that reduced or held even all accounts that legally could be held down. While health and human services accounts took a significant share of the pain, they were by no means the only targets. Voke also proposed "level funding"—or no additional funding—for "local aid" to cities and towns, widely considered the most politically sacrosanct part of the state budget. Dukakis had proposed $194 million in new local aid in his budget plan, but contingent on approval of his $604 million tax package. Voke proposed other high-visibility cuts to drive home the severity of the growing fiscal crisis, including the elimination of all state funding for arts programs, after years of generous hikes.

Immediately, affected interests began intense lobbying to restore funding increases promised to them in the Dukakis budget proposal. News stories told of senior citizens faced with the loss of homemaker services, school systems threatening layoffs and elimination of programs, mayors warning of the loss of vital municipal services, and more. Particularly aggressive were the arts advocates, who labeled Voke a "Philistine" for his zero-funding proposal and who came to the State House in droves to buttonhole their local reps to restore funding. But among no-new-taxes supporters, Voke became an instant folk hero, heralded on Jerry Williams's drive-time program and by Barbara Anderson, the head of Citizens for Limited Taxation. Anderson had been chiefly responsible for passage of the 1980 property tax limitation initiative (Proposition 2 1/2) that had set in motion the unquenchable thirst of city and town officials for state aid. Now she publicly nominated Voke for "Emperor of the Universe." Williams and Anderson were hugely disliked by most legislators. Thus it was with discomfort and anger that we heard Voke on Williams's program urging listeners to call their reps to support his budget plan.

Voke and I had shared a cordial relationship since my entry into the House in 1985. He helped me get my priorities through his committee (such as my 1987 legislation to reform the state's lead poisoning prevention laws), and I supported his initiatives on the floor. In late 1988, at my request, he supported my effort to win a seat on his important Ways and Means Committee. As a result he expected me to follow his lead. But I found myself uncomfortable with his approach and tactics on the emerging problems in February 1989. My instinct was to figure out what was driving the fiscal crisis. My own review of the budget led me to conclude that six hard-to-control accounts (out of more than twelve hundred) were driving the crunch: Medicaid, debt service, public transportation, health insurance for state workers, rental assistance, and pensions. These six accounts made up 32.7 percent of the proposed Voke budget but ate up fully 83.3 percent of the growth. Cutting the rest of the budget without getting at the root problems in these accounts and without new revenues in the meantime to avoid damaging the rest of the budget, I thought, would not help.

At a town meeting sponsored by human service advocates in my neighborhood of Jamaica Plain on February 27, more than a hundred angry constituents were not interested in my esoteric analysis of state budget dynamics. This was a liberal-progressive community that wanted to fight cutbacks to human services and local aid. "We expect you to stand up and fight these cuts and to make the case for new taxes, even if you are the *VERY LAST REP* standing there," my friend and supporter Tom O'-Malley yelled at me to tumultuous applause. I wrestled hard in my mind wondering what was the right thing to do: support Voke (who had helped me get a seat on his committee) in his attempt to change the pace of state spending and lower expectations, or support my constituents who expected me to stand up for those who would be hurt by the cuts. Community versus Voke: either way, I would be seen as a coward by one and a stand-up guy by the other.

Two days later, a small group of progressive legislators met inside the State House. We agreed to put together a list of budget amendments to fix what seemed to be the harshest cuts to human service accounts. We called our plan the "survival budget" and ourselves the "survival caucus." I agreed to be the point person and leader.

MARCH 1989

On March 5, an op-ed article I wrote, "Why Cuts Won't Solve a Revenue Crisis," appeared in the *Boston Sunday Globe* outlining my analysis of the six high-spending accounts and making a case for new taxes. No one noticed as the budget debate in the House of Representatives dragged on through the entire week. More than a thousand amendments had been filed by the 160 representatives. Normally, legislators file amendments to help projects in their own districts or programs that are important to them. This time, though, hundreds of amendments also were filed to cut various programs as members attempted to reposition themselves as budget cutters. But the cuts most often affected programs directly connected to others' legislative districts, not their own. Most were accepted or defeated on voice votes: legislators often like to take credit just for filing amendments, regardless of the effort or result.

Every single item in our "survival budget" was defeated overwhelmingly on the floor. Members did not like the cuts but they disliked new taxes even more and appreciated Voke's hard-line stance more than we realized. Voke took special delight in debating against an amendment to restore funding for arts programs, mimicking a falsetto patrician accent to devastating effect. At the end of the long week, several other members who opposed our survival budget proposals had their amendments accepted by voice vote to restore funds to some of the same accounts we had tried to fix. I came to recognize this as a familiar pattern in budget debate: those who hewed close to the leadership's agenda during the course of debate were quietly rewarded at the end of the process. As for me, Voke was pissed—and didn't speak to me or even make eye contact for months.

Living in the midst of the 1989–90 fiscal crisis was like being on a small island in a storm without communications equipment. Was this a brief squall, a serious storm, or a full-blown hurricane? How long would it last? Were we in the eye or on the periphery? How extensive would the damage be? We had no idea. The fiscal monitoring technology of the time gave us only limited understanding of our precarious and slowly emerging position. The giant Massachusetts-based computer companies (Wang, Digital, Prime) that employed tens of thousands had totally missed the personal computer revolution of the mid-1980s and now faced massive layoffs as demand for their mainframes disappeared. The end of the Cold War blew a massive hole in the demand for the products of massive defense companies such as Raytheon. Banking industry behemoths such as the Bank of New England faced collapse as huge, risky loans went sour. Commercial real estate development—which always had at least several new downtown Boston office towers under construction during the 1980s—went dry. Within months, Massachusetts went from having one of the lowest unemployment rates in the nation to one of the highest. Though many other states from Connecticut to California faced similar distress, the morphing of the Massachusetts Miracle to the Massachusetts Mess held a poignancy few could miss. Unwittingly, we had become the nation's synecdoche for state fiscal distress and mismanagement.

Neither Richard Voke nor I had it right, but Voke was far closer to the truth than I was. Dukakis's proposed $12.9 billion in FY90 spending was reduced by Voke to $12.3 billion in the House budget plan. Human service advocates fervently hoped that the State Senate in its upcoming budget proposal would rescue programs that had been cut by the House. They were disappointed in late March when Senate Ways and Means Chairwoman Patricia McGovern announced that the House figure would have to be cut by at least $250 million more because of rapidly dropping revenue estimates. Was this, at last, the bottom, or just today's estimate that would be far worse tomorrow? How bad could it get? How deeply would we have to cut? No one knew.

One of the fiercest reactions came from Boston Mayor Ray Flynn, once described as "Boston's Lech Walesa," the legendary Polish electrician, union leader, and post-Communist president. Flynn announced that it was "lucky I didn't put my foot through the television set" watching Mc-Govern's press conference, repeatedly characterizing cuts in local aid as "bullshit." His administration now projected more than a thousand city worker layoffs in response to the budget cuts. The state education commissioner announced at the same time that more than twenty-four hundred teachers, administrators, and support staff statewide had already received layoff notices in anticipation of the budget reductions.

.   .   .

Anger at legislators often had little to do with support or opposition to new taxes. Representative Frank Hynes voted against most new taxes. A moderate from the South Shore, he received a telephone call from a Boston firefighter who lived in his suburban Marshfield district. Not only was his job directly dependent upon local aid to cities and towns, the man had an autistic child who lived in a state-funded residential facility for the developmentally disabled. "Don't you dare raise my taxes," he yelled at Hynes. "Don't you see," asked Hynes, "how you are personally affected by what happens to the budget?" "They can't lay me off because I have too much seniority," he replied. "But don't you dare cut funding for the retarded either."

.   .   .

APRIL 1989

It was becoming increasingly clear that the Commonwealth's budget problems were not confined to state fiscal year 1990, which would begin on July 1; the state was spending far more in the current fiscal year, FY89, than it was bringing in revenues to finance, hemorrhaging red ink at an alarming rate as numerous state agencies began running out of funds to pay the final three months' salaries. That realization had driven Mc-Govern's comments from several weeks earlier. Voke would have none of it, telling his committee members at a public session that Senate leaders were surreptitiously laying the groundwork for a tax increase by focusing attention on the current year's growing deficit.

Municipal leaders began discussing launching a state ballot initiative to guarantee them a set portion of annual state revenues as data were released showing that more than 100 of the 351 cities and towns relied on state aid for more than 40 percent of their budgets. School officials in Arlington announced that $1.5 million in education cuts would be implemented by closing a junior high school, laying off teachers, and eliminating many school sports and computer classes. State and county corrections officials warned at a Senate budget hearing that jail breaks, disturbances, and "another Attica" were likely if new money was not appropriated soon to ease prison overcrowding. Dukakis's human services secretary, Philip Johnston, indicated that funding for the massive Medicaid program had been underprojected in both the governor's and the House budgets by about $385 million. A special legislative commission warned that Massachusetts roads and bridges were in dangerously poor repair and would require about $37 billion over the coming ten years to bring up to shape—as construction industry leaders began working on their own ballot initiative to earmark all gasoline tax revenues for this need.

MAY 1989

Speaker of the House George Keverian quietly supported Voke during the drive for a no-new-taxes budget in the House. They were close friends, Voke having been one of Keverian's most trusted lieutenants during the latter's 1984 drive to become Speaker and having been rewarded with the coveted Ways and Means post. They were fellow poker players and came from the adjacent working-class cities of Everett and Chelsea. Keverian had been a popular Speaker who relaxed the tight reins held on the House by his predecessor. He openly referred to the House as "my family" and treated rambunctious and unruly members like a doting 1950s TV dad. Keverian also had promised to stay no longer than eight years as Speaker, a commitment his loyal majority leader, Charles Flaherty from Cambridge, badly wanted him to keep. The state treasurer's job would be up for grabs in the November 1990 elections, and Keverian had already decided to run for it. He disliked persistent rumors that Voke was also eyeing the office. He also was increasingly worried about the deteriorating situation for fiscal years 1989 and 1990.

On May 10, Keverian publicly broke with Voke, telling reporters that new taxes would be needed to resolve the state's deepening budget problems. A week earlier, Senate President William Bulger had made similar comments, meaning that leaders of both chambers were now on record, along with the governor, in support of a tax hike. Other legislators began floating their own proposals for budget cuts, tax increases, or combinations of both. Tax talk was in full swing as the signs of distress and breakdown continued on numerous fronts.

Oyster growers had to let thousands of bushels of oysters and other shellfish go bad because state fishery inspectors had been laid off. A 7.7 percent tuition hike was approved for all state colleges and universities. Permits to build on wetlands, hook into sewers, and release emissions into the air that had taken months to obtain were now being delayed for up to two years. Job openings at state-run pools, beaches, and parks were delayed or canceled. Pharmacists and other providers for the state's Medicaid program had payments delayed for months for amounts totaling $100,000 and more. Each of these developments, coupled with thousands of similar actions, generated waves of angry calls to legislators. At the same time, two-thirds of Massachusetts voters told pollsters that they wanted cuts in government spending and no new taxes.

On May 16, I was invited to appear on the *10 O'Clock News,* the educational TV station's nightly news program, to debate the state's leading antitax advocate, Barbara Anderson, a quick, sharp, and articulate critic of state government. The host, Christopher Lydon, warned me ahead of time, "Don't let Barbara intimidate you. She's a real pro at this." She walked all over me. I was terrible, and I knew it. I realized later that Barbara—as good as she was—had the added advantage of daily practice and that there was nothing I could say that she had not heard numerous times before. She had her best answers ready for whatever I would say. I chalked it up as a good learning experience. That night she said one thing in particular I had not heard before: she would use the ballot initiative process against any tax increase the legislature might approve, allowing the voters to have the opportunity in November 1990 to rescind any hike.

.   .   .

Paul Eustace, an airline mechanic and union leader who had become Dukakis's secretary of labor, was an outspoken defender of the administration. He remembers visiting his father in a nursing home one afternoon and walking into the recreation room to see a banner hanging on the wall: "*No New Taxes!*" Eustace knew that his father and friends listened daily to talk radio, but this was incredible. His father eyed him, shook his fist, and yelled, "You're breaking us with these taxes." Eustace scratched his head: "Wait a minute. You're all on Medicaid, for Chrise sakes! You claim more of the state budget per person than anyone in the state. And you don't pay a dime in taxes, to boot! How can you complain like this?" he asked. "These taxes are killing us!" his father exclaimed. "You've got to stop it!"

.   .   .

JUNE 1989

Two higher sources weighed in on the growing fiscal emergency this month. Protestant and Catholic church leaders wrote to legislators asking them to raise taxes to preserve essential public services. "All of us, through some involvement as active participants in our communities, have seen evidence of problems caused by inadequate public funds," noted the Massachusetts Council of Churches. The four Roman Catholic bishops stated: "While the widely felt resistance to taxes can be seen as a helpful incentive to appropriate efficiencies in the administration of government, it should not keep us from fulfilling our social responsibilities." The financial gods of Wall Street also joined in, dropping the Commonwealth's credit rating two notches, returning it to the level of the last state recession in 1975, second only to Louisiana as the lowest rating in the nation. "Wall Street is hitting the state over the head with a two-by-four to get its attention," said the state's bond counsel. "They wanted to do something dramatic." Besides the psychological wound, the downgrading ensured that borrowing costs for the state, already high, would become even more oppressive.

The State Senate approved its version of the FY90 state budget in a twenty-five-hour marathon session. Like the House, the Senate included no new taxes in its budget, which called for $12.47 billion in spending, contrasted with $12.3 in the House version. A budget bill is many things, but chief among them, it is a bill, a piece of legislation that moves inexorably through the legislative process like any other. A committee of conference (including three senators and three representatives, two Democrats and one Republican from each branch) is appointed to resolve differences between the two legislatively approved versions and produce a single conference report, which is then brought before both branches for final up or down votes. On the final day of the fiscal year, June 30, the legislature approved a $12.6 billion spending plan that House and Senate leaders acknowledged was imbalanced. While the budget did not contain new taxes, leaders agreed to begin work the following week to craft a tax package to fill the budget holes.

Midmonth, I had another round with Barbara Anderson before a luncheon forum for about two hundred fifty employees of the John Hancock Mutual Life Insurance Company on the sixtieth floor of their glass-mirrored tower in Copley Square. Anderson's organization, Citizens for Limited Taxation, was already organizing a ballot initiative to keep the state income tax at 5 percent, rescinding any and all tax hikes that the legislature might approve up to the November 1990 election. This time I was better prepared and felt more confident in debating her. When it was over, workers swarmed around Anderson to congratulate and thank her. No one came to me, and I quickly left.

JULY 1989

July 13 was the first of several "D-Days" when the full political and economic weight of the fiscal crisis hit ground zero. Two major events occurred on this same day. First, Governor Dukakis vetoed $491 million in FY90 spending, including $210 million in local aid to cities and towns and $97 million in human services programs. Standing before a deep blue curtain in a packed State House auditorium, he said that "the first $250 million hits bone and will cause real pain. The balance hits raw nerve and will be devastating to people and to communities." Dukakis received expected criticism from interests that bore the brunt of the cuts: cities and towns, human services, education. But he received no reciprocal praise from those who criticized his earlier unwillingness to make cuts. Instead, claiming that he deliberately and unnecessarily cut popular parts of the budget in order to bolster the case for new taxes, they vowed to seek to override his veto of local aid. The villainization of Dukakis was now complete: damned when he did, and damned when he didn't.

The villainization of the legislature was not far behind. Later that same day, the House and Senate gave final approval to a new $743 million tax package that would raise the state income tax from 5 to 5.75 percent for eighteen months; the revenue from the increase would be used to repay bonds issued to cover the FY89 debt as well as hundreds of millions in outstanding Medicaid bills from prior years. Voke now trimmed his prior no-new-taxes stance to opposition to new taxes to support the FY90 budget, while he reluctantly agreed to increases for the other two purposes. The new statute set the income tax to return after eighteen months to 5 percent.

The final vote in the House was favorable, 82 to 78. Keverian and his majority leader, Charles Flaherty, worked intensely to line up the votes. Keverian had a fondness for colored markers that he personally used in his numerous legislative redistricting assignments to create impressive, colorful maps displaying proposed new boundaries. He took them out again to keep track of lobbying efforts: one color for solid "yes" votes, another for leaners, one for solid "noes," another for "no" leaners, yet another for "maybes," and still one more for those who might take a walk. Among rank-and-file legislators, we had our own categories: those who voted for new taxes and budget cuts, those who voted for new taxes and against cuts, those who voted against new taxes and for cuts, and those who voted against cuts and against new taxes. We took comfort knowing that in the next life, the fourth group—substantial in number—would be consigned to the lowest circle in hell.

The dedication of the new tax revenue to pay bills from the FY89 fiscal year and before confirmed in much of the public's mind the belief—bolstered by Dukakis opponents—that the entire crisis was a result of fiscal shenanigans to boost the governor's failed presidential bid. Largely unreported was the fact that by August 1, thirty states across the nation had raised taxes in 1989, three of them—Illinois, Connecticut, and Georgia—by amounts greater than in Massachusetts.

Within the space of several weeks, legislators had done the two things elected officials most despise: raise taxes and cut spending for popular programs. As the legislature wrapped up its work on July 22 and headed into the summer recess, we knew that we had suffered severe political damage. But it was fourteen months until the September 1990 primary elections: lots of time to heal the injuries and win back the public's goodwill. Thank goodness, we thought, that the worst was finally over.

AUGUST–SEPTEMBER 1989

It wasn't. The July tax increase was designed with the belief that the FY90 budget—especially after the $491 million in Dukakis vetoes—was based on a realistic projection of revenues and expenditures. It wasn't. By September the administration estimated that the state was running a current-year deficit of $295 million; Senator McGovern disagreed, pegging the deficit at closer to $350 million. The economic recession gripping the region was picking up speed, not abating. The summer tourist industry experienced its first drop, 5 to 10 percent, in memory. Unemployment continued to rise as layoffs, public and private, accelerated, though many criticized the Dukakis administration for its slow pace in reducing the state workforce. Battered-women's shelters, hospitals, families of mentally retarded, seniors in need of homemaker services, teachers, prisoners, the mentally ill homeless, community colleges, all had their TV moments detailing the harm of budget cuts to their abilities to meet basic needs.

One small story, in particular, caught my attention. The State Department of Public Health announced that it would soon stop providing free vaccines—for measles, mumps, rubella, whooping cough, and more—because of funding cuts and unanticipated new costs. Across the nation, the numbers of children contracting these diseases had been rising at alarming rates in recent years. In Massachusetts, only 6 children caught measles in 1988; by early fall 1989, the number was already over 50; 17 children caught mumps in 1988, with 47 by fall 1989; 82 caught whooping cough in all of 1986, and 208 by the fall of 1989. Medical officials made urgent pleas for action. As the larger fiscal picture seemed overwhelming and insolvable, making sure that kids got immunized was one thing I could relate to. In September, I filed a bill to increase the state cigarette tax by a few cents to generate more than $12 million in funds for the immunization program. Given the fiscal situation, it seemed foolish to try to restore funds without a revenue source, and cigarette taxes had not been raised in years. Including funding in the bill—while politically risky outside the building—enhanced the proposal's credibility with budget writers inside the State House. As a member of both the Health Care and Ways and Means Committees, I sat on both committees that would review the bill. I couldn't predict the outcome but felt that I had found a worthy and winnable issue.

·   ·   ·

Speaker George Keverian frequently traveled to all corners of the state to attend the fund-raisers of his members. He took special joy riding in his car that carried license plates emblazoned with the words "The Speaker." During the heady days of his early Speakership, he would regularly get beeping horns and thumbs up from passing drivers. More recently, he got a heavy dose of beeping horns and raised middle fingers. Like many of his members who had proudly displayed "House" plates on their cars, he had his car plates changed at the end of August to display an unidentifiable number.

OCTOBER 1989

The Health Care Committee held a hearing on my immunization bill on October 3. The new public health commissioner, David Mulligan, told the committee that all vaccine supplies would be exhausted by early December and that help was needed to avert a crisis. I said: "This is one of the last things you let go in state government. You put out all the lights and put all the desks out on Boston Common before you let kids go without immunizations." I had not spoken with Ways and Means Chairman Voke in six months and knew that action would require his help. He had always been especially good on children's health issues, personally launching one of the nation's first public assaults on infant mortality in the mid-1980s, and I hoped this issue would be an icebreaker between us. He was friendly and helpful. Too much was happening on too many fronts for him to freeze me out any longer. The July tax increase had made him an enemy of the no-new-taxes camp. And even though he opposed more tax increases now, he wanted all the friends he could get to deal with a budget fiasco growing worse every day. He assigned me to work with his budget director, David Mateodo, to develop a workable plan to fix the immunization program. If we could find a solution, he would fold it into the larger budget-cutting legislation now under discussion in the House and Senate.

By now, estimates of the current year FY90 deficit had grown to $500 million, accompanied by an excruciating political stalemate in the House. Dukakis and Keverian agreed on October 3 that the only solution involved both new sizable spending cuts and major new taxes. But Keverian, whose leadership style rested on persuasion and not coercion, found himself unable to convince enough of his members. Some feared the consequences of voting for new taxes twice in the same year; others felt the groundwork had not been laid with dramatic cuts in state government; others opposed any tax increases while providing only token ideas to cut spending. A sizable number of Keverian's appointed committee chairs openly ridiculed his tax proposals, giving ample political excuse to rank-and-filers seeking cover. Early in the month, Keverian and Dukakis called for combinations of tax hikes and spending cuts. By midmonth, Keverian, in an unusual appearance before the House Ways and Means Committee, urged a line-item-by-line-item review of state spending to find reductions before consideration of new taxes. By the end of the month, Keverian was prepared to bring to the House a combination plan of $855 million in new taxes and additional cuts. In an emotional meeting with his leaders and chairman on October 30, Keverian asked those opposing him to raise their hands and was stunned to find Voke's hand among them. "And you, too, Richard?" he asked, ashen-faced, paraphrasing Caesar's response to Brutus in *Julius Caesar*. Facing a rank-and-file revolt on the floor, Keverian withdrew his bill, indicating that he would reintroduce a cut package in the near future.

NOVEMBER 1989

Each month, tax revenues were coming in at lower and lower levels than had been predicted by the economic experts. At the beginning of the month, the deficit was pegged at $730 million, but by the end of the month, the official estimate rose to $820 million. Failing in his effort to win support for a tax package, Keverian directed all factions in the House to work together on a cut package. On November 6, Voke produced a $401 million package, $270 million of which were not cuts but nontax revenue increases in fees and assessments; by the time the full House finished work on it on November 17, it had dropped in value to $308 million. After the lengthy debate, Keverian told his members to prepare for a tax package to close the gap.

Earlier that month, Senator McGovern released a widely publicized report detailing five state budget accounts increasing at an alarming rate and consuming all the growth in state revenues: Medicaid, health insurance for state workers, public transit, debt service, and pensions. She labeled them "the budget busters" and focused a growing spotlight on issues driving them. I could not help noticing that all five were outlined in my March *Globe* column that had gone completely unnoticed. I discerned two lessons from this: first, the importance of *who* releases information; and second, the value of naming things.

During debate on the House budget cut package, homeless advocates held a twenty-four-hour round-the-clock vigil in the cold outside the State House; twenty demonstrators were arrested trying to set up an "emergency winter shelter" inside the capitol building. As budget cuts idled the state's fishery patrol boats, fights and assaults broke out offshore. Pediatricians expressed alarm at the impact of cuts and lengthy waiting lists on the "failure to thrive" program for at-risk infants. A forty-one-year-old Vietnam veteran died of a drug overdose after being denied admission into a post-traumatic stress disorder clinic because of budget cuts. Meanwhile, the U.S. Congress repealed the Medicare Catastrophic Coverage Act it had passed only the year before, leaving the state with unexpected Medicaid obligations in the current year of $60 to $70 million.

Throughout the month, Voke's budget director, David Mateodo, and I met privately with health insurers and others to find a way to get them to contribute to the cost of providing vaccines, something that had been provided free of charge by the Commonwealth up to now. Unfortunately, the insurers had a point: there was no database that could be used to fairly apportion the costs among the various payers. And time was running out.

•   •   •

In one of his many drives to assemble eighty-one votes in favor of a tax package, Keverian reached out in late November to Sal DiMasi, a likable, wisecracking attorney and rep from the North End section of Boston. DiMasi had recently been released from the hospital after suffering a heart attack and was recuperating at his home, only a five-minute drive from the capitol. Keverian called to ask if he would consider making a special trip to the State House to vote for the tax package. "You don't understand, George," he said. "I had a heart attack, not a lobotomy."

•   •   •

DECEMBER 1989

On Friday, December 1, the House leadership brought to the floor a $626 million tax package that proposed raises in half a dozen tax categories, including capital gains and sales. Antitax legislators assaulted the plan with crippling amendments, several of which were successful. By the end of the day, Keverian admitted defeat and sent it back to the Committee on Ways and Means. House leaders, desperate to shift the spotlight to the Senate, said they would take no action on taxes until the other chamber acted on the cut package sent to it in November by the House. Within a week, McGovern unveiled her own package of $348 million in cuts and nontax revenue increases and called the state "broke." On December 28, the legislature sent to the governor the $350 million package including $230 million in new nontax revenues and only $120 million in cuts—$75 million of which was spending that had already been frozen by the Dukakis administration.

A tiny section of the bill authorized the transfer of $8 million in fiscal years 1990 and 1991 to a new Vaccine Trust Fund from the pool that reimbursed hospitals for bad debt and charity care costs. The funds paid into the pool were generated by health insurers, so the use of the monies was—in a policy sense—valid. The hospital industry did not appreciate the move but was in no position to argue against vaccines for children.

They were furious with me for not telling them beforehand, but I knew they would try to kill it if they could. For me, we fixed a small but important problem during a desperate period, and I had shown Voke that he could rely on my help on difficult and sensitive issues.

It was my own personal silver lining in an abysmal situation. The excruciating year ended in a painful war of words and finger-pointing among leaders of the House, the Senate, and the administration. Could 1990 be worse? No one dared to make a prediction, except that it was far from over.

JANUARY 1990

For elected officials, every year is a political year, but none more so than an election year. Ours had now begun, and it was already shaping up to be special. Major initiative questions, including the CLT Tax Cut, had generated enough signatures to qualify for the ballot. The continuing round of cuts and tax hikes had already convinced a record number of twenty-four legislators not to seek reelection and had shaken any feelings of invincibility from the rest. At center stage, the race to succeed Michael Dukakis as governor was not yet fully formed but moving fast. On the Republican side, House Minority Leader Steve Pierce from western Massachusetts had an early lead and a built-in advantage from daily State House media coverage of the fiscal crisis; former federal prosecutor William Weld had made a deal with moderate State Senator Paul Cellucci to run as a team, the former for governor and the latter—who had planned to run for the top job—for lieutenant governor. While Weld's most noteworthy proposal was to remove all televisions from state prisons and to "reintroduce inmates to the joys of busting rocks," it was not clear how well his patrician style would play in this populist year. The Democratic race was most noteworthy for the strong contenders who had declined to run: former U.S. Senator Paul Tsongas, who currently chaired the higher education Board of Regents and had harshly criticized Dukakis and the legislature; the well-liked Congressman Joseph Kennedy; and Boston Mayor and working-class hero Ray Flynn. In the race were liberal Lieutenant Governor Evelyn Murphy; former Attorney General and Lieutenant Governor Frank Bellotti, a moderate early favorite; and a wild, wild card, Boston University President John Silber, sharp-tongued, authoritarian, and idiosyncratic. In late January, when Dukakis released his budget proposal for fiscal year 1991, which would begin July 1, Silber said that state spending could be reduced by $1.2 to $1.6 billion: "I suspect that there is at least 10 percent waste in the state budget."

As the political clouds gathered, the fiscal storm clouds darkened further. The state revenue commissioner announced on January 2 that tax collections for December (always one of the year's most lucrative months) were 13.2 percent lower than those for the year before: $763 million collected in December 1989 versus $879 million in December 1988. Speaker Keverian continued his pilgrimage in search of a tax package that could win approval. Every possible combination of increases in income, sales, gasoline, alcohol, cigarette, and new service taxes was put forward to members. A $300 million package was reported by the House Ways and Means Committee on January 13 but was soundly rejected by House Democrats in a stormy caucus on January 16. I recall one member's complaint that it was the House that always went first: "Why can't the Senate go first?" Nice idea to a lot of us, except that the state constitution requires all tax bills to originate in the House.

Dukakis, meanwhile, had learned a lesson from his January 1989 budget proposal for FY90 that included $600 million in new taxes; his FY91 proposal, at $12.6 billion, included major reductions in all discretionary parts of state government as a "wake-up call" to those skeptical about the need for new taxes. "We will probably lose some citizens of the Commonwealth," he said, because of cuts in services to the poor, the sick, the homeless, and the elderly. Stories of dangerous prison overcrowding and the soaring rates of cocaine-related infant deaths didn't matter. Dukakis's credibility with the public had vanished, and nothing he said seemed to matter anymore.

·   ·   ·

For many years, Representative Steve Angelo, from north suburban Saugus, had a Saturday morning volunteer ritual helping constituents unload newspapers and bottles from their cars for the recycling program at the town landfill. It had always been a popular, friendly scene that allowed Angelo to see and be seen by many constituents. But after the first major round of budget cuts and tax increases, he noticed increasing numbers of cars that refused to stop to let him unload their recyclables. They would sit in their cars with the doors locked, refusing to look at him, waiting for another volunteer to be free so they could avoid contact with their rep.

·   ·   ·

FEBRUARY 1990

Senator McGovern had ably focused blame on five "budget buster" accounts, but one dwarfed them all: Medicaid. Nothing else came close. Between FY89 and FY91, when the total state budget rose by $1.03 billion, the Medicaid budget rose by $733 million, or 71 percent of the total, even though the federal-state medical program for the poor had represented only 14 percent of total spending in FY89. Medicaid was "the eggplant that ate Chicago," pushing aside everything else that state government did to satisfy its insatiable appetite for dollars. The intense political controversy generated in 1989 by items such as departmental press secretaries and use of state cars was comically trivial by comparison.

At the same time, because of its unusual funding structure, it was a most difficult account to slow down. For every dollar the Commonwealth spent on Medicaid, the federal government gave us fifty cents. If the state was providing a human service at full cost, it could, by moving that service to Medicaid, provide the same assistance at half the state cost. Thus, in 1988, the state began aggressively "maximizing federal revenues" by shifting large numbers of state services into Medicaid, artificially and dramatically inflating the program's bottom line to the benefit of other agencies. Unfortunately, that was not the only cause of the program's explosive growth. Medicaid was administered in an open-ended, fee-for-service arrangement that permitted providers—nursing homes, hospitals, home health agencies, and others—to retroactively bill state government to capture the full "cost" of services years after they had been provided. Thus, a significant portion of the program's annual budget—as well as the 1989 tax package—went to pay prior-year Medicaid bills. Finally, these were years of hyperinflation in medical spending for all public and private health payers, with staggering annual price increases of 20 percent or more. Like it or not, Medicaid was an integral part of an out-of-control health system.

Fresh from the childhood immunization victory, I was back in Chairman Voke's good graces. When his budget director and health care expert, David Mateodo, resigned in January, I recruited a replacement for him, Paul Romary, who had worked as research director of the Health Care Committee when I first entered the House in 1985. I persuaded Voke that in order to get to the root cause of fiscal instability, we had to make a major assault on Medicaid in the FY91 budget. He agreed to set up a Special Committee on Medicaid with three reps (Democratic Representative Carmen Buell from Greenfield, liberal Republican Representative

Barbara Gray from Framingham, and me as chair) and four outside health care experts, all of whom had intimate knowledge of Medicaid. In late February, we began twice-weekly closed-door meetings, three hours on each Tuesday and Thursday morning. We met with everyone and anyone who offered to help, and we planned to have recommendations ready by April.

Also this month, Voke stated that the Commonwealth would need a $400 to $500 million package of "permanent" new taxes to dig out of the crisis. CLT Director Barbara Anderson publicly warned that if the legislature raised taxes again, her ballot petition to roll back taxes and fees to their 1988 levels would "win very, very big." Meanwhile, the state's welfare caseload rose to its highest level in seven years. Department of Social Services officials reported a sharp rise in child deaths due to parental drug use, physical abuse, AIDS, and other causes. The state-appointed foster parents of a twenty-two-year-old severely mentally retarded man attempted to leave him at the office of Governor Dukakis when their state financial support was eliminated. Without mentioning specifics, Republican gubernatorial candidate William Weld told a TV program that he could cut 10,000 employees from the state payroll without cutting state services.

MARCH–APRIL 1990

As our Medicaid Special Committee met feverishly throughout the early spring, the fiscal crisis continued to worsen. Despite the $350 million cut package approved and signed into law in January, the FY90 deficit in early March was back up to about $750 million, about where it was before the passage of the package. By early April, after a dismal March corporate tax collection, both McGovern and Voke predicted that the current year's deficit would top $1 billion. Wall Street, in the form of Moody's Investor Services, dropped the Commonwealth's bond rating to number 50, the lowest of any state, below Louisiana and Mississippi. Investment officials warned the state that the continuing deficits as well as the CLT Tax Cut ballot initiative forced them to value the state's bonds at only one level above junk bond status. Economic indicators gave no hope for change: jobs continued to decline, building permits fell 40 percent from the year before, and a new round of teacher layoff notices had begun.

Tax talk continued—but only talk. Keverian mounted his fourth effort of the fiscal year to find a tax increase package that could muster majority support, a quest that continued to be an exercise in futility. Democratic gubernatorial candidate John Silber endorsed a 20 percent temporary increase in the income tax to stabilize the state's finances. Also, a coalition of some of the state's largest businesses endorsed higher state taxes as long as the new money would be earmarked for public schools, a move that suggested an emerging shift in the corporate community's antitax stance.

On April 3, the State House opened its new Great Hall, a former dank airshaft positioned like the hole in a square doughnut, transformed into a lavish public reception space with an Italian marble floor, a splendid skylight three stories up, and a gaudy "public art" clock immediately dubbed the "birdcage" by building denizens. The $2 million renovation had been commissioned during the heady, long-forgotten days of the Massachusetts Miracle. The opening in the spring of 1990 gave numerous political candidates one more opportunity to draw the public's attention to a State House culture that appeared alarmingly out of touch.

·   ·   ·

Representative Robert Emmett Hayes, a rising star in the House, was a moderate Democrat who represented the historically Republican town of Whitman, south of Boston. Major water cleanup legislation was called the Hayes Law in acknowledgment of his leadership role. He was also the only House committee chairman from his region to vote for taxes. Knowing that his votes to cut spending and raise taxes would make him politically vulnerable, Hayes began knocking on doors in his district in 1989. Initially, he had one or two doors slammed in his face daily. As the campaign heated up—along with continuing tax and budget fights— he had five to eight doors slammed in his face daily. At one torturous House Democratic caucus in the spring of 1990, he silenced everyone: "Look," he said in a voice nearly breaking, "you don't understand how angry people are. They will take it out on us. I'm already gone. But there is still time for you to save yourselves. We have to get this finished. We're making it much worse by the way we just keep dragging this out."

·   ·   ·

MAY 1990

With Voke needing to release his FY91 budget proposal to the full House, it was time for the Medicaid Special Committee to report. Throughout the spring, in hallway and sidewalk conversations, numerous legislators from both parties and all political persuasions urged me repeatedly to be "tough" and to tame the destabilizing giant. We concluded that it was essential to require change from every sector touched by the program. We had a long report and set of recommendations to restructure not just Medicaid but the entire health infrastructure of Massachusetts government. The following items were among our key recommendations.

First, we would require Medicaid to enroll all recipients into managed-care/HMO plans by January 1992. With an up-front HMO payment for a Medicaid recipient's services, the process of huge and unpredictable retroactive payments to providers would stop. We would put the program's administrators in a more powerful position to control future spending. Though this recommendation would have no short-term savings, we saw it as an essential long-term reform.

Second, knowing that nursing home costs claimed the lion's share of Medicaid expenditures (75 percent of Medicaid budget increases in recent years were for long-term care) and that large numbers of middle- and upper-class seniors "impoverished" themselves by shifting assets to family members before they entered a nursing home, we proposed to count the value of a recipient's home as an asset when determining eligibility—except when a spouse or dependent lived in the home or there was a possibility that the individual might return. As a new incentive, individuals who purchased long-term-care insurance would not be subject to the rule if their private benefits were exhausted. We estimated annual savings from this change at $30 million.

Third, we recommended combining about twenty state government health agencies (Medicaid, Public Health, Group Insurance for state workers, the Division of Insurance, the licensing agencies, and others) now spread across four cabinet secretariats into a single Department of Health under the leadership of a "health czar" who would have powerful tools to control spending and create efficiencies. The mega-agency would be situated within the Secretariat of Human Services. Cost savings from this move would be realized over time.

Fourth, we recommended limiting growth in all provider contracts to no more than 3 percent, down from the current 10 percent average, for a $90 million annual savings.

Fifth, we recommended deleting a number of recipient benefits that were optional under federal law, including adult dental services, chiropractic care, Christian Science nursing services, and others, for annual savings of $24 million.

Sixth, in order to demonstrate that *no one* would go untouched, we recommended cutting in half the "personal needs allowance"—the money provided to nursing home residents to purchase personal items—from $60 to $30 a month, for a $7 million savings.

I was personally uncomfortable with a number of these proposals, especially adult dental services and the personal needs allowance. But these and other changes were in the context of an FY91 budget that still would increase the Medicaid line item by $350 million. The three reps on the Special Committee—Carmen Buell, Barbara Gray, and I—spent time with Voke and House leadership members to test the viability of our recommendations. We offered to change anything they felt inappropriate, unwise, or politically out-of-bounds. They changed nothing, thanked us for our work, and encouraged us to move ahead.

On May 7, Voke unveiled a $13.3 billion budget proposal, $500 million more than the current fiscal year ($350 million of which was for Medicaid) and $1.1 billion out of balance if the House failed to pass a new tax package. The effects on the budget from Medicaid and state workers' health insurance costs—as well as the Special Committee's recommendations—were the centerpiece of his budget presentation. Our Special Committee's report, released with the budget, concluded: "State government is not in control of our health system's costs. . . . We believe instead that health costs are controlling state government—to the detriment of all other vital state systems." In a May 13 *Boston Globe* story on our findings, I said, "A fiscal crisis is an opportunity to do things you could never do otherwise."

In 1989, as noted earlier, CLT's Barbara Anderson had nominated Voke to be "Emperor of the Universe" for his no-new-taxes stance. Now, with Voke a leading advocate of a permanent tax hike, Anderson withdrew her nomination. Under House rules, members had to be given the Ways and Means budget proposal at least a week before floor debate could begin. During the interregnum, the House leadership prepared for major action on new taxes to fill the budget gap. On May 9, the House approved a $1.2 billion tax plan composed of permanent increases in income and gasoline taxes. Income taxes would rise from 5.75 percent to 6.75 percent in 1990, then decline to 6.5 percent in 1991, and permanently to 6 percent in 1992 and beyond (once the bonds from the 1989 tax hike had been paid off), while the gasoline tax would rise by ten cents over two years. The final vote on May 10, 92 to 66, was not close. Whatever the consequences, a solid majority now accepted the need for new taxes and cuts to solve the crisis. Keverian, Flaherty, and Voke worked members hard and delivered. After months of agonizing stalemate, the tax issue was before the Senate, not the House.

Senate leaders acted surprisingly quickly, releasing on May 18 their own $1.6 billion plan that increased the income tax permanently to only 5.5 percent but extended the state's 5 percent sales tax on goods for the first time to every imaginable service—legal, professional, and business— literally thousands that no one could enumerate. Extending the sales tax to services had been an idea favored by progressive and union groups, but it was fraught with unknown and unexplored problems. At 2:30 A.M. on Saturday, May 19, only about thirty-six hours after releasing the plan, the Senate approved it, 24 to 14. Both chambers had now approved major tax increases, yet both had chosen markedly differing paths.

The House budget debate that began on Monday, May 21, went on for ten contentious, angry, and arduous days. In the midst of debating needed expenditures for the coming year, legislators spent hours debating an amendment by Representative Tom Finneran, the chairman of the Banking Committee, to bar the state's Arts Council from providing support to any individual or group that produced, promoted, or displayed "obscene" art, a response to a public exhibition of the works of gay photographer Robert Mapplethorpe. It passed, 98 to 51.

Surprising to me, the recommendations of the Special Medicaid Committee were mostly noncontroversial, with one major exception. The proposal to count a nursing home patient's home as an asset for Medicaid eligibility triggered a major debate. Representative Chester Suhoski from Gardner, a sincere, self-effacing guy who was facing a serious reelection battle, filed an amendment to eliminate the provision. Chet organized opposition from senior groups and sent a memorable letter to all his House colleagues that concluded: "If we allow this proposal to take effect, attached below is what you will be doing to your senior citizen constituents." Taped to the bottom of the letter was a gold-colored screw.

I made a strong defense on the House floor, displaying large charts showing the real and projected increases in Medicaid spending and the large proportion attributable to nursing home costs. I personally lobbied and pleaded with members to stay with the proposal. One conversation with a Republican floor leader who had voted against taxes and against budget cuts was memorable: "Listen," he told me, "these are middle class people who paid taxes their whole lives and haven't asked us for anything. If they want to be able to pass their estates onto their children to preserve their dignity, that's OK with me." I had a sinking feeling after that, knowing I would go down to defeat no matter what I did. After several hours of debate, Suhoski's amendment passed, 86 to 62. I suddenly realized that when many members had asked me to "tame" Medicaid, they meant only as it related to poor mothers and children—who accounted for only about a quarter of program spending—not to middle- and upper-class seniors.

The House finished its budget debate on May 30 by a vote of 84 to 72. More than $200 million had been added by members to the bottom line, now at $13.5 billion. Newspapers called it a "feeding frenzy." Many members who themselves added—or voted for—amendments increasing the bottom line also voted "no" on the final roll call to indicate displeasure with the House's inability to constrain spending. If they felt a contradiction in their actions, they kept silent about it.

JUNE 1990

Luckily for the House, the embarrassment of the budget process was quickly surpassed by the public humiliation of the Massachusetts Democratic Party's nominating convention in Springfield, which began on Friday evening, June 1, and lasted all day the following Saturday. As delegates arrived for the endorsement proceedings on a hot Saturday morning, they were greeted by Springfield police union pickets blockading the city's Convention Center. Crossing a union picket line is something no self-respecting Democrat can do, especially when seeking statewide office, so all candidates directed their supporters to respect the line. But this was no ordinary picket. The police union had publicly endorsed George Bush in his 1988 presidential race against favorite son Michael Dukakis, and Bush's political director, Ron Kaufman, had been seen around town during the proceedings. This had the stench of a high-level political dirty trick to humiliate the state party and its candidates. After four hours of standoff, the picketers retreated, and the delegates entered a sweltering hall with broken air-conditioning. An afternoon and evening of sweaty intrigue gave former Attorney General Frank Bellotti the gubernatorial endorsement but also Boston University President John Silber the 15 percent vote he legally needed to have his name appear on the September state primary ballot. The convention became the season's favored image of a Democratic Party that seemingly could get nothing right.

Back at the State House, House and Senate leaders set agreeing on a tax plan as their first priority. But Voke and McGovern were engaged in a bitter stalemate over their respective plans. McGovern publicly castigated the House plan as inequitable and one that would give Massachusetts the highest state income tax in the nation. Voke ridiculed as complex and burdensome the extension of the sales tax to thousands of services. The Senate had completed action on its version—from unveiling to final vote—in thirty-six hours. As business groups deciphered the impact of the plan, they flooded the House with pleas of opposition. The leaders' infrequent meetings were rancorous and unproductive. Meanwhile, Speaker Keverian and Senate President Bulger barely spoke with each other.

While they squabbled, Standard & Poor's, one of Wall Street's major bond rating firms, placed Massachusetts government on its credit watch list, thus warning potential investors that the state's lowest-in-the-nation bond rating could soon be lowered to junk bond status with the real possibility of default. A new economic report, commissioned by the Massachusetts Bankers Association, predicted a regional economic turnaround in 1991 or 1992 but warned that conditions might get much worse before then. Newspaper reports named forty senators and representatives preparing to run in the fall elections who had declined their customary right to have their names listed on the fall ballot as "candidate for re-election."

Sensing no movement on the tax front, McGovern released her $13.6 billion FY91 budget proposal on June 25. Very little of the House Medicaid recommendations could be found—only a proposed study of the health agency consolidation. However, late in the Senate's floor debate on June 30, the Medicaid "house as an asset" proposal was added on a voice vote as part of a larger leadership "bundle" of amendments. Senate leaders knew if they had included the provision in their original version, it would have been fought and defeated on the floor. Slipping it in late in the process enabled nervous senators to say it had been done without their knowledge.

·   ·   ·

Representative Sue Tucker, a liberal Democrat with a passion for public education, represented another traditionally Republican district centered in the town of Andover. Like most legislators, she had received many hundreds of constituent letters opposing any tax increase and threatening political retribution. One letter, received right before the final 1990 tax vote, stood out. It included a cartoon of someone lying in a coffin. A xeroxed photograph of Sue's head had been carefully cut out and glued onto the cartoon character's head. The caption simply read: "Your political death." Seeing it convinced her that voting for a tax package would cost her job. She remembers walking out of the House chamber after voting for the tax bill with a sinking feeling in her gut that she would not survive.

.   .   .

JULY 1990

The new fiscal year began on July 1 without a budget and without a tax package to pay for the deficit. On July 5, House and Senate negotiators released a $1.6 billion compromise tax plan. The gas tax would go up ten cents. The income tax would rise from 5.75 percent to 5.95 percent for 1990, to 6.25 percent for 1991, and go back to 5.95 percent for 1992 and beyond, permanently. The extension of the sales tax would apply only to four professional services—legal, accounting, engineering, and architectural—as well as a miscellaneous collection of business services, and would not kick in until mid-1991. In the early hours of Saturday morning, July 7, the House approved the bill, 80 to 76, and the Senate later approved it, 21 to 16. Four House members who had previously voted against taxes were not present. Just barely, the leadership once again delivered. The prevailing feeling among the eighty was an eerie kind of fatalism, recognizing the deep political risks involved in a "yes" vote and also sensing an inevitability that the CLT ballot petition—now known as Question 3—would pass overwhelmingly, negating two years of excruciating work.

But the work was not done, and finishing the FY91 budget was equally difficult. Media descriptions of the legislature and the process during the final two weeks of July were harsh: water torture, Keystone Kops, Animal House, Porky's Revenge, unruly mob—to name a few. Representative Suzanne Bump from Braintree said, "You keep thinking it can't get any worse, but then we do something to top ourselves." After weeks of stalemate, Senate and House negotiators produced a $13.7 billion budget on July 26 that they admitted was at least $300 million out of balance—even with the expected revenues from the new tax package. The budget package included most of the elements proposed by the Medicaid Special Committee, including managed care for recipients, counting the house as an asset, and health agency consolidation into a new secretariat instead of a new department.

Meanwhile, the release by the Revenue Department of a list of 594 business services that would be subject to the new sales tax extension produced such a torrent of public anger and opposition that House and

Senate leaders, as well as Dukakis, openly discussed redoing the just-passed tax package to eliminate the sales tax portions.

House members revolted on July 26, rejecting consideration of any new tax bill as well as the out-of-balance budget plan in an unprecedented rebuke. A number of members also bitterly complained that House leaders agreed to the Medicaid "house as an asset" provision after it had been rejected by a sizable margin on the House floor. Two days later, on a long, hot Saturday, negotiators returned a $13.4 billion budget, pared by requiring a 4 percent across-the-board cut of $264 million in all discretionary spending accounts. Also removed from the final budget plan was the "house as an asset" requirement. In his veto message, delivered a week later, Dukakis vetoed the health agency consolidation. In the end, the only portions of the Medicaid Special Committee's work that survived were the managed-care mandate for welfare recipients and the rate slowdown for providers.

·   ·   ·

On July 18, I was a member of a *Boston Globe* panel questioning the Democratic gubernatorial candidates on health issues. It was routine and dull until one panelist asked the candidates what they would do about the cost of nursing home care in the Medicaid budget. Recalling Shakespeare, candidate John Silber said: "Ripeness is all. . . . When you've had a long life and you're ripe, then it's time to go." My seatmate Steve Tringale and I looked at each other in disbelief. Did he really say that? The candidate felt a need for clarification. "And anyone who has ever bothered to read Aldous Huxley's *After Many a Summer Dies the Swan* will understand exactly what I'm talking about." That night, I scoured area bookstores and libraries until I found a copy I immediately read. I still didn't get it.

·   ·   ·

AUGUST–DECEMBER 1990 (AND SLIGHTLY BEYOND)

Of all the principals in the fiscal crisis, Dukakis, Bulger, Voke, McGovern, only one, George Keverian, faced the statewide electorate in the fall of 1990 as a candidate for the Commonwealth's treasurer. He was defeated in the September primary election by another Democratic House member, William Galvin, who was defeated in the November final by Republican outsider Joseph Malone. The Speaker who saw the House as his "family" felt deserted by members he had personally aided through many years. The man who stood publicly for new taxes and budget cuts to weather the fiscal crisis felt crucified by an ungrateful and confused public. After days of meandering and frustrating sessions in mid-December that included futile attempts to address yet another growing budget deficit, he faced his members in the chamber late one night and said, "I'll see you later," and walked out, permanently cutting off any and all contact with former friends and associates.

Keverian was not the only political loser in the fiscal crisis. In the House, sixteen Democrats and two Republicans were defeated for re-election, among them Emmett Hayes, Sue Tucker, and Chet Suhoski. Among the defeated were legislators who voted for and against taxes, liberals and conservatives. It was the incumbent tag that seemed to hurt the most in 1990. In spite of these losses, Republicans realized a net gain of only 8 seats, from 30 to 38, in the 160-member House, though their Senate numbers shot up from 8 to 16 of 40 members.

Yet another major loser was Citizens for Limited Taxation. Their tax-cutting initiative, Question 3, went down to defeat on November 6 by a resounding 60-to-40 margin (80-to-20 in my own Boston district). Voters clearly disliked the manner in which state leaders had responded to the crisis but refused to accept the assertion that government could cut its way out of the massive hole that Question 3 would have created.

For Republican gubernatorial candidate William Weld, elected governor over Democrat John Silber by a narrow 51-to-49 margin, it was an outcome too good to be true. Weld sustained his dyed-in-the-wool, no-new-taxes stance by supporting a "yes" vote on Question 3 and yet never had to live with the consequences. He entered the governor's office in January 1991 able to use more than $1 billion in revenues from the 1990 tax package to finance his own first budget, always rhetorically opposing the tax hike that made it balanced.

To be sure, more cuts—in the form of another cut package—were needed in the spring of 1991 to balance the FY91 and FY92 budgets. But Weld was helped not only by the $1 billion tax package he opposed but also by a windfall of more than $500 million in onetime federal Medicaid "disproportionate share hospital" payments he was able to negotiate from the Bush White House in early 1991. As was true for his predecessors, it was a combination of new revenues, cuts, and reorganization that held the Commonwealth's fiscal house together until the economy finally began to turn around in 1992. Weld's major tax cut came in the spring of 1991 as the legislature agreed to rescind the controversial sales tax on services that had been enacted but not yet implemented.

·   ·   ·

Most of the time, we act in ways that are consistent with, or at least not contrary to, our self-interests. Within the confines of our narrow personal spaces, we construct rationales and perspectives that permit our actions to make perfect sense from both public- and self-interested points of view. At varying times, most of us take calculated risks for principle, for the protection of current assets, or for potential future gains. For most of us, most of the time, serious conflict between our personal needs and public obligations rarely occurs.

This is different from the rational choice perspective outlined earlier in this chapter. According to the rational perspective, individuals' actions are driven mainly by their self-interests. Elected officials, to this thinking, make their priorities, choices, and votes not just cognizant of their self-interest but driven by it. According to the rational choice view, parties and politicians make policy to win elections, rather than win elections to make policy. Reality is more complicated. Oftentimes, political leaders do make choices for political advantage and electoral concerns. And often they do not. Most politicians, from my close observation, are concerned with "making good policy" and "doing the right thing." The fact that they also pay attention to the potential political consequences of their actions does not diminish that concern.

For me, the events of 1989 and 1990 were frustrating, painful, and demanding. I took many different roles and positions over the two-year ordeal. I tried my best to meet the challenges and obligations of the time, including the need to push for politically unpopular and risky changes or "reforms." While I advocated positions that created anger and conflict directed at me, at no time did I genuinely feel that my political office was at risk. In short, at no time did I consider myself—or most of my colleagues—political "profiles in courage."

The House did, however, have a few. Representatives Emmett Hayes and Sue Tucker—along with others such as Representatives Pat Fiero, Augie Grace, and Fran Alexander, all of whom were Democrats representing traditionally Republican districts—cast repeated votes to increase taxes and cut spending, fully understanding that their actions placed their political careers in dire jeopardy. All of them were defeated for reelection on November 6. (More than a few other legislators in similar circumstances ducked, ran for cover, and developed carefully couched rationales to justify their "no" votes on new taxes and budget cuts.) Their explanations were simple: their consciences dictated their actions, regardless of the political cost. In my thirteen years in the Massachusetts legislature, they stand out as genuine articles, true profiles in courage.

I would also place Speaker George Keverian in this category. His style proved a difficult match for the times, and his indecisive maneuvers were often maddening. Yet despite having to face the statewide electorate in the fall of 1990, he never retreated from his determination to bring the Commonwealth through its turbulent fiscal problems. In his legislative actions as well as his failed campaign for treasurer, he always sought to explain rather than to exploit the crisis. In the end, he deserved better than he got.

We are all a mix of motives in our lives and in our actions. At any point in time, any of us is capable of acting with the highest of ideals or the basest of motivations. We can always find ample supplies of both. We constantly seek the mixture of both that feels "right" to each of us. That mix will vary, from person to person, from situation to situation, and from time to time. In political conflict, it is always essential for the participants to think about and to understand their personal mix of motives, as well as those of their allies and competitors. Understanding each other's motives may or may not lead to conciliation and consensus, but it is rarely a waste of time to try.

CHAPTER FIVE

Representation, Relationships, and Campaign Warchests

O world! World! Thus is the poor agent
despised. O traitors and bawds, how earnestly are you
set a-work, and how ill requited! Why should our
endeavor be so loved, and the performance so loathed?
Shakespeare, Troilus and Cressida

A professional pollster friend of mine once asked his subjects what they most look forward to in their daily lives. The most common answer surprised him, but not me: the mail. I have always *loved* getting mail. My appreciation of the daily post was fortunate, because legislators get lots of mail, at the capitol and at home, of all sorts, mostly unsolicited. One spring day in 1996, in my mail pile at home, I found an envelope with an optometrist's return address. No surprise, I assumed, it's another lobbying letter for legislation to expand their scope of practice, a bill bitterly opposed by their aggressive rivals, the ophthalmologists. Sure enough, the letter from the president of the state optometrists' association asked me to use my influence to pry their bill loose from the House Committee on Ways and Means where it had been bottled up for many months. Enclosed with the letter was a check for $500 made out to my campaign committee.

The letter did not mention the check—it was just included without comment. This was not illegal, though had the check been sent to my State House office, that would have violated our campaign finance laws. This was not really improper, either, because I was already on record in support of the bill the optometrists were seeking, and there was no hint of a quid pro quo regarding my support (though the optometrists' president clearly assumed the check would spur my nagging of the Speaker and the House Ways and Means chairman). No one but the two of us would know that the check and the optometrists' advocacy had been so intimately intertwined. Had the association sent me the letter, and sent the check separately to my campaign committee, I probably wouldn't have felt odd at all. But I did. That night, I wrote a letter to my correspondent indicating my support for the bill and returning the check. He never mentioned it to me, and I never spoke of it to him, or to anyone else.

Only later did I come to recognize and understand better the source of my discomfort. I did not want this individual and his organization to feel in any way that I would be their *agent*, their *representative*. Friend, ally, compadre—these were OK, but accepting the check would have implied a sense of obligation I did not want to incur, a relationship I did not want to allow.

In the previous chapter, I explored the self-interest/public interest duality, a constant which permeates nearly every political choice. In this chapter, I explore another ever-present duality, the duty of representation versus the power of relationships. Representation refers to the manner in which people's views and interests are advanced by their elected or appointed officials. Tension inevitably arises between the duty to reflect the preferences of a constituency (the delegate model) and the obligation to one's conscience (the trustee model). What does an elected official owe the citizens whose ballots elect him or her, particularly when there is conflict between their views and the official's? This is a related though different dynamic from the self-/public interest duality. Standing with one's constituency can easily be portrayed in a self- or public interest light, as can sticking with one's personal preferences.

But representation is not all there is. It is, in fact, but one distinct form of another crucial political dynamic: relationships. In politics, as in the rest of life, relationships are fundamental. They form the core from which nearly everything else follows. Some are based on bonds of friendship, love, trust, respect, and loyalty, while others rely more on power, employment, coercion, and fear. Often, the tug of district representation collides head-on with the power of other relationships. While some relationships in politics are collegial and partnership-based, most involve some degree of inequality: someone is on top, someone is on the bottom, or else the parties are struggling with each other to figure it out. Someone plays the boss, and someone plays the worker, the drone, the peon. Another way of looking at it is, someone plays the *principal*, and someone else plays the *agent* whose job is to carry out the principal's will.

The first section of this chapter explores the dynamics of representation and relationships. I examine representation through the writings of

Hannah Pitkin, Alan Rosenthal, and others who present a variety of ideas to explain this dynamic. I discuss relationships by focusing on a model called agency theory. I then attempt to tie these two dynamics together to clarify the role of each in understanding politics. The case story involves consideration of legislation to overhaul the Massachusetts campaign finance and ethics laws in 1994. This story illustrates both the real nature of representation and the power of relationships in politics. Through these two lenses, we see how complicated relationships and overlapping lines of authority can become in the crafting of laws and public policies.

REPRESENTATION AND RELATIONSHIPS

REPRESENTATION

At first glance, there should be no problem. A constituency chooses an individual to represent it in a legislative assembly. The individual is sent to reflect the policy preferences and biases of the electorate. But problems quickly emerge. On some issues, such as abortion, gun control, or affirmative action, one's constituency may be sharply divided. On others, the legislator may have far more information about a matter than the voters do, and the media often fail to communicate the issue's true complexity. Sometimes, the chamber's party leadership or the governor may hold the key to passage of other legislation more important to the member, and often will press hard for a favorable vote on an issue less crucial to the district's needs. At other times, the member may find the district's expressed preference morally untenable or practically infeasible. Still other times, a portion of the district—not a majority—may fervently prefer a direction the rest of the district less intensely opposes. Lots of other times, a legislator has to vote on an important matter with little or no input from the district. This list of problems goes on.

The traditional view of the representation dilemma presents a bipolar choice. A member can represent the views of the electorate (the *delegate* model) or can reflect his or her own conscience (the *trustee* model). The sense of an either/or choice is reinforced by the oft-quoted statement of Edmund Burke to Bristol electors in 1774:

> [H]is unbiased opinion, his mature judgment, his enlightened conscience, he ought not to sacrifice to you. . . . Your representative owes you, not his industry only, but his judgment; and he betrays, instead of serving you, if he sacrifices it to your opinion.

Political scientist Hannah Pitkin reconceptualized the dynamic away from an either/or choice toward a continuum. In real life, legislators do not make a stark either/or choice between district and conscience. Instead, they constantly weigh a balance between the two, placing themselves at their most comfortable and compatible place on the continuum between delegate and trustee. "Which should prevail depends in each case on why they disagree and which is right. . . . Both formulations distort."[1]

Aside from what legislators should or should not do is the reality of their lives. Alan Rosenthal, the dean of political scientists who study state legislatures and legislators, confirmed the notion of a representation continuum in his discussion in the mid-1990s with seventeen Florida legislators. On a scale from 1 to 10, with 1 indicating complete agreement with the delegate notion and 10 representing agreement with the trustee model, five Florida legislators placed themselves at points 5 or 6, in the middle, while twelve put themselves at points 8 or 9, toward the trustee model.[2] While each individual legislator finds an overall posture, his or her position on the continuum will not be firmly fixed. Rosenthal and others observe that new legislators ordinarily lean in the delegate direction, while longer-serving and more experienced members gravitate toward the trustee end. Moreover, each member's respective position on the scale may easily shift from issue to issue. Matters that generate controversy and feedback from the district will move members toward the delegate end, while matters that do not generate feedback will be treated in more of a trustee pattern.

I draw another distinction. Some issues relate closely to personal values, such as a woman's right to choose to have an abortion, capital punishment, and civil rights. On those issues, I always would vote my conscience as best I could (the trustee model), hoping I was in sync with my district's views. But if not, they had the choice to get rid of me because I would not change my vote. Distributional or taste issues, though, were different and tilted toward the delegate notion. On the distribution of state aid dollars to municipalities, I was always a strident advocate for cities in general and Boston in particular because I saw it as my responsibility to get as much as possible for my community, knowing that most other legislators did the same. Another example: throughout my tenure in the legislature, my district obsessively debated the choice between street buses and trolleys on a public transportation line called the Arborway. There were lots of arguments pro and con, with many people passionate in their views. When the question was asked, in a public referendum and elsewhere, two-thirds of the community always supported the trolley. To me, it was a choice between vanilla and chocolate ice cream, not one of principle, and I respected the expressed view of my constituents on the matter, whatever my personal feelings.

John Kingdon, in his study of the behavior of U.S. Congress members, identified ten key sources of influence on voting behavior: 1. The constituency; 2. Like-minded colleagues; 3. House party leadership; 4. Committee leadership; 5. The party; 6. Interest groups; 7. The administration or executive branch; 8. Congressional staff; 9. The media; and 10. The legislator's own policy attitudes or ideology. While finding constituency to be a consistently important factor, Kingdon concluded that like-minded colleagues were the most consistent influence on voting behavior, though "no one actor in this set is preeminent in congressmen's decision making."[3]

The representation discussion places heavy emphasis on the voting aspect of a legislator's role. In fact, the job of representation is far more varied and complex than simply voting on bills. Members speak out and educate on policy issues, seeking to develop, nurture, and promote proposals long before they reach the voting stage. They intervene with the bureaucracy in behalf of district interests and individuals. They engage in home-based problem-solving activities. Rosenthal identifies four basic ways "representatives represent" their constituencies: 1. Being "one of them" by staying in close touch with the district; 2. Providing services through legislative casework; 3. Acquiring resources through legislative and executive branch activity; and 4. Expressing their policy views and interests through votes and public statements.[4] Focusing only on the voting aspect of the role misses many important functions. Many citizens dislike their legislator's voting record, yet still support his or her reelection because of the member's skill at winning resources for the district.

While a multitude of influences weigh upon each member's voting and other activities, numerous studies over several decades have found "staying in touch" with the district to be a key priority for legislators. Richard Fenno, in his classic study, *Home Style,* found members of the U.S. Congress, while exercising a variety of styles and practices, absorbed with the interests of their district. Three goals are paramount for most members: winning reelection, accumulating power, and making good public policy. To achieve those goals, members engage in activities to win the trust of their constituents; trust is the currency which gives them freedom of action to pursue their priority goals.[5]

How can we reconcile the requirement to represent with the reality that on the vast majority of issues and votes, legislators must vote or act with no significant input from their constituents? Hannah Pitkin provides a useful way to understand this dilemma:

> There need not be a constant activity of responding, but there must be a constant condition of responsiveness, of potential readiness to respond. It is not that a government represents only when it is acting in response to an express popular wish; a representative government is one which is responsive to popular wishes when there are some. . . . We can conceive of the people as "acting through" the government even if most of the time they are unaware of what it is doing, so long as we feel that they could initiate action if they so desired.[6]

We can draw several conclusions here. The representation responsibility is a mix of both delegate and trustee activities, and will differ among different legislators, and even within the same legislator over time and from issue to issue. While voting is a key way legislators represent, it is only one, and not necessarily the most important from a constituent's point of view. Legislators have a mix of goals—reelection, power, policy—that do not always place the interests of a district first but must be reconciled if the individual hopes to remain in office for long.

We conclude this section by returning to the words of Edmund Burke. His remarks repeated above about the responsibility of a legislator are well known. But several sentences in that speech to the Bristol electors show him to be far more respectful of the interests of his constituents than the previous excerpt implies. Before those words, he said of his constituents:

> Their . . . wishes ought to have great weight with him; their opinion high respect; their business unremitted attention. It is his duty to sacrifice his repose, his pleasures, his satisfactions, to theirs—and above all, ever, and in all cases, to prefer their interest to his own. . . .

Anyone who has served in public office, federal or state, for any length of time can appreciate the reality of those sentences. The requirement to "be one of them" is onerous, draining, time-consuming, and relentless. There are always far more events, meetings, and conferences to attend than one human can accomplish. The act of representing is complex and varied, and can't be reduced to a single dimension or act.

RELATIONSHIPS

I think of representation as a subset of a much broader dynamic, relationship. Representation is a way of structuring and understanding the relationship between an elected delegate and the constituency he or she is chosen to represent. The many styles of representation reflect an infinitely greater number of relationship forms. In politics, as in most aspects of life, relationships are central and crucial. This can be understood in a negative way: it's who you know, or in a more positive light, your word is your bond. One way to think about relationships is to distinguish between those that are equal and those that are unequal. Friendship, collegiality, rivalry, and other dimensions characterize relations among equals. But in politics, as in the rest of life, many relationships are characterized by inequality, an imbalance of power between two actors. This second set is of greater interest here.

The patient and the physician. The client and the attorney. The seller of a house and the real estate broker. The passenger and the airline pilot. The golfer and the caddy. The buyer and the supplier. The board of directors and the CEO. The CEO and the workers. The local school board and the school superintendent. The school superintendent and the local school principal. The voter and the elected official.

A common thread binds each of these relationships. The former in each example is the *principal* who, with a particular goal in mind, delegates the latter as an *agent* to take actions on his or her behalf. The length of time involved in the relationship doesn't matter, be it a two-minute stop at the physician's office or the thirty-eight-year tenure of a senior United States senator. Whether written or unwritten, formal or informal, expressed or implied, a contract is created that binds the principal and agent together for a specific purpose. The *contract*—written or unwritten, expressed or implied—is the metaphor describing the relationship. Only two conditions must be met to set the relationship in motion: the agent must be willing to accept the contract and must be willing to comply after accepting. *Agency theory* is a construct that helps to understand and explore these complex relationships. In its broadest sense, agency theory applies whenever one person or group engages another to perform some task that involves delegation to an agent.[7]

When the goals of the principal and the agent are in perfect alignment, there is no agency problem. (The organization itself may be going to hell in a handbasket, but that's another subject.) Agency theory assumes that most of the time, there will be some degree of conflict among the players and that the desires and aspirations of the agents will not be in perfect sync with those of the principals. For example, a friend who served as the commissioner of inspectional services for the city of Boston was disturbed to pick up a copy of the *Boston Herald* one morning to see a front-page photo showing several of her housing inspectors sitting in a parked car in a South Boston parking lot taking a nap. In other words, she was having an *agency* problem.

When agents act contrary to the terms of their contract, they engage in behavior called *shirking*. The principals, facing agents who fail to provide the degree of agreed-upon effort, experience *moral hazard*. Agency theory relies on three assumptions about human behavior. First, agents will generally act in their own self-interest, leaving principals at risk when the former fail to keep their end of the bargain. In any conflict between an agent's and a principal's needs, the agent will be tempted to shirk. Second, everyone involved faces limits based on the adequacy of information at his or her disposal, a limitation sometimes referred to as *bounded rationality*. While one may seek to act in ways that are rational, lack of adequate information hinders the ability to make a truly rational choice. Third, agents usually will be more risk averse, or unwilling to take chances, than their principals. This fact influences the choices facing principals when structuring their relationships with their agents.

Information about the activities of agents is crucial. Without it, principals cannot know whether agents are shirking until it is too late. While good information is usually obtainable, it always comes at a price. For example, following the newspaper exposé, the Boston inspectional services commissioner obtained better information about the behavior of her inspector agents by paying a private detective firm to tail them during working hours. Information at a price! All principals make a trade-off between their need to know and the cost of knowing. Principals have a variety of ways to obtain information: more supervision, reporting procedures, budgeting—but all at a cost.

Agency theory offers guidance for principals to create contracts that will ensure optimal behavior by agents. Principals need to identify the most efficient contractual arrangements to manage relations with their agents. They have three basic options.

The first option is to establish *behavioral-based* contracts. These set micromanagerial standards for agents' daily activities—for example, how many forms should be completed, how many customers should be serviced, how many patients should be screened, per hour, per day, per week. These process-style requirements are accompanied by heavy management oversight and significant investments in information collection. In general, the more programmable the task, the more attractive behavioral-based contracts will be because information about agents' behavior can be more easily monitored and tracked. These contracts work best when principals are able to know exactly what agents do—such as workers on a shop floor who can be monitored with comparative ease.

The second option is to create *outcome-based* contracts. These are more appropriate when the collection of information required to monitor agent behavior becomes too expensive or difficult to obtain. An outcome-based example would involve paying a sales agent a per-sale commission rather than an hourly wage. In this case, the principal needs far less information about the agent's activity and the outcome can be more easily defined and measured. This kind of contract shifts a significant burden of risk from the principal to the agent, thus curbing the potential for agent opportunism. A health plan that pays a physician a capitated payment for care of a patient, rather than a fee-for-service payment for each procedure, would be another good example. A key difficulty with this form of contract is that outcomes are not always a function of behavior: a poor outcome can occur despite an agent's superlative efforts, and a good outcome can occur despite inadequate efforts. Because agents tend to be risk averse, this kind of arrangement can lead to agent manipulation, for example, avoiding sales territories that require more effort or patient skimming.

The third option involves the creation of *social control* contracts that seek to align agents' interests with those of the principal through mechanisms such as selection, training, and socialization. Providing workers with stock options to create a greater stake in a company's overall performance is one approach. Another approach requires investments in training and education to transform agent beliefs and attitudes in the direction of the principal's. An example of this is the introduction of total quality management (TQM) programs that seek to align executives, managers, and workers with an agreed-upon mission statement. TQM programs seek to reorient all participants willing to change, and to eliminate those who won't adapt to the new order. An example of social control I encountered involved a company's sales agents, each of whom was required to take a Myers Briggs personality test, a battery of questions categorizing individuals into personality "types." Managers identified which personality types were most associated with their successful agents, fired the rest of the agents, and only hired replacements with high scores in the winning personality cells, a unique form of employment discrimination!

Each contracting approach has advantages and disadvantages relative to the specific arrangement under consideration. In general, principals seek to control the behavior of their agents through a mix of behavioral-style oversight activities and outcome-based incentives. Agents can be expected to use their own advantages, including discretion and information, to resist the control by principals. The degree to which agents respond depends on the effectiveness of the control mechanisms available and the willingness of principals to use them.

Agency theory's roots trace back to efforts in the 1960s to understand the relationships between corporate boards of directors and executives, as well as relations between executives and their managers. Since then, it has been used in a variety of fields, including accounting, economics, finance, marketing, organizational studies, sociology, psychology, and political science. The concept of agency has deep roots in legal theory as well. It is a useful construct to explore relationships in many different fields, including two that are central to this book, health care and government.

In health care, the fundamental principal-agent relationship is seemingly straightforward, the patient as principal and the physician as agent. We can observe how managed care has altered that relationship by asserting its own financial authority, challenging the providers' undivided loyalty to the patient. Once again, information becomes a critical flash point: for plans spending huge sums to develop elaborate information systems; for consumers seeking legislative requirements for the disclosure of information about provider-plan relationships; and for providers seeking to protect the confidentiality of information. Much of the debate over regulation of managed care involves competing efforts by consumers and plans to assert their respective roles as principals.

In government, principal-agent relationships abound and go well beyond the basic voter–elected official bond. The Medicaid program, for example, which provides health services for many poor Americans, is a federal-state partnership with Washington as the principal and state governments as the agents. The federal government—through Congress and the Health Care Financing Administration—sets the rules as conditions for its generous financial payments; state governments must conform or lose federal financial participation. Within this relationship, we can observe substantial shirking on the part of state governments as they respond to local demands and values. For example, some states resisted the Bush administration's attempts to prevent Medicaid providers from counseling patients about abortion options; other states resisted the Clinton administration's attempts to require states to provide abortion coverage through Medicaid.

In each of these examples, agency theory provides a mechanism to explore relationships, to think about the role of information, and to identify the kind of contractual relationships that could work best. Often, political exigencies restrict the range of possible relationships. But referral to agency theory can often expand the range of potential solutions.

REPRESENTATION AND RELATIONSHIPS

Seeing the concept of representation as a specific relationship form helps drive home an essential point: in politics, relationships are vital, whether based on equality or inequality. Representation, while important, is secondary to the power and requirements of relationships at all levels. The bond between the voter and the elected official, while vitally important, is only one of many to be balanced by the public official. One is tempted to say relationships are everything, but that goes against the grain of this book. Nonetheless, it is difficult to think of much that is as critical as relationships, of all forms, at every level, among individuals, among organizations, and between individuals and organizations. Just as in life, they take work and commitment on a consistent basis. They are as varied as the individuals who find themselves embroiled in political conflict.

Agency theory is not a perfect fit to understand power relationships. But it provides a guide to analyze critical features: the need for information, the structure—or lack thereof—of contracts, shirking, lines of authority. The following case story explores a different field of political conflict I briefly entered in 1994, an attempt to win approval of comprehensive campaign finance reform legislation. In this story, the challenges of representation and relationships are central. Principals and agents abound; shirking, moral hazard, and risk aversion are ever present. And information was a priceless commodity.

WARCHESTS AND CAMPAIGN FINANCE REFORM LEGISLATION

THE JUNKETEERS

This story begins with shirking. Fresh from a vigorous and highly successful 1992 campaign season, a group of seven House members and one senator, led by House Speaker Charles Flaherty, signed up to attend the December conference of the Council of State Governments in San Juan, Puerto Rico. During a busy lame-duck legislative session with major unresolved issues, the House suspended formal sessions for the week of the conference for the benefit of the high-level attendees. Instead of going to the conference, however, the legislators spent their week at the posh Palmas del Mar resort at the other end of the island. They were accompanied on their jaunt by nine lobbyists for insurance, beer, hospital, utility, racing, physician, and other interests. Unbeknownst to them, they were also accompanied by a _Boston Globe_ photographer posing as a tourist who was part of a team investigating influence peddling between legislators and lobbyists.

Starting on Sunday, May 23, 1993, the paper began a four-part front-page series: "Beacon Hills' Money Game: A Hidden World of Tropical Junkets, Easy Cash, and Sweet Deals." The photographer obtained photos of bathing-suited, bare-chested, beer-drinking, cigar-smoking legislators and lobbyists and documented the latter group's picking up the tab. The reporters also followed Senate President William Bulger to a legislative conference in Honolulu, Hawaii, all expenses paid by a charitable foundation sponsored by a bevy of corporations; Bulger also was displayed bare chested in his bathing suit. Monday's report was even worse: "Caucus in the Caribbean: Flaherty, Pol Friends Enjoy Secret Spree with Lobbyists." Flaherty "traded in his gavel for a cold beer and fat cigar. He was playing hooky from a December legislative conference being held in San Juan, relaxing on the other side of the island with an invitation only group of fellow legislators and doting lobbyists. . . ." The series documented a range of special interest bills and amendments that were tied to the priorities of the lobbyist partygoers.

The _Globe_ had wanted to set off a firestorm, and it got its wish. Within days, the State Ethics Commission, the secretary of state, the state attorney general, and, most ominously, the U.S. attorney all began a series of investigations, probes, and inquiries into legislators and lobbyists. Agents from the Federal Bureau of Investigation were observed poring over lobbyist filings; rumors spread through the State House of unannounced FBI sweeps of various offices; seemingly at random, members were summoned to appear before State Ethics Commission investigators and ordered to turn over date books, telephone logs, and boxes of records with no indication of the alleged offense under review. Members were warned by leaders not to appear without legal counsel, the cost of which ran easily to more than $2,500 per day.

During that same summer and fall of 1993, volunteers from the "good government" reform group, Common Cause, began gathering the first set of required signatures to place their "Act for Accountable Politics" as an initiative question on the November 1994 ballot. They presented themselves as citizen principals attempting to create more effective means to control the behavior of their unruly agent, the legislature. The hurdle they needed to jump was high: more than 70,000 signatures of registered voters from across the state. But in the wake of the *Globe* series, their volunteers found willing endorsers lined up at the shopping malls waiting to sign. By the early December deadline, they had more than 80,000 in their pockets. Common Cause leaders had been trying to convince legislators to pass their Accountable Politics Act since the early 1990s and turned to the ballot only after becoming convinced that the House and Senate would never act without a genuine outside threat. In May 1993, before the publication of the *Globe* series, the legislature's Joint Committee on Election Laws, cochaired by liberal State Senator Stan Rosenberg and moderate Representative Richard Moore, reported favorably to the House a version of the Common Cause bill that the organization liked. But the chairmen had acted without their respective leadership's approval, and every indication suggested the bill would move no further in the legislative process.

The gloomy prospects for the Common Cause bill were not difficult to understand. Few could see how House leaders would ever endorse the far-reaching plan to lower the existing annual individual contribution limit for all state officials from $1,000 to $100 and severely restrict use of those political funds, along with a mountain of other changes, some reasonable, some outlandish. Nonetheless, Representative Warren Tolman pushed aggressively for House leaders to take up the legislation. As the pressures from multiple outside investigations began to mount, Speaker Flaherty and others decided that the bill presented a dual opportunity: first, to make some modest campaign finance changes that would convince Common Cause to drop its ballot initiative, and second, to make changes in the state ethics statutes that would force that aggressive enforcement agency to tone down its investigations. In two stormy closed caucuses of House Democrats in the fall of 1993, members railed against their enemies in the U.S. attorney's office, the Ethics Commission, the attorney general's staff, and the Office of Campaign and Political Finance, which regulated the use of campaign funds. Pugnacious Ways and Means Chairman (and future Speaker) Tommy Finneran denounced the regulators and received wide and enthusiastic applause for suggesting legislation to end any and all restrictions on legislators' use of campaign funds, including personal use, and simply to require full disclosure.

To me, it was a stunning disconnect: on the one hand, the public's growing disgust with media-driven perceptions of influence peddling, luxuriant junkets, and inappropriate deal making; and on the other hand, the members' intense persecution complex, feelings of being underpaid ($30,000 was the annual base salary, while committee chairs received bonuses of $7,500 and up), underappreciated, and underrespected. This disconnect led to an intense political crash in late December 1993.

YULETIDE GREETINGS

Five days before Christmas, Speaker Flaherty brought to the House floor legislation to revamp the state laws regulating campaign finance and governing the ethics of public officials, especially us. The two forces that brought the House to address these topics—considered loathsome by most legislators—were widely recognized. First, the government watchdog group, Common Cause, had collected sufficient signatures to place its initiative question on the November 1994 state ballot, threatening to change dramatically the campaign finance and ethics statutes; legislators wanted to do their own milder version to thwart the ballot question. Second, the continuing series of probes, subpoenas, and inquiries into legislator-lobbyist influence peddling convinced many legislators that the State Ethics Commission, the entity charged with addressing misconduct by public officials, was a rogue elephant out of control and needed to have its powers clipped.

As frequently happened with controversial issues, the bill was provided to House members only at the start of the day's debate, accompanied by a summary outline of "key" sections. Most complex legislation is indecipherable by itself and requires concurrent reading with existing statutes and other materials to minimally comprehend. Only a small number of members keenly versed in the complexities of the dense ethics and campaign finance statutes had any idea what was in the actual bill. That small group who understood the bill filed enough procedural and substantive amendments to prolong the debate on the Monday of Christmas week for seven hours. The final House version was approved by a vote of 116 to 31.

Campaign finance and ethics issues had never been among my priorities. I considered myself "agnostic" on the issue, recognizing the need for regulation but also understanding that any reforms would be subject to gaming and its own set of unintended consequences. I attended the two angry and interminable caucuses of House Democrats during the fall, and listened to scores of members complain about intimidation and unfair treatment by Ethics Commission investigators. I knew many had been ordered to produce their calendars, schedules, and boxes of materials for investigators who then went "fishing" for potential offenses. The playing field on this issue was already crowded, and I felt I had nothing special to add. After my first campaign, I faced only token opponents and never tried to raise a lot of campaign money for its own sake; I stayed away from the lobbyist watering holes that attracted my less careful colleagues. During the floor debate, some of my friends warned me that the bill was "a real stinker." But I figured that it would be substantially changed if it moved to the Senate, didn't want to see the issue die without any action, wanted to show some sympathy for some of my colleagues who were under the gun, and had been trying of late to be less of a rebel. Besides, I was about halfway through my part-time doctoral studies at the University of Michigan and felt I didn't have much time to engage. Nobody pushed or tried to convince me to go one way or the other. When the moment to vote that night arrived, I thought back and forth for a few minutes and then pushed the green "yes" button on my desk in the House chamber.

In the succeeding days, the full scope of the approved House legislation become clear. The bill stripped the Ethics Commission of its power to subpoena anybody for anything, prevented it from keeping informants anonymous, and gave accused officials full access to everything, emasculating the commission's investigative powers. While ostensibly limiting lobbyists' ability to give officials gifts, the bill also permitted them to spend up to $100 per legislator each year on "food and beverages." It also permitted officials to use campaign funds for personal use and limited the cases in which officials convicted of crimes would lose their pensions. In short, it was a real stinker.

An instantaneous uproar arose across the state. "The State Ethics Commission, which is intensifying its probe of state lawmakers' ties to Beacon Hill lobbyists, would be stripped of key powers under a bill rammed through the House yesterday," reported the *Boston Globe* on page 1. "Cynical and vindictive" was the judgment of their editorialists. "Ugly and appalling," said the editorialists at Channel Five. "Crass pols," intoned the tabloid *Boston Herald*. Talk radio callers screamed in outrage for days. Attorney General Scott Harshbarger accused the House of "gutting our watchdog agencies." Even ethically challenged Republican Governor William Weld, after a week of avoiding comment, promised a veto should the bill reach his desk. Within days, it became clear that the bill was dead on arrival in the State Senate and would never again see the light of day. The principals screamed, loudly, and their agents responded. The legislative session ended without a Senate vote, and the bill died.

Many members who voted for the bill were chagrined at the humiliation. "The worst vote I've cast in my three years in the Chamber," my pal Jim Marzilli from Arlington told the *Globe*. Called by the same reporter, I tried to save an ounce of face for the institution, referring to "witch hunts and fishing expeditions" that precipitated the House overreaction. My office was besieged with a torrent of calls from outraged citizens—though not one from constituents in my district. Inside the House chamber, a number of members came up and quietly thanked me for not joining the self-flagellatory orgy. The consensus was that efforts to enact ethics and campaign finance reform legislation were dead, that the bill had backfired, and that the citizenry would do it themselves on the November 1994 ballot. We had a chance to do it ourselves, but we really blew it, I thought. Too bad.

OPPORTUNITY IN CRISIS

In late 1992, after years of waiting, I had finally been placed on the House "leadership track," having been named vice chairman of the Committee on Post Audit, generally recognized as one of the least active and significant leadership posts.

"What does this mean?" I asked Speaker Flaherty when he called to inform me.

"It means you're in leadership," he replied.

"Oh."

It was OK for me. I needed the extra pay and as much spare time as possible for my doctoral studies, and so this became a welcome kind of in-House sabbatical. In the fall of 1993, Flaherty promoted me to another meaningless post, House chairman of the Committee on Counties. It had a nicer office, and I got more staff, with no additional work. It also meant that I was included in the infrequent chairman meetings in Charlie's office. Each member's relationship with the Speaker was crucial to his or her ability to advance. If he liked you, great things were possible, and if he disliked you, there was little you could do to advance but curry favor with the likely next Speaker. After missing an opportunity to move up when Flaherty became Speaker in early 1991, I was being considered more often now.

On a Monday afternoon in mid-February 1994, I got a telephone call to come up to Charlie's office. This was not unusual for members of his leadership team. These summonses came unexpectedly, usually to talk with some of his guests about an issue before my committee.

When I arrived at Charlie's office on that afternoon, I was surprised to find myself alone. Charlie sat behind his large desk that was, as usual, piled high with letters, reports, memos, and more. "What's up?" I asked.

"I'm going to make you chairman of the Committee on Housing and Urban Development," he said.

"Ummm, . . ." I said.

This was a complete surprise. I knew that the former Housing chairman, Ray Jordan, had just got a federal job. He and the House chairman of the Election Laws Committee, Dick Moore, were early supporters of President Bill Clinton and stuck with him through the gloomy sex scandal days of Gennifer Flowers during the 1992 New Hampshire primary. In early 1994, they both were rewarded with federal jobs, thus creating two committee chairmanship vacancies in the Massachusetts House. But because I had been appointed to Counties just three months before, I assumed it was not my turn.

But now I did a split-second political and career analysis: housing had been a nothing issue in the state since 1991 when Republican Bill Weld became governor and Tommy Finneran took over the House Ways and Means Committee; while they passed a housing construction bond bill every few years, that had just been done in 1993 and wouldn't happen again for a long time. I really wanted to be House chairman of Insurance or Health Care and feared that I could easily get stuck at Housing for a long time. Meanwhile, the Election Laws Committee, usually just a pit-stop chairmanship, had a potentially huge and interesting challenge ahead of it in the form of the campaign finance and ethics imbroglio.

"Gee, thanks a lot, Charlie. This is a terrific honor. I wasn't expecting this at all. But, uhh, could I make a possible suggestion?"

"Sure. What?"

"Well, it seems to me that the Election Laws Committee has a major challenge in front of it because of the campaign finance and ethics situation. I have credibility with Common Cause, the *Globe,* and other players on that side. But I voted for your bill, I understand the concerns of the members, and I may be able to play a role in bridging the two sides with a compromise that could stop the ballot question—if you're interested in pursuing that."

Charlie stared at me inscrutably for five long seconds. Was he going to call me an ingrate and throw me out of his office? "You know," he said, "that's a good idea. I think I'm sending you to Election Laws instead."

"Whew!" I thought as I walked out. "This could be really good!"

STAN & ME

It was almost March, and the legislature would be in business only until the end of July. The point of no return for the Common Cause ballot question, though, would be reached by early July; after that, it would be nearly impossible to withdraw. Four months to structure a deal and get it through the legislature seemed awfully tight but doable. The starting point was my new responsibility, the Joint Committee on Election Laws. Each joint committee was made up of six senators and eleven representatives. But the House and Senate cochairs controlled the agenda as well as the committee staff, giving them effective control. Rank-and-file members on active committees often played key roles. But Election Laws was considered a sleepy backwater that rarely had a major issue in its lap. Luckily for me, this would be one of the active years. The rest of the committee membership largely ignored our work. I kept them informed and they thanked me and left me alone.

The relationship between committee cochairs is critical. Two chairs who do not get along can often create stalemates on important issues. Bills that pass one branch easily get held up in the other as the rivalry intensifies. On the other hand, cochairs able to establish a positive relationship get a strong head start in passing legislation as they work together to craft bills that can pass muster in both chambers.

On this point we were off to a great start. I had a strong personal relationship with my new cochair, Stan Rosenberg, a state senator from the western Massachusetts university town of Amherst. Stan and I became friends when he served in the House between 1986 and 1991, at which point he won an open seat in the State Senate. Earnest, hardworking, bright, and likable, Stan sometimes chafed at the way other members had stolen issues from him on which he had worked hard. He was one of the organizers of the legislature's foster child caucus, made up of four former foster children serving in the legislature. He had been Senate chair of Election Laws for about two years and had engineered passage of a complex "motor voter" bill in 1993 that eased voter registration procedures. A former staffer for the State Democratic Committee, he was comfortable with the label "liberal" and rubbed his hands together when he first saw me after my appointment. "At last," he exulted, "the liberals are in charge!" Personally, I preferred the label "progressive."

We both agreed the consensus of opinion was that our efforts were doomed to failure. Yet our own analyses convinced us otherwise. Conversations I held with key House leaders and with Common Cause Executive Director Nathan Gibson convinced me that a substantive bill could be crafted to appeal to both sides. Stan and I clearly understood our respective roles. We were agents, not for our districts, not for our institutions, certainly not for Common Cause or the media, but rather for the House and Senate leaders who appointed us and gave us the green light to proceed. Stan's first principal was Senate President William Bulger who delegated his authority to his own primary agent, Senate Ways and Means Chairman Tom Birmingham, a working-class, chain-smoking Rhodes scholar and labor lawyer who was the fast-rising star and power in that chamber. Effectively, Stan was the agent for Birmingham and Bulger, his principals. It was more direct for me. My principal was Charlie Flaherty. I touched base and consulted with many other members, but I reviewed each decision, point by point, alone with Charlie, in his darkened, wood-paneled office. Stan and I both spent enormous amounts of time listening to and learning from our respective members to gain their confidence and support. Yet we both recognized our primary principals. Achieving progress on this issue was first and foremost about relationships: issues of representation came later.

One of the first things we did was to develop a matrix to keep track of the host of issues involved in the controversy. We identified all the major categories of concerns: campaign donations, public financing, ethics issues, lobbyist matters, and more, and then broke each category down into more specific issues. One column listed relevant provisions of existing law, another the provisions of the proposed ballot initiative, and a third column listed the relevant provisions of the aborted House bill of December 1993. The fourth and final column on the right was blank, to be filled in as Stan and I negotiated our bill. The matrix became a valuable, consistent tool in all our discussions, and as members would complain about our suggested provisions, it enabled us to easily compare each with the more onerous features of the Common Cause proposal.

What was in this for Stan and me, aside from an interesting challenge? We both wanted to move up the chairmanship ladder in our respective chambers. Key to achieving that was establishing strong relationships of trust with our respective principals. Winning passage of a bill that would be acceptable to both chambers and the governor and yet be strong enough to convince Common Cause to back off was a "mission impossible" challenge in the eyes of most. Carrying this off successfully would set us both up for future advancement.

Stan had one representation concern different from mine. In his liberal, university-based hometown of Amherst, he had to deal with an active, grassroots "Pro-Democracy Campaign," a guerrilla theatre–style group that organized to win support for full public financing of all political campaigns. Stan felt a need—as their official "agent"—to represent their interests and to place something in the bill that would begin to address their demands for broader public dollars to run political campaigns.

Stan and I decided to assemble an unusual meeting of our principals and key participants prior to negotiations with Nathan Gibson of Common Cause. We met in late March in the dark-wood-paneled office of House Majority Leader Richard Voke, who, like Birmingham, was from poor working-class Chelsea. Voke, who had already begun lining up support to succeed Flaherty as Speaker, had tried to steer a middle course in the House during the 1993 debacle, felt badly burned, and doubted prospects for passage of a bill. Tom Birmingham joined us, as did his legal counsel, David Sullivan, a former Cambridge city councillor and good friend of mine for about fifteen years. While David watched out for the interests of the Senate, he was also the former general counsel for the State Ethics Commission. He understood the campaign finance and ethics statutes intimately and by no means viewed them as enemy terrain. Stan's and my key staff members, Steve Long and Ray Ausrotas, joined in. Stan and I presented the plan: we would negotiate with Gibson and bring every recommendation back to our principals for their assent. We confidently assumed our ability to strike a deal acceptable to all parties.

"Don't assume that you will be able to make a deal with them," Birmingham cautioned. "You should keep in mind that you may have to move a bill forward without their approval." I regarded his comment as predictably pessimistic. Nonetheless, the leaders gave Stan and me the green light we wanted. That was enough for now.

On March 22, 1994, the John Hancock Mutual Life Insurance Company announced that it would pay over $1 million in fines to state and federal regulators in a settlement to avoid prosecution against the company. Hancock confessed to spending, between 1986 and 1993, over $31,000 in illegal wining and dining of more than twenty-four legislators; the activities included "lavish" meals at tropical resorts, purchase of skybox sports tickets, and golf rounds at luxury golf courses. Over the ensuing weeks, a succession of legislators signed consent agreements with the State Ethics Commission, admitting to violations of the conflict-of-interest statute and consenting to pay fines and other damages. The noose was tightening, and the atmosphere growing increasingly tense.

Sightings of FBI agents in the State House were becoming routine, as many wondered where the probe would end and how high up the leadership chain it would progress.

On March 23, the *Boston Globe* ran an editorial calling on the legislature to adopt campaign finance reform ourselves instead of forcing the voters to do it for us. While their editorialists always wrote anonymously, I knew the author of this piece well. Political writer Bob Turner had an intense interest in campaign finance reform and public financing and talked several times a week with me, Stan, Nathan Gibson, and others to check on our progress. The *Globe* had a big stake in this issue, would not walk away, and would not let us forget that fact. I welcomed the intervention, feeling that Turner would only strengthen our hand in pushing the House and Senate to act.

Stan's and my first substantive decision recognized that a bill combining campaign finance and ethics reform was too broad. A lot of work had been done by many to understand the campaign finance issues, while the ethics issues had been far less developed. We recommended that a special commission be formed to undertake a thorough review of all complaints connected with the ethics statutes—including complaints that the commission was too harsh as well as too lenient. Parties on all sides—our House and Senate principals, as well as Common Cause—agreed. The leadership of the State Ethics Commission, with whom Stan and I secretly talked, breathed an audible sigh of relief. We had just withdrawn the gun pointed at them. Meanwhile, our workload was cut in half, and some of the most intractable issues were taken off the table. From now on, we were just doing campaign finance reform.

STAN & ME, AND NATHAN

We initiated an intense series of meetings with Nathan Gibson and his assistant. Gibson had been an organizer in the successful 1992 campaign to raise the state's cigarette tax by twenty-five cents to fund antismoking programs. His mother, Mary Jane, was a former longtime member of the House from Belmont, liberal, soft-spoken, and universally beloved. Nathan, as befit his role, could be acerbic and critical in castigating legislators for failing to heed the Common Cause agenda. Predictably, he was as widely disliked among legislators as his organization. I found him smart, likable, flexible, and a good negotiator, recognizing that he—like Stan and me—was an agent. His principal was a board of thirteen citizens who had to sign off on whatever he negotiated. His negotiating power was 80,000 certified signatures that would place his question on the November ballot unless we enacted a deal into law by early July.

Over several weeks, we made progress on many difficult points. We agreed to place aggregate limits on the amount of money any candidate could accept from political action committees. We agreed to ban "candidate PACs" that legislative leaders formed to curry favors and IOUs from members (in his "in your face" humorous style, Charlie Flaherty named his PAC "CODDLE"—Committee of Democrats Dedicated to Legislative Excellence). We agreed to require contributors of $200 or more to disclose their occupation and employer. We agreed to limit the aggregate amount any individual citizen could annually contribute to all state election candidates to $12,500. We agreed to restrict the practice of *bundling,* whereby lobbyists and other influence peddlers gathered and personally delivered stacks of contribution checks to candidates. We agreed to require individuals who lobbied the executive branch to register as "executive agents." We agreed to strengthen prohibitions against employer reprisals for employee political activity. To address Stan's agenda and his local pressures, we expanded the scope of public financing for candidates for statewide office such as governor and attorney general. On and on, we agreed to dozens of changes in election laws, winning consent from our respective principals for each of them. I was amazed at how easily Charlie agreed to each of these changes, especially the banning of candidate PACs, making only slight modifications.

Gibson pushed us to agree to an item in the Common Cause ballot question that flatly prohibited any public official from accepting gifts of any size from lobbyists. Stan and I resisted because it would have required making changes to the state ethics laws, a statutory territory we had earlier agreed to avoid. Opening the ethics statutes to this change would risk opening them to a wide assortment of changes on the floors of the House and Senate, something we earnestly and sincerely cautioned Gibson to avoid. We finally agreed instead to amend a different set of statutes dealing with the registration of lobbyists by requiring that a legislative or executive agent could purchase *nothing* of value for any public official or else face the loss of his or her lobbying license. We recognized the contradiction: a substantial penalty would face a lobbyist who bought something for an official; however, the official would only be in trouble if he or she broke the existing limit by accepting something worth more than $50 in value. But the principle would be established, we felt, and the contradiction could be remedied through the later work of the proposed Special Commission on Ethics. "Not a cup of coffee, not a stick of gum" were the metaphors Stan and I used to detail the impact of this recommendation. It became one of the signature issues in our bill. This would impose a huge culture change, we thought, in the relationship between legislators and lobbyists in the State House, and I expected Charlie to reject this proposal out of hand. Instead, he easily agreed as long as no new penalties would befall legislators.

Other issues were harder to resolve. One of the cornerstones of the Common Cause ballot petition would have restricted campaign funds for strictly political uses connected with electoral campaigns. The current law prohibited the use of campaign funds for any personal use but permitted use for the "enhancement" of the candidate's political career, a broad definition that officeholders used to justify buying meals for friends in fancy restaurants, gifts for constituents and supporters, and a lot more. Those who used it included several of the Puerto Rico vacationers who were subsequently ordered by the Office of Campaign and Political Finance to reimburse their campaign committees for these expenses. Yet I also knew many legislators who used campaign funds for a wide variety of noncampaign purposes that seemed entirely valid—Representative Paul Caron from Springfield, for example, used his political funds to pay for the costs of running his district office. I had become actively involved in a group called the National Academy for State Health Policy, the premier group for state health policy wonks. There was no state money to support my participation, and I couldn't afford it on my salary. So I used my campaign funds to support my involvement. I also knew that House members fiercely opposed establishing a new layer of regulatory oversight on their campaign committees. But Gibson also was adamant.

Then I told Gibson and his assistant a true story. My legislative district included parts of Boston that had been besieged in the early 1990s by gang violence, drug dealing, gun running, and the like. Kids killing kids was a weekly occurrence. In 1991, one young boy from the Academy Homes housing development in Roxbury was shot and killed on his way home from school. As I did on the occasion of every shooting in my district, I visited the bereaved family and offered my sympathy and support. Usually they thanked me for the offer and asked for nothing. This time, the mother tearfully told me that she didn't have the money to pay for her son's funeral expenses, and the funeral director would not proceed until he got paid. "Could you help us?" she asked. I went to the funeral director and gave him a check for $1,500 from my campaign account.

"Every elected official worth his or her salt," I said to Gibson, "does things like that at various times. They have no direct campaign connection—but do you really want to stop us from doing them? How is that in the public interest?"

They stopped pressing that concern, and we dropped it.

We left the hardest issue for last. The existing law allowed any individual to donate up to $1,000 to a candidate each year. The Common Cause ballot question proposed reducing that maximum to $100, something that even Bob Turner regularly criticized as unrealistic in his *Globe* editorials. Stan and I convinced our principals to agree to a two-part compromise: a $500 annual limit, plus a $200 contribution limit for legislative and executive agents. Gibson was surprised and pleased with the offer—but some of his board members felt strongly that the $100 limit was the heart and soul of the ballot initiative. He came back to us willing to accept the compromise, but *only* if we also would agree to prohibit something known as "warchests."

Powerful and ambitious officeholders commonly use their positions to extract campaign donations from everyone in sight, far more than necessary to counter imminent electoral threats. Some do this to amass reserves for a future run for higher office. Others do it to amass power and influence in their current positions and to discourage potential challengers. One political scientist once found that the best explainer of a politician's behavior lay in his or her future plans—whether running for higher office, moving up within one's legislative body, going into the private sector, or whatever; this observation definitely applies to fundraising behavior as well. Most legislators, myself included, view fundraising as a necessary evil, raising only what is needed for the current cycle and no more. But more ambitious politicians get hold of the secretary of state's quarterly listing of more than 500 legislative agents and their employers and mail each of them an invitation to their "times." One of my good friends in the House, Joe McIntyre from New Bedford, told me he did that—only once. "After they gave me money, they were all over me like fly-paper, like they owned me. It was really gross." Arguments against warchests, I knew, had some legitimacy—to a point.

But there were weaknesses in the Common Cause position. The key United States Supreme Court decision on campaign fund-raising—the 1976 *Buckley v. Valeo* case—found that campaign spending by candidates is a form of speech protected by the First Amendment. A state may limit the amount an individual can contribute to a candidate in order to prevent a contributor from gaining excessive influence, but it cannot limit the total amount a candidate can raise from all legal sources. It was widely believed, and affirmed in several lower court cases, that restrictions on the amount a candidate can "carry over" from one election cycle to another also would be found unconstitutional under the Supreme Court's rationale. Gibson and Common Cause recognized this problem. Their proposed ballot initiative did *not* include a warchests provision because the attorney general's office had informed them in the summer of 1993 that such a provision would be unconstitutional and would lead to their question being disqualified from the ballot. Nonetheless, Gibson now pressed us to include the provision as the trade-off for setting the individual contribution limit at $500 instead of $100.

"How can you ask us to include a provision which we have every reason to believe is unconstitutional and which you didn't put in your ballot initiative?" Stan and I pressed.

"Put it in and let's have another court test on the matter," Gibson replied.

Easier said than done. Neither Stan nor I ever had a direct conversation with our primary or secondary principals about whether to accept Nathan's offer. It wasn't necessary. We knew the provision was objectionable on any basis—and not just with House and Senate leaders. Since early April, we had been meeting with key staff for Governor Weld and Attorney General Harshbarger, both public endorsers of the Common Cause ballot question but both private and vociferous objectors both to the $100 limit and to any limits on campaign warchests. Stan and I knew that including a warchests provision would lead to certain abandonment of the legislation by our principals, and the end of our efforts.

Unable to make headway with Gibson, Stan and I agreed to meet on the evening of April 21 with the board of Common Cause. We decided ahead of time that Stan would play the good cop and I the bad. We had a spirited, engaging discussion for several hours that went nowhere. But it was useful to me to have the opportunity to eyeball these folks. They were all white, middle and upper-middle class, suburban, and hugely ignorant of the realities of running for office and legislating. With one exception, I had never heard of any of them. They certainly were not folks I was used to working with on issues such as health care access, affordable housing, safe streets, and economic justice. Sitting with them I wondered, were these the true principals who spoke for "the people," or rather a narrow and self-appointed slice? I knew I did not feel beholden to them and that they had no right to tell me what to do. In the final analysis, my observations didn't matter. They had more than 80,000 bona fide signatures, and that was all that mattered. That is why Stan and I were there with them.

It was late April and we still did not have a bill in motion. Time was growing short, with little more than two months until it would be too late for Common Cause to withdraw their ballot question. Turner pushed us in a May 3 *Globe* editorial: ". . . if they fail to show leadership, the voters will fill the breach." But we were stalemated. Accept Gibson's offer and the legislation would never pass. Reject it and watch our efforts come to nothing if Common Cause went to the ballot. Stan and I decided to call the organization's bluff. We would put a bill before the Election Laws Committee with all the provisions on which we had reached agreement, including the $500 contribution limit and the $200 limit for lobbyists, and not including a warchests provision. Flaherty, Birmingham, and the other principals gave us the green light. The governor and attorney general gave us their private support.

On Wednesday, May 11, Stan and I put our bill before the Election Laws Committee and won unanimous approval. We had briefed reporters from the *Globe* and the *Herald* the day before to assure favorable press. Gibson was quoted as saying that the bill "doesn't go as far as we would like" and "leaves incumbents with an overwhelming advantage in fundraising." But Turner was considerably more positive, editorializing on Monday, May 16, that Stan and I "deserve considerable credit for crafting a credible multifaceted proposal," while stroking Common Cause by noting, "It's obvious that the legislation would not have come this far had it not been pushed" by the organization.

"Geesh," I thought to myself. "This is beginning to look easy."

THE SENATE

My principal, Charlie Flaherty, insisted on only one thing from the start: "We always end up going first on these things. We test the waters and take the hits. Those damn senators sit back and wait, and then look like god damn diplomats! I want this package to go to the Senate first. Let them take some grief."

"Yes, sir," I said. I had hoped for this, feeling that the Senate would be more careful than the House because of Stan and Birmingham.

Stan and the Senate leaders were entirely agreeable. The bill was reported favorably by Tom Birmingham's Senate Ways and Means Committee on Friday, May 13. We were heading for the floor of the Senate on Tuesday, May 17. Knowing that David Sullivan would be deeply enmeshed in the Senate process gave me added comfort that nothing would go wrong. What none of us counted on was an unexpected move by a friend, Senator Shannon O'Brien.

When a piece of legislation comes out to the full Senate or the full House, lots of things can happen. Members can move to amend the bill, report it back to any committee they choose, postpone debate, substitute an entirely different bill, and more. Legislative leaders can cajole, prod, and pressure, but ultimately, individual members are free agents to do whatever they choose. From the proponent's viewpoint, the only helpful thing they can do with a bill is approve it and move it to the next stage in the legislative process. That was our goal.

The Massachusetts State Senate is made up of forty members. Republicans have been badly outnumbered since the late 1950s and in 1994 had nine members compared with thirty-one Democrats. But all was not peaceful on the majority side. Senate President William Bulger had presided over the chamber since 1978 and had a public reputation of ruling through bullying and intimidation. In truth, while he held an intense interest in a small number of concerns such as permitting state aid to parochial schools, he largely delegated day-to-day control to Tom Birmingham and several others. In 1993, a group of six Democratic senators openly broke allegiance with Bulger and announced their intention to organize support to oust him as Senate leader in January 1995. Their leader was suburban Senator William Keating, hence their nickname, "the Keating Six." Their approach was to exploit any and every opportunity to embarrass Bulger and to demonstrate the need for new leadership. By mid-1994, when the campaign finance reform bill hit the Senate floor, their revolt was sputtering into irrelevance, and they were anxious to find new openings to weaken the President.

Senator Shannon O'Brien was not one of the Keating Six. She was a bright, hardworking, and articulate legislator from the western Massachusetts community of Easthampton looking to run for statewide office. By May 1994 she had already announced her plans to run for state treasurer in the fall elections against the incumbent Republican treasurer, Joe Malone. Outside the building, Malone's image was that of a squeaky clean reformer who had mopped up a patronage-soaked mess in his office and restored integrity to the post. Inside the building, Malone was fiercely disliked as a sanctimonious phony by Democrats and Republicans alike. Malone was also an aggressive fund-raiser who had amassed a considerable warchest during the three years since his 1990 election. O'Brien was looking for opportunities to find and exploit Malone's weaknesses.

Learning of Common Cause's interest in banning campaign warchests, and anxious to demonstrate that she was not a Bulger insider, she thought she had found an answer.

O'Brien filed an amendment to prohibit officeholders from raising more than a certain amount of funds in nonelection years ($30,000 for state reps, $60,000 for senators, $125,000 for statewide officeholders except for the governor, who would be subjected to a $250,000 cap). She told Stan she did not expect the amendment to be approved. She would file it, speak for it, and then agree either to withdraw it or to have it voted down on a voice vote. She knew it would mess up the bill if approved, but her target was Joe Malone, not our legislation. She even asked one of Stan's staff members to write the amendment for her. She gave the amendment to the Senate clerk, expecting a quick rejection.

But O'Brien and Stan were both startled when Republican Senator Richard Tisei stood and demanded a roll call on her proposal. The Republican nine and the Keating Six quickly united in a gleeful effort to upend and embarrass the Senate Democratic leadership. O'Brien introduced her amendment at 4:45 P.M. At 4:57, the President declared a recess for the purpose of majority and minority party caucuses—the preferred approach in that chamber to dealing with delicate and messy issues. At 6:12 P.M., they reassembled, debated for several minutes, and declared another recess for another caucus at 6:25 P.M. Behind the scenes, Stan and Birmingham were working hard to thwart the O'Brien amendment, but the Republican and Keating fifteen wouldn't let go and were joined by other neutral and Bulger-supporting Democrats who were fearful of being portrayed on the wrong side of what had instantly become the pivotal issue in the debate. At 6:52 P.M., they reassembled and debated the amendment until a vote was taken at 7:39 P.M.

The amendment passed by a vote of 25 to 12, and the bill was given final Senate approval a few minutes later, then sent to the House in amended form for its consideration. Many of the twenty-five privately told Stan they were opposed to the amendment. Stan was furious, refusing to send out press releases his staff had already prepared heralding the passage of the bill. O'Brien was deeply apologetic for her miscalculation. I shared their chagrin: House members would be equally skittish to reject a popular warchests provision—even if it meant scuttling the entire bill. Keating was exultant: "The public broke down the walls of the Senate today." Common Cause suddenly was reenergized on an issue it had thought lost. Bob Turner, the *Globe* editorial writer who had praised Stan's and my efforts, was ecstatic in his Thursday editorial: "Redemption on Beacon Hill." I had several long conversations with him explaining that the warchests amendment was patently unconstitutional and politically radioactive, guaranteeing nothing would pass. His response came in an editorial on Monday, May 23, as I worked with House leaders to prepare our strategy. "The House Menu" intoned:

> Campaign finance reform took another path last week when the Massachusetts Senate turned a decent piece of chuck into a choice T-bone. . . . This week, House members should resist any effort to trade back to a lesser cut or to grind the issue into sausage meat. . . . No logic equates a warchest carryover to spending limits.

THE HOUSE

Carrying a major and controversial piece of legislation on the floor of the cavernous House of Representatives is an exhilarating experience. Opponents most often wait until the last possible moment to reveal their strategy. Weakening attempts often emanate simultaneously from different ideological directions. Debate can be vapid or sharp, deadly dull or fiercely engaging. Most of the time, floor debate is only the playing out of controversies that have been sorted out and settled in the committee process. Woodrow Wilson wrote in 1885 that "Congress in session is Congress on public exhibition, whilst Congress in its committee rooms is Congress at work." This is true in state legislatures as well. Sometimes, though, all does not get settled in committee, and what happens on the floor can be tantalizingly unpredictable. The House campaign finance debate on Thursday, May 26, was one such case. And it was my bill.

House leaders met several times to review strategy devised by me and my aide, Ray Ausrotas, a young and energetic self-starter from Flaherty's working-class Cambridge neighborhood. We both met on Tuesday, May 24, in the Speaker's office with Flaherty, Majority Leader Voke, House Ways and Means Chairman Finneran (the Senate-approved bill had been referred to his committee), and the House legal counsel, Lou Rizoli. I explained that we could easily remove the warchests provision from the Senate bill in Finneran's committee but knew that we would then face attempts to put it back on the House floor by amendment. At my request, we had received a formal letter from the attorney general's office on Monday declaring that the Senate warchests provision "would likely be struck down under the First Amendment." The letter gave us a rationale for our three-pronged strategy: first, to excise the warchests provision from the bill in the House Ways and Means Committee; second, to bring the excised provision to the House floor as a new, separate bill; and third, to refer the new bill to the justices of the state's Supreme Judicial Court for an official opinion on its constitutionality (Massachusetts is one of only several states where the highest court will review a piece of legislation for its constitutionality before it becomes law). Besides asking for their opinion, the move would give House members political cover in keeping the warchests provision out of the House version of our campaign finance reform bill. Additionally, by the time the SJC justices gave us their opinion, the legislative fight would be long over, one way or the other.

The maneuver did one more crucially helpful thing. By completely removing any reference to warchests from the larger bill, if a member tried to reinsert the provision by amendment on the floor, I could make a point of order that the amendment was now "beyond the scope" of the current bill and thus not properly before the body. Flaherty, or whoever was in the chair at the time, appropriately would rule the point of order was well taken and lay the amendment aside. Any member could then "doubt the ruling of the chair," forcing a time-limited debate and roll call, but "doubting" motions nearly always became party line votes in a chamber where Republicans were outnumbered about 125 to 35.

The clerk of the House of Representatives, a gentle, wise, and intensely proper man named Robert MacQueen, had advised me years before that challenging unfriendly amendments as "beyond the scope" was one of the least-used and most legitimate tactics in debate. In the Massachusetts legislature, we have two kinds of bills. Appropriations bills (or budget bills) are wide open for any and all amendments on the floor, which is why members frustrated in trying to bring their own bills to the chamber will often propose anything, from the death penalty to abortion, during budget debates. Regular legislation, without any appropriation sections, can only be properly amended on the floor by proposals that hew closely to its prescribed purposes, unless no one objects.

At the Wednesday, May 25, session, Chairman Finneran reported the warchests provision from Ways and Means as a separate piece of legislation, with an accompanying recommendation that it be referred to the SJC for an official opinion. I waved the attorney general's letter in the face of anyone who had questions about our plan. Not understanding our game plan, no one in the House objected, and the legislation was so referred. Finneran then went down to his office and reported out of his committee the remainder of the campaign finance legislation—sans warchests—for House action the following day.

Later that day, Flaherty called a meeting of the House Democratic caucus to have me explain the provisions of the bill that would be coming to the floor the next day. This was the same forum that had been so excruciating in the fall of 1993 and that had led to the December debacle. It was a useful dry run for me and went without a hitch. The most memorable moment occurred when Representative Anne Paulsen, a savvy liberal from Belmont who had succeeded Nathan Gibson's mother in the House, stood up to say, "I have just one question—is there anything in this bill that is going to embarrass us?" I stood confidently and replied, "We have poured Clorox and bleach [a redundant metaphor, I know] all over this bill. There is nothing in here for anyone to worry about."

The Thursday House debate went on for about four hours. Fifty-five amendments were filed by members that went in two directions: mostly Republicans filed amendments to make the bill stronger, amendments they knew would not pass but could be used later to embarrass House leaders; mostly liberal Democrats filed a series of amendments to weaken the bill, for example, by permitting groups such as "Emily's List," which bundles donations from across the nation for progressive women candidates, to be exempt from the bill's restrictions on bundling. Sometimes the amendments and my conversations with the sponsors were surreal, as was one with the maker of an amendment to disallow lobbyists from making any campaign donations at all.

"Umm," I said. "We have a problem with your amendment because it's patently a violation of the First Amendment to prevent an individual from exercising his or her right to support a candidate. We can limit it, but we can't eliminate it."

"Well that's even better," he responded. "We can do it and get credit for it, and it will never have to take effect. That's great!" I looked at him cross-eyed and walked away.

The first controversial amendment was offered by Representative Bill Constantino, an idiosyncratic member from Clinton who wanted to bar any lobbyist from soliciting political donations for candidates. I never had any lobbyist solicit anything for me, but his proposal opened up whole new fronts of ambiguity we were trying to minimize, and so I debated against him. But members did not want to appear as though they were defending lobbyists, and we barely defeated the amendment, 72 to 74. This was too close for comfort, especially for the first amendment on which we were trying to set a positive, in-control tone. I went up to the Speaker and begged him to bring his leadership team to the floor to help me corral the votes that we needed.

Constantino filed the next two amendments as well, first barring any bond underwriters from contributing to any candidates and next prohibiting anyone who worked for a human services agency with state contracts from donating as well. The debate was already dragging down into foolishness. We had more than four dozen amendments pending and needed to pick up the pace. We accepted both amendments in modified form, knowing we could eliminate both in the upcoming conference committee. That is one of the strongest powers of a committee chair, knowing he or she gets another bite at the apple to rewrite bills a final time in the conference committee. I appreciated that power now.

The Republicans' smart, articulate, and aggressive floor leader, Peter Forman from Plymouth, introduced the warchests amendment along with four Republicans and one renegade Democrat. Republican Governor Weld and his lieutenant governor, Paul Cellucci—already amassing funds in preparation for a gubernatorial run in 1998—were adamantly opposed to any warchests limitation. I worked closely with their key legislative operatives to prevent the House Republicans from introducing a warchests amendment, all to no avail.

As soon as the clerk read the amendment, I stood at my seat, called for recognition, repeating the rote recitation I had heard too often.

"Mr. Speaker!"

"Mr. McDonough of Boston. For what purpose does the Gentleman rise?"

"Point of order, Mr. Speaker."

"The Gentleman will state his point of order."

"Mr. Speaker, in light of the House's action yesterday sending this same matter to the Supreme Judicial Court for an opinion, I believe that the amendment before the body is beyond the scope of the legislation."

A lengthy off-the-record argument on the rostrum ensued. Our side already knew what the result would be. The Speaker conferred with Mac-Queen and ruled in my favor. The Republicans and their allies had not seen this coming and squealed in anger, doubting the ruling of the chair. Their leader, Peter Forman, took the rostrum to debate me: ". . . dangerous precedent . . . horrendous ruling. . . . If this ruling is allowed to stand, we are giving the Speaker a whole new array of authority to limit debate."

I gave a pathetically weak response, reading the attorney general's letter and reminding members of their decision the previous day to refer the warchests matter to the SJC for an opinion. Members were concerned about the use of a parliamentary maneuver most had not seen before, and I had not sufficiently prepared myself to argue to that point. As I spoke, I saw some of my good friends shaking their heads at me, and I lost the cocky confidence I had held to that point. I was desperately relieved that debate was limited to fifteen minutes. I pleaded with House Majority Whip Joan Menard, who was presiding at the time, to give me a hand rounding up votes. We survived, upholding the Speaker's ruling by 100 to 50. It was messy, but we did it. Bloodied and bruised, we successfully kept warchests out of the House-approved version.

Stan Rosenberg's key aide, Steve Long, joined my aide, Ray Ausrotas, in rapidly analyzing and figuring out my response to each of the fifty-five amendments. Some we would accept, deciding they were bona fide improvements, some we accepted knowing we would eliminate them in the conference committee and didn't want to fight at that time, some we convinced sponsors to water down for acceptance, and some we convinced the sponsors to drop. Some we debated, winning most and losing only a couple. Exhilaration gave way to weariness after about four hours. One of my liberal woman colleagues had filed yet another pro-bundling amendment to weaken the bill to the advantage of the Emily's List agenda. Fearful that Gibson and Common Cause—seated in the House gallery during the entire proceeding—would go off the wall if we accepted it, I developed a fierce case of legislative road rage. I raced up to her, surrounded by several of our common friends, in the chamber: "This amendment is going to send Common Cause off the wall, and we'll have no chance of getting them to drop their initiative. If you insist on pressing for it, go ahead, but I'll take the microphone and explain to everyone that you're trying to gut the bill to benefit your friends and cronies. I suggest that you withdraw it!"

I held her amendment in my hand, outstretched to her. Shaken, she took it. I stormed back to the front of the chamber. Walking back, I remembered a recent conversation with Representative Chris Hodgkins, one of the more outrageous and rebellious House members who, like me, was on the slow leadership path under Flaherty. "I remember being here in my early days," he said, "and watching from my seat as the top leaders would huddle on the rostrum trying to finagle something through. Then a few months ago, as I was standing up on the rostrum with Flaherty and his lieutenants, I realized all of a sudden, I had *become* what I once abhorred! I was now one of *them*."

There was more than a little truth in that. Back in the early 1980s as a tenants' rights advocate, I watched in dismay as savvy and experienced legislators used the rules and the process to derail our proposals that didn't fit with their plans. In 1994, I was still here in the State House, except now *I* was the one doing it.

At the end of the long debate, the bill was approved, 148 to 1.

As I was leaving the State House several hours later, I ran into that woman rep on the street. I walked over to her, shook her hand, and sincerely apologized for the way I had spoken to her. She smiled and told me to stop worrying. But I couldn't, and I remembered that incident for the rest of my time in the House.

THE CONFERENCE, THE GOVERNOR, AND COMMON CAUSE

Bob Turner was not pleased. As we prepared to meet in conference committee the following week, he made a final editorial stab on June 4: "The Conference Committee should move beyond the House version in leveling legislative campaigns. If it does not, Common Cause will be encouraged to seek voter approval of its much tougher ballot initiative." But the conference was easy sailing for us. Each chamber makes three appointments, two Democrats and one Republican each. To win conference committee approval, at least two members from each branch had to sign the final report. Because conference committee appointments were the complete prerogative of the presiding officer, we had a lock on sufficient cooperative appointees. Stan and I served as committee cochairs. It was my first and only time as a member of a conference committee.

We had about twenty major differences to iron out and had no problem with any. A last-minute controversy erupted over an amendment approved during the House floor debate that had been offered by Representative Joan Menard, then the third-ranking leader in the House and the chair of the State Democratic Party. Her amendment permitted the Democratic and Republican national committees to "transfer" unlimited amounts of money to the Massachusetts affiliates for the purpose of "administration, overhead, or party building activities," though not for the direct support of party candidates. Without recognizing the consequences, we had opened up the "soft money" loophole that plagued the Democratic National Committee in the late 1990s. We responded to the complaints by further narrowing the scope of her amendment. The controversy thus abated, a brief squall.

The Republican members of the conference committee put up a fuss arguing for the warchests provision. But it was all for show. They knew that we could pass the measure without them. The conference committee agreed to a report on Tuesday, June 7. On Wednesday, the bill returned to the House and Senate for two sets of votes, the first on accepting the conference committee report and the second on enactment, the final vote on a bill before it heads to the governor's desk.

After all the brouhaha over this issue, dating back to the *Globe* Spotlight Series in May 1993 and before, I expected my final remarks on the floor would be closely listened to by most members. After the bruising process we had endured, I spent time preparing remarks that I assumed would be widely heard. A half hour before the start of the session, I took a brisk walk around the Boston Common to relax the butterflies in my stomach. When I began my remarks on acceptance of the conference report, I quickly realized that barely anyone was listening. It was normal treatment for House speeches: members chatting together in their seats, lining up to buttonhole this or that leader to pry loose their pet bills, reading papers and writing letters at their desks. I remember having to raise my voice to be heard over the din. And then I understood. This was an issue no one wanted, and now, thankfully, it was done, and we could move on to other business. I cut my intended remarks by about two-thirds and sat down. The bill received House approval by a 146-to-1 vote, and Senate approval, 33 to 1.

The day Governor Weld signed the legislation into law, Wednesday, June 15, Bob Turner wrote one last *Globe* editorial on the issue, "Common Cause for Satisfaction," noting that "landmark improvements in the financing of political campaigns are scheduled to become law today" and further urging the Common Cause board of directors to back off from its ballot initiative. The Massachusetts Public Interest Research Group, a Ralph Nader–inspired organizing entity that fought bitterly most of the time with the legislature, issued a report calling the new law "the toughest campaign finance reform law in the nation." When the Common Cause board met on the evening of Thursday, June 16, they voted 12 to 1 to abandon their ballot question.

AFTERMATH

In January 1995, Senator William Bulger easily beat back the revolt of the Keating Six and was reelected President of the Massachusetts Senate. Within a year, he resigned his seat to become president of the University of Massachusetts. Senator Tom Birmingham won a tough fight to succeed him as President and named Stan Rosenberg as the new chairman of the Senate Committee on Ways and Means. Critical to Stan's appointment was the relationship he established with Birmingham during the campaign finance reform process. Also in January 1995, Speaker Flaherty named me to be the new House chairman of the Joint Committee on Insurance, one of the two committee posts I most coveted; later that year in August, he named me chairman of the Joint Committee on Health Care, the spot I had always most wanted.

The passage of the 1994 campaign finance law ended the legislative battle that erupted in the wake of the spring 1993 *Globe* investigatory series, but it did not end the federal probe into the House generally, or Charlie Flaherty in particular. The U.S. attorney's office kept up a relentless search through every aspect of Charlie's political career until it could find something to stick. It eventually discovered that in 1990, Flaherty had spent some unreimbursed time in the Cape Cod condominium of an individual with an interest in the Big Dig, the massive Boston highway construction project. Though the U.S. attorney's office could not identify a quid pro quo given for the favor, it applied enough pressure for Flaherty to plead guilty to a minor tax violation from the 1980s and resign his position as Speaker in April 1996. He did not run for reelection and left the House after thirty years at the end of 1996. Many House members, myself included, felt he had been railroaded out of office by overzealous prosecutors.

Most of the provisions of the campaign finance law were implemented as intended, including the reduction in the campaign contribution limits, the requirement for reporting the occupation and employer of donators, the limitations on political action committees, the prohibition on gifts from lobbyists to public officials, the registration of executive agents, the restrictions on bundling, and more.

One provision that did not play out as intended was the law's change in the provisions addressing the public financing of campaigns. Prior to the new law, taxpayers could "check off" a one-dollar donation on their annual state tax returns that would go into a fund to be distributed to statewide candidates. The checkoff would add one dollar to the taxpayer's tax liability. Over the years, only about 1 percent of filers voluntarily contributed to the fund, leaving little in public financing for distribution to candidates. The 1994 statute changed the law so that the one-dollar checkoff became a liability to the Commonwealth's General Fund and not to the taxpayer. If about 20 percent of filers checked off the box—at zero cost to themselves—there would have been sufficient funds to support major public financing for statewide races in the 1998 cycle. Instead, only about 10 percent of taxpayers did so, thus ensuring an inadequate amount of public financing support. The citizenry as principal gave a mixed message at best concerning its support for public financing.

Nonetheless, in the 1998 election cycle, Common Cause joined with a coalition of other liberal and progressive organizations to initiate a ballot question to permit broad public financing of all statewide and legislative races, modeled after previous successful public financing campaigns in Maine, Vermont, and other states. Candidates who accepted public financing would have to agree to $100 contribution limits from individuals as well as strict overall spending limits. Voters approved the initiative by a two-to-one margin.

The Special Commission on Ethics, on which Stan and I served, made its final report to the House and Senate in June 1995, recommending a series of complex changes to the ethics statutes, some making the laws tougher and some making them easier and less onerous for public officials. The legislature never acted on the recommendations, demonstrating once again that outside pressure is a critical factor in pushing the House and Senate to address sensitive issues involving themselves.

·   ·   ·

While the public viewed this debate as one about issues of representation—to what extent state government heeded the public's desire for political reform—in fact it was much more an illustration of relationships. Those relationships were multiple, among them: Flaherty and me, Birmingham and Stan, Nathan Gibson and his board, Stan and me and Nathan, Stan and my respective relationships with our colleagues and caucuses, the *Boston Globe*'s relationship with all of us, and lots more.

Stan and I knew unambiguously who our principals were, Tom Birmingham and Charlie Flaherty. To the extent that we were able, we steered the bill in directions we wanted. We pushed our respective leaders on expanding public financing, lowering the contribution limits, banning gifts from lobbyists to public officials, and more—all items that we personally supported and thought that we could sell to our institutions. The meetings in my office in March and April with Stan, Nathan Gibson, and me were pivotal: three agents finely attuned to the desires of our principals and the points at which they would cease negotiations, yet coconspirators in our common desire to see a worthy bill pass that would end the ballot campaign. Stan and I had only the most informal of contracts with our principals—outcome-based agreements with a dash of social control. Charlie Flaherty and Tom Birmingham didn't want to regulate our day-to-day behavior, but they wanted absolute veto over the results.

To achieve their desired outcomes, they picked two agents who understood and respected their needs. Understanding their desires and respecting the reality of our relationships with them were critical to our success.

Representation is a puzzling concept in the context of this story. During the long process, for example, I never had a single call or letter from a constituent commenting on my votes, my role, or the issue. The people, the citizenry, were overwhelmingly unengaged after the December 1993 House fiasco. The Common Cause board represented a slice, not the whole, of public opinion. The internecine quarrels about warchests, bundling, checkoffs, legislative and executive agents, and the rest were carried on without any genuine public engagement. Hannah Pitkin's writing on representation most comes to mind at this point: "There need not be a constant activity of responding, but there must be a constant condition of responsive*ness,* of potential readiness to respond. . . . We can conceive of the people as 'acting through' the government even if most of the time they are unaware of what it is doing, so long as we feel that they could initiate action if they so desired."[8] When it mattered to them, the people spoke. When the discourse became too technical and complex, they tuned out, as long as no one felt the need to reawaken their interest. Such is the reality of much of representation, American style.

POSTSCRIPT

For a while, I actually believed Stan and I had helped to change the culture of the institution. I understood the real limits of that change only several years later during a formal House session when a senior member beckoned me in the chamber. Holding a fistful of at least a dozen envelopes, the member handed me one.

"Here, buddy, this is for you. Keep up the good work."

I thought it must be one of those silly birthday greetings some members send to each other and stuffed it inside the pocket of my suit coat.

Some time later, standing in the outside lobby, I opened the envelope. A piece of the member's official stationery, without any message, was inside. Attached to the blank page was a campaign check for $250 made out to me from a health-related lobbying group.

Many senior members funneled campaign contributions to rank-and-file members as a way to curry favors and future support. But our 1994 campaign finance law had banned so-called candidate PACs. It took several years for members to figure out a way to circumvent the prohibition. The solution was for senior members to collect campaign checks made out to specific rank-and-file members directly from lobbying groups and then to deliver the checks in a way that made the senior member's solicitation visible to the recipient and invisible to everyone else. They did nothing illegal; they just spit on the spirit of the 1994 law.

Something else, though, was more immediately disturbing. Ever since my first day as a rep in 1985, I had been warned *never* to deal with campaign funds inside the walls of the State House. Yet here was a senior member handing me a campaign check inside the House chamber. I went to see an associate well versed in campaign finance law, and we checked the statutes together. It turned out, as the statutes were written, anyone who *accepts* a donation within the confines of the State House breaks the law, while the *giver* commits no offense.

I went back to my office and wrote a note to the member returning the check. The member's office was already vacant. I slipped the envelope under the darkened door. We never spoke of the matter to each other.

PART THREE

Models

To this point, I have discussed basic ideas and themes about politics that resonate in almost any politicized situation. In this next section, I describe and use two models that bring together many of the elements described thus far. Basic ideas and themes can be helpful in making sense of a situation. But integrative models can do much more: they can serve as comprehensive tools to understand something that has happened. More importantly, they can also serve as guides to enable activists to plan future activities and campaigns more effectively.

In this section, I present only two of these models in full (several others are described in part). Countless models have been developed which can be useful in political analysis. I chose these two—the punctuated equilibrium model in chapter 6 and the agenda-setting model in chapter 7—for two reasons. First, I find both enormously helpful in making sense of the case stories that follow. Second, I find them extraordinarily useful models in their own right. In chapter 6, I use one model retrospectively to help make sense of something that already occurred. In chapter 7, I show how I used another model prospectively to guide my activities in the House.

The two stories are more central to my political life than any others in this volume. They are also the two most clearly related to health care policy and politics. Together, they spanned my thirteen years as a member of the House.

CHAPTER SIX

Punctuated Equilibrium and the Fate of Hospital Rate Setting

A stand can be made against invasion by an army;
no stand can be made against invasion by an idea.
Victor Hugo

In the wake of the 1993–94 national health care reform catastrophe, some suggested the real loser in the debacle was the concept of comprehensive reform, while the true winner was the notion of incrementalism. The system, it was argued, just can't handle change too big all at once. Both the stunning failure of the Gingrich Congress in 1995–96 to achieve its own ambitious plans to reinvent Medicaid and Medicare and the more recently stalled initiatives to overhaul Social Security and Medicare provide further evidence for this view. Step-by-step makes the most sense and actually works, goes the argument, even if it proves less exciting and provocative. Noted political scientist Charles Lindblom even came up with a term for it in the 1950s: "the science of muddling through."[1]

The problem with elevating incrementalism too highly is that big-time, comprehensive change does indeed happen in American politics and policy. The U.S. welfare system underwent a radical transformation in 1996, moving in a dramatically different direction that some characterize as reform and others as destruction. Whatever the judgment about its value, it clearly happened. In 1986, the U.S. tax system was transformed in a major fashion that stunned observers who were expecting "business as usual" and only minor tinkering. Over the past twenty years, entire regulatory structures have been dismantled, beginning in the late 1970s with airlines, telephone, and trucking and continuing into the 1990s with utilities, telecommunications—and health care. To go back further, the creation of Medicare and Medicaid in 1965 and the invention of Social Security and Unemployment Compensation in the 1930s could in no way be characterized as incremental changes.

Sometimes incrementalism carries the day and is the only possible and logical vehicle for change. But at other times, broad revolutionary change is not just possible but seemingly inevitable. Facing this moment can be a troubling experience. While pushing too far may ruin a chance to achieve solid yet incremental progress, not pushing far enough may miss a real opportunity to achieve fundamental change. Is there a way to recognize the difference between these two situations, especially before something big may happen? The political model we consider in this chapter, known as the punctuated equilibrium model of policy change, seeks to explain the difference. It has roots in theories of science, paleobiology, organizational theory, and more. It is a challenging model that complements the dynamics of John Kingdon's agenda-setting structure described in chapter 7.

The case story involves a moment when big-time, nonincremental change in the Massachusetts health care environment seemed distinctly realistic. In 1991, both the Commonwealth's and the nation's health care systems were considered to be in a state of crisis. Widespread dissatisfaction was evident with the state's hospital rate setting system, a complex and bureaucratic regulatory structure that had been created during the state's prior fiscal crisis in 1975 to control the growth in hospital and health costs. With the inauguration of a new governor in January 1991 as well as a continuing state fiscal crisis, radical change to the status quo was not only conceivable but encouraged. The question was, what kind of change: expanded government control through a single-payer financing system or less government through deregulation and reliance on market dynamics? Had I known and understood the punctuated equilibrium model at the time, answering that question might have been a lot easier.

PUNCTUATED EQUILIBRIUM

Throughout modern history, dating back to the Renaissance and Descartes's development of the scientific method, our ancestors assumed that knowledge of the world increased in a linear and progressive way. Each successive generation "stood on the shoulders" of those who came before and added to our base of knowledge on behalf of those who followed. Progress was thought to be continuous and unending, a "development by accumulation" process resembling a straight line moving ever upward on a graph where the x-axis represents accumulated knowledge and the y-axis represents succeeding years.

In the early 1960s, Thomas Kuhn of MIT found this model of the history of science inadequate and developed a new concept he called "scientific revolutions." "Normal science," as he described it, is based on past scientific breakthroughs that formulate what become basic and accepted ideas of how the world works. "Normal scientists" spend their careers engaging in "mop up operations" that extend knowledge on the basis of these prior, breakthrough ideas. In this process, the growth in knowledge resembles the linear, progressive form that characterized earlier beliefs. An example of normal science can be found in the work of astronomers who followed Ptolemy's geocentric computations of planetary positions indicating that the Sun and the other planets revolved around Earth. Development of his core ideas, once revolutionary, became "normal science" and proceeded for 1,500 years in a linear, cumulative fashion, succeeding generations expanding and elaborating his central concept with increasing detail and complexity.

Over time, Kuhn observed, scientists unearth problems and unanswerable questions that cast doubt on the original breakthrough construct. Older and more established practitioners of the discipline are typically the most resistant to acknowledge the gravity of the challenges and the most dismissive of those who cast doubt on the validity of the original core idea. Younger and newer members of scientific disciplines are usually—within the political economy of their careers—more willing to examine the problems with a fresh eye, often facing great resistance: "Normal science often suppresses fundamental novelties because they are necessarily subversive of its basic commitments," wrote Kuhn.

Eventually, a new theory emerges that not only does not build on the original one but requires its rejection: "Its assimilation requires the reconstruction of prior theory and the re-evaluation of prior fact, an intrinsically revolutionary process," Kuhn asserts. Copernicus's new theory claimed that Earth and the planets revolve around the Sun, a revolution in astronomical thinking. The old order does not change its thinking in the face of this fresh challenge but resists mightily. For a time, the two sets of ideas may coexist (for example, the theory of the miasmic origin of disease versus newer germ theory). Eventually, the defenders of the older idea die off, and their ideas with them. The new order, in the aftermath of the Copernican revolution, then enters its own equilibrium phase, and a new era of specialization begins, built around the innovative organizing theory. At the core, it is the emergence of the new *idea* that makes the revolution possible: no new idea, no revolution.

Kuhn found this dynamic repeated in many branches of the physical sciences and outlined them in his pathbreaking book, *The Structure of Scientific Revolutions.*[2] Whether Copernicus and astronomy, Newton and the theory of light and color, Lavoisier and the oxygen theory of combustion, Einstein and the theory of relativity, or others—in each instance their new ideas "necessitated the community's rejection of one time-honored scientific theory in favor of another incompatible with it. Each produced a consequent shift in the problems available for scientific scrutiny and in the standards by which the profession determined what should count as an admissible problem or as a legitimate problem-solution."

Kuhn makes clear his view that the social sciences are markedly different from the natural sciences because of the latter community's ability to give near-universal acceptance to organizing *paradigms,* "universally recognized scientific achievements that for a time provide model problems and solutions to a community of practitioners." It is beyond dispute that no such broadly accepted paradigms currently exist in the social sciences. However, near the end of his volume, Kuhn toys with the thought that his ideas might help to illuminate the dynamics of political as well as scientific revolutions:

> Political revolutions are inaugurated by a growing sense, often restricted to a segment of the political community, that existing institutions have ceased adequately to meet the problems posed by the environment that they have in part created. . . . In both political and scientific development the sense of malfunction that can lead to crisis is prerequisite to revolution. . . . Political revolutions aim to change political institutions in ways that those institutions themselves prohibit. Their success therefore necessitates the partial relinquishment of one set of institutions in favor of another. . . .[3]

Kuhn's work had an extensive impact on many intellectual disciplines beyond science and politics. In the 1960s and 1970s, many intellectuals eagerly applied and adapted his ideas and construct to the study of history, philosophy, economics, art, religion, social thought, American foreign policy, sociology, psychology, literature, education, and more. Some credit "Kuhnian" ideas as seminal in the development of postmodern thought, a contention from which Kuhn distanced himself. As intellectuals began to see "paradigm shifts" everywhere, the term itself became an overused cliché. Many writers from varying disciplines found reasons to assault Kuhn's thesis, bored large holes in it (one writer counted twenty-two different definitions of the word *paradigm* in Kuhn's book), and identified various countertheses.[4] Kuhn answered many of these critics in a 1969 *Postscript* to the original text challenging many of the revolutionary interpretations of his 1962 book. Nonetheless, Kuhn's legacy is the abandonment of the idea of simple linear intellectual progress in the sciences and other disciplines. Others had observed nonlinear phenomena prior to Kuhn, but none had his dramatic impact across a host of intellectual disciplines.

One continuing strand of Kuhn's thought can be found in the term *punctuated equilibrium*. Though Kuhn never joined these two words together in his book, the concept closely tracks his ideas. Researchers in other fields have found the dynamic of punctuated equilibrium Kuhn described to have relevance to their own studies. In the early 1970s, paleobiologists Niles Eldredge and Stephen Jay Gould used the concept to explain long periods of stability punctuated by random, infrequent, and dramatic spurts in the evolutionary record over millions of years.[5] In the early 1980s, Michael Tushman and Elaine Romanelli applied the concept to organizational theory to describe a firm's progress through "convergent periods punctuated by reorientations which demark and set bearings for the next convergent period." The reorientation periods are "episodes of short, discontinuous change where strategies, power structures, and systems are fundamentally transformed toward a new basis of alignment."[6] A more recent variant of this dynamic can be found in Intel CEO Andrew Grove's description of "strategic inflection points."[7]

In the 1990s, two political scientists applied this construct to political change. Frank Baumgartner and Bryan Jones introduced the "punctuated equilibrium model of policy change" in 1993 to describe the process of revolutionary versus incremental change in political systems.[8] They observed that new institutional structures and arrangements most typically form during distinct periods when new issues, ideas, and "policy images" emerge into public view. These new structures then can remain in place for years or decades, creating a false illusion of stability and "equilibrium" until new issues or images emerge to destroy the institutions, replacing them with new ones or radically transforming the old ones. A new equilibrium period then ensues during which changes are once again of an incremental sort, building on or refining the existing idea rather than challenging it—until the next round of fundamental change begins. Three important sets of ideas are rooted in this "political" punctuated equilibrium model (all three are derived from themes and concepts already explored in earlier chapters):

→ 1. *The Structure and Scope of Conflict in the Policymaking Process:* While many observers of the policy process see stability and consensus building as driving dynamics, Baumgartner and Jones view conflict and the ever-present possibility for upheaval and instability as more significant characteristics. As discussed in chapter 3 on the nature of conflict in political systems, "at the root of all politics," according to Schattschneider, "is the universal language of conflict . . . politics is the socialization of conflict." It is through conflict that new ideas are advanced to topple existing regulatory and institutional structures. These structures are created and then guarded by interests and officials who benefit from their existence and become, in Baumgartner and Jones's terms, a "policy monopoly" seeking to control participation, dialogue, and conflict to preserve the basic structure.

⌐→ 2. *The Role of Ideas in Policymaking:* All policy monopolies, without exception, exhibit two characteristics: first, a definable institutional structure to shape and manage participation; and second, a powerful supporting *idea* that justifies the structure. To Baumgartner and Jones, existing policy monopolies are not toppled by competing interest groups, however powerful, but rather by competing policy ideas that undermine and eventually delegitimize the prevailing one. While interest groups are important, they are powerless to challenge an existing system without a strong and compelling replacement idea. Kuhn found this to be a critical dimension in the success of scientific revolutions: "The decision to reject one paradigm is always simultaneously the decision to accept another."[9] Interests are important—but ideas make the critical difference.

⌐→ 3. *The Nature and Pace of Change in Political Systems:* Some observers, such as Lindblom and Carl Van Horn,[10] have found the slow, incremental pace of change to be a key feature of politics, or at least of American politics. Others, such as William Riker, reach the opposite conclusion, that "disequilibrium, or the potential that the status quo can be upset, is the characteristic feature of politics" and can occur whenever political actors introduce new dimensions of conflict—or expand its scope—thus destabilizing a previously stable situation.[11]

Baumgartner and Jones synthesize these perspectives into one coherent framework that recognizes both dynamics at work during different periods of the punctuated equilibrium cycle. Policy systems and structures can operate in seemingly stable environments for long periods of time without effective challenge or opposition, during which time the policy

reform process resembles the incrementalist model advanced by Lindblom and others. But when new ideas are advanced by new players who
consciously seek to challenge and topple an existing policy structure,
Riker's instability is indeed the system's characteristic feature.

Thus, while the punctuated equilibrium model of policy change is a
construct derived from other fields of inquiry including the history of
science, biology, and organizational theory, it is also a model built on
ideas that have been central to the study of politics and policy change
for a long time. It helps to shed light on those brief, rare moments when
big change is not only possible but almost inevitable. The model does
not assume that the new system with its accompanying structural
changes is necessarily better than its predecessor, only different. One final
point: policy systems not only refer to the behemoths such as Social Security, welfare, or Medicare; in fact, policy subsystems are ubiquitous,
perched in larger secretariats or agencies, rarely seeing much light of
public attention—except when major structural change affecting them
reaches the public agenda.

The following case story examines a potential moment of substantial
institutional change in the Massachusetts health care system in 1991, a
challenge to the Commonwealth's hospital rate setting system that had
been set up in 1975. Also at issue was what kind of change would become the alternative organizing idea: more government involvement or
less. With this story, we can observe the punctuated equilibrium model
at work, including (1) the development of a new idea (rate setting) accompanied by its own institutional structure; (2) the efforts to defend
and maintain that structure by interests that favored it; and (3) the emergence of alternative policy ideas that challenged it, accompanied by interests working to bring down the once new and now old idea.[12]

HOSPITAL RATE SETTING

It was a beautiful, balmy September day in 1987 on the Boston Common across from the elegant, red-bricked Massachusetts State House designed by Charles Bullfinch in 1798. A lot of the heat that day came not
from the sun but from a loud demonstration of about 10,000 hospital
workers—nurses, physicians, orderlies, administrative staff, aides, and
others—who had been transported by their executives to the steps on the
Common beneath the monument to the Massachusetts Fifty-Fourth Reg-
iment, the first African American Union battalion of the Civil War. The
demonstrators held placards and banners, some identifying their re-

spective institutions and many others with a variant of their immediate message, "Cost Containment Has Gone Too Far." While a number of state legislators addressed the rally and accepted cheers and applause, I stood on the other side of a heavy, black, wrought-iron fence bordering nearby Park Street and watched. I shook my head both at the political mess that had engulfed a regulatory system designed to control the costs of the world's most expensive hospital system and at the jeopardy the controversy posed for our efforts to win passage of legislation to guarantee universal health insurance coverage for all Massachusetts residents. I didn't know it then, but this single rally—more than any other event—signaled the inevitable end of hospital rate setting. By what crazy, messed-up route did we get to this point? . . .

State regulation of hospital rates of payment—in Massachusetts and about thirty other states—had not been created casually or without struggle. It was a change in business as usual that represented a genuine threat to health care providers comfortable with a prior financing and insurance system that paid whatever they billed and asked no questions. During the decades following the conclusion of World War II, hospitals and the health system operated with a blank-check mentality regarding costs. George Annas writes that the prevailing metaphor for the system created by the survivors of the world conflict was military.[13] Thus we waged "war" on cancer, heart disease, and other critical ailments, suggesting, as in war, that costs were a secondary consideration as we mounted a "technological arms race" to conquer disease. The insurance industry—Blue Cross and commercial payers—regarded themselves largely as financial pass-through agents. Employers, taking advantage of the favorable tax treatment of health benefits established during the war period, raised few objections to rising premiums (except for the cost of caring for their elderly retirees during the 1950s and early 1960s before the establishment of Medicare). Consumers did not see the rising costs hidden in their paychecks.

The creation of Medicare and Medicaid in 1965 changed the landscape by adding two new players who quickly became committed to controlling rising costs in the medical sector: the federal government and the state governments. As the national economy ended its extraordinary postwar growth epoch in the late 1960s, private employers joined government to seek ways to control rising health care costs. Employers, who purchased health insurance in blank-check, fee-for-service arrangements, had no effective means at their disposal to stem cost increases. (The emphasis, until the 1990s, was always on holding back the *rate of increase* in costs, never on reducing the real level of costs.) The solution, developed gradually and in many distinct forms beginning in the late 1960s, was public sector regulation, and the key target of this regulation was the hospital.

The rationale for targeting hospitals was the Willie Sutton justification for robbing banks: because that's where the money is. Representing more than 40 percent of the health care dollar in the 1960s, hospitals were viewed as the heart and lungs of the health care colossus, the physician's playhouse that consumed progressively larger portions of the gross national economy. In 1961, Cornell's Milton Roemer in an influential study found that increases in the supply of acute-care hospital beds were always accompanied by proportional jumps in inpatient hospital utilization, leading him to formulate what became known as "Roemer's Law": under a policy of full-cost reimbursement, "a built bed is a filled bed." In economic terms, the health sector was considered to be a compelling example of "market failure": the prevalence of insurance, the inability of consumers to act as prudent purchasers, the lack of useful information, and the unique nature of medical care all combined to violate the assumptions necessary for the operation of an efficient, competitive market.

A panoply of regulatory mechanisms was invented to address the cost problems in the health sector, most aimed squarely at the hospital. A Democratic Congress and Republican President Richard Nixon agreed in the early 1970s to require states to establish so-called certificate of need systems, compelling hospitals to follow an extensive and elaborate public review process before they could expand their physical plants, add new beds, or incorporate new and expensive technologies. The same Congress and president also decided to require states to establish elaborate health planning structures, bringing health providers and consumers together on public boards to review proposals for hospital capital spending and devise plans to slow the growth in hospital costs. The same Congress and president concurred in 1973 in passing a law to encourage the formation of "health maintenance organizations," a revamped form of prepaid group practice that had existed on a small scale in some parts of the country since the 1930s with the establishment of the prepaid Kaiser Health Plans.

Finally, the same Congress and president decided in 1972 to encourage states to develop new systems to regulate hospital budgets, known as *prospective rate setting*. The concept sought to alter fundamentally the financial incentives faced by hospitals. Prior to rate setting, hospitals simply billed insurers and other payers after treatment to collect whatever their charges happened to be. Thus the hospital's incentive was to increase charges as much as possible. Rate setting sought to correct that set of perverse incentives by determining rates of payment in advance, thus forcing hospitals to be more cost conscious and efficient. In more ambitious forms, some rate setting programs determined ahead of time the total amount of charges a hospital could collect from *all* payers during a given period of time, hence the term *all-payer rate setting*. Federal officials did not dream up the idea of prospective hospital rate setting on their own. Officials in a number of states, especially New York and Maryland, had succeeded in establishing their own structures prior to the 1972 federal act. But cost-conscious federal policymakers of both parties wanted desperately to act and encouraged other states to follow the pacesetters' examples. Importantly, while hospitals protested and chafed under the new regulatory strictures, there were *no* voices during this formative decade arguing for market competition as a more effective means to control health spending. Employers who paid attention to health care costs nodded their approval of the new, governmentally sponsored regulatory controls because their perceived choice was between prospective payment regulation and an out-of-control and unaffordable fee-for-service model.

Ultimately, the federal laws dealing with hospital capital expansion, health system planning, and health maintenance organizations were repealed or substantially scaled back and judged well-intentioned failures. (HMOs began their membership explosion in the early 1980s not because of federal support—the Reagan administration suspended that support in 1981—but because of recession-driven employer discontent and an injection of private sector capital when plans began to convert to for-profit status.) The experience with prospective payment, however, was more promising. By 1980, more than thirty states had established their own hospital rate regulation programs, and a core of more progressive and industrialized states began to experiment successfully with more sophisticated and aggressive models. Officials in Maryland, New Jersey, New York, and Massachusetts developed all-payer, prospective rate setting systems that regulated hospital payments by all four major payers: private commercial payers, Blue Cross plans, state governments through Medicaid, and the federal government through Medicare. Officials in New Jersey were the first to experiment with a new prospective payment model called *diagnostic related groups,* or DRGs, that provided hospitals with a lump-sum, per-case payment based on a patient's primary diagnosis. During the hyperinflation years of the late 1970s, President

Jimmy Carter made his major health initiative an attempt in 1978 and 1979 to establish a national prospective payment system for all acute-care hospitals, an effort the national hospital lobby was able to thwart in Congress. Nonetheless, federal officials liked the prospective payment scheme so much that in 1983 they adopted it as the model for Medicare's payment structure for inpatient hospital services.

Beginning around 1980, health services researchers started to produce empirically based studies documenting a lower rate of increase in hospital costs in states that adopted aggressive forms of prospective rate setting. Most studies examining the rate setting states from a variety of perspectives throughout the decade found similar results. The authors of a 1985 study provided this assessment: "[T]he verdict is unanimous: no matter how cost is measured, every study in this group found that mature rate-setting programs, taken together, constrained hospital costs; and all but one of these findings were statistically significant."[14]

It was also during the early 1980s that voices began to emerge on the national scene arguing that competition and the market would be more effective vehicles than regulation in holding down rates of increase in health care spending that were still far outpacing national economic growth. A 1984 article in the journal *Health Affairs* by Jeff Goldsmith argued that because of managed care, DRGs, employer self-funding of health plans, the Blue Cross break with hospitals, and the development of alternative delivery systems, "the economic power of providers nurtured for decades has begun to shift from those who provide care to those who pay for it."[15] The regulatory response, he argued, didn't fit with the new reality and actually held back the kind of change necessary to deal with it. The article was titled, presciently, "Death of a Paradigm."

MASSACHUSETTS REGULATION

Though limited forms of hospital rate regulation in Massachusetts can be traced as far back as 1953, it was the severe economic recession of 1975 that precipitated major controls. Democrat Michael Dukakis had been elected to his first term as governor in 1974, defeating liberal Republican Frank Sargent by making a "lead-pipe cinch" guarantee that he would not raise taxes during his first term in office. But a perilous fiscal crisis forced him to renege on that promise in mid-1975, his first year in office, an about-face voters remembered in 1978 when they denied him reelection. Chief among the out-of-control costs of state government at the time was the Medicaid program, which generated huge amounts of red ink and attention. Dukakis tried to rein in program spending by freezing increases in all hospital charges, not just Medicaid's, a move the hospital lobby successfully blocked in the state legislature. But legislative leaders agreed to create new regulatory controls over Medicaid and Blue Cross charges as an alternative to the Dukakis freeze.

State officials understood that Medicaid was only a minor—and stingy—payer to hospitals and that effective control of hospital spending required clamping down on more than just Medicaid in order to force hospitals to become more efficient. Blue Cross's participation, because of its huge size and subscriber base, ensured that the system would command serious attention and results from the hospital community. Regulatory duties for the new system were handed to bureaucrats at the Commonwealth's Rate Setting Commission (RSC) who worked diligently to create the new structure by 1977. The principal motivation behind the establishment of rate regulation was clear: to provide an effective means to control the growth in Medicaid hospital costs.

During these years, health care and hospital finances were often compared to a "Chinese pillow"—push down on one side and the other side of the pillow rises. The metaphor was apt: while Medicaid and Blue Cross officials saw some rate relief during the early rate setting years, private, unregulated commercial insurance plans became recipients of huge cost shifting by hospitals. The practice for large commercial insurers such as Prudential and Aetna was to develop a broad national subscriber base, but one that had thin penetration in any local market. This left these plans without local leverage and vulnerable to cost shifting by hospitals who saw their Blue Cross and Medicaid payments reduced. A lengthy, legislative brawl involving hospitals, Blue Cross, commercial carriers, administration officials, and legislators resulted in the creation in 1982 of an all-payer rate regulatory system that controlled the growth of nearly all inpatient hospital spending: Medicaid, Blue Cross, commercial plans, and (with special federal approval) Medicare.

The new all-payer system (known as "Chapter 372") did several important things: first, it limited hospital inpatient revenue to what each hospital earned in 1981, plus a growth factor; second, it limited the growth factor to the national rate of medical inflation each year, minus one percentage point in order to put economic pressure on hospitals; third, it required that nearly all purchasers of hospital services (government, private insurers, self-insured businesses and labor unions, and self-pay patients) pay a fixed percent of approved hospital charges; and fourth, it required special recognition by payers for each hospital's "uncompensated care" costs in caring for patients with no insurance coverage. In a significant detail that escaped the attention of most observers, the state's tiny population of health maintenance organizations was left outside the regulatory structure, free to negotiate their own special rates of payments with hospitals (most other states with rate setting required HMOs to play by the same rules as all other payers).

At this point around 1982, we can observe several key features of the punctuated equilibrium model in the Massachusetts rate setting story. First, the new regulatory system was established because of intense dissatisfaction with a prior financing model—fee for service—that no longer met the needs of important stakeholders in the system, chiefly state government, business, labor unions, and insurers. Second, the creation of the new system was driven by an idea, that the only way to correct "market failure" and to restrain the growth in health system costs was through governmentally imposed regulation of hospitals and hospital charges. The choice was not perceived to be regulation versus market forces, but rather regulation versus unfettered price setting by the hospitals.

The third key element was the establishment of a so-called policy monopoly that guarded and managed the new structure. The state legislature had attempted in 1980 to create such a group by setting up a special commission to develop recommendations for improvements to the rate regulation system. That commission disbanded in 1981, unable to come to agreement on the outlines of a new system. Into this vacuum stepped Nelson Gifford, the CEO of a large manufacturer and the chairman of the Health Care Task Force for the Massachusetts Business Roundtable. Gifford formed what became known simply as "the Coalition," a nongovernmental, nonofficial group he handpicked to include the heads of the Massachusetts Hospital Association, Blue Cross of Massachusetts, the Life Insurance Association of Massachusetts, the Massachusetts AFL-CIO, the Massachusetts Medical Society, and the Commonwealth's Executive Office of Human Services, with Gifford as chairman representing the business community. The group was later expanded to include a representative of the Massachusetts Association of HMOs, though consumer groups were denied their request to join.

The creation and enactment of the 1982 all-payer system (Chapter 372) was the result of the Coalition's lobbying clout as the incomprehensible enabling legislation sailed through both the State Senate and the House of Representatives without dissent. Between 1981 and 1986, the Coalition wielded effective veto power over all aspects of the rate regulation system, deciding in its closed sessions which changes to accept and which ones to reject. During my first year in the House of Representatives, in 1985, the legislature approved significant changes to the rate regulation system (establishing a statewide pool to reimburse hospitals for uncompensated care costs, removing the federal Medicare program from the all-payer system, and more) without debate. The legislation had been agreed to by the Coalition, and legislators were asked not to mess up their fragile consensus. The desire to maintain consensus was driven by a sense that the system was achieving its cost containment ambitions. For example, a 1988 study found that rate setting systems had "reduced inflation rates by 16.3% in Massachusetts, 15.4% in Maryland, and 6.3% in New York, compared with the control hospitals in 43 states."[16]

For progressives such as me, the goal of cost containment was compatible with my own goal to expand coverage to the growing number of citizens who lacked any health insurance. The more hospital costs went up, the more expensive health insurance became, leading employers to drop coverage and workers to become uninsured. All the data and studies available confirmed this process. Thus, holding down costs, starting with hospitals, was seen as crucial in moving to universal coverage. HMOs, which sought—at least rhetorically—to hold down costs by improving quality and providing preventive services, were viewed as important allies and positive contributors to this effort.

Nelson Gifford was not, by nature, a pro-government regulator. He said on several occasions that he viewed the Massachusetts rate setting structure as only a transitional arrangement until conditions were ready for genuine market-based competition for health care and hospital services. As a result, the Coalition always recommended rate setting laws with a life span of only several years, forcing interest groups and state government to revisit the structure every few years. Thus, the 1982 system was designed to sunset at the end of September 1985 (the systems were always designed to begin on October 1 because it was the common start for hospital fiscal years, as well as for the federal government); the 1985 system, "Chapter 574," while making important modifications to the Chapter 372 model, maintained the basic features but was given a life span of only two years, until the end of September 1987. The Coalition wanted to move the system in a more competitive direction in the near future, and activist legislators (myself included) and consumer advocates took advantage of these legislative reviews to push the Commonwealth to commit to meeting a goal of universal health insurance coverage for all the state's residents. A new "special commission" was established in late 1985, as part of the Chapter 574 law, to pursue these twin objectives.

While the hospital industry is commonly seen in monolithic terms, the reality is quite different. Academic teaching hospitals, community hospitals, urban public hospitals, and rural institutions compete within each group and with each other. As rate regulation's effective pressures began to be felt by the Commonwealth's hospitals, more and more of them began to reach out to their local legislators to seek redress and special treatment, singly or in groups. One segment of community hospitals, for example, felt they were unfairly disadvantaged by the 1982 (Chapter 372) structure which established 1981 as the base year for rate setting calculations. Because all institutions were permitted to increase their charges by the same percent, hospitals that had charged less in 1981 than their competitor institutions received smaller annual revenue adjustments than hospitals with fatter budgets. Several of these hospitals, feeling pinched, hired consultants to run numbers, identified all hospitals in a similar situation, formed the "Low Cost Hospital Coalition," and hired legislative lobbyists to press their case for special adjustments to their member hospitals' rates. Legislators, unable to fathom the arcane complexities of the rate setting model, and wanting to please their local institutions, pushed through a special legislative adjustment in 1987 (this was the only occasion in my thirteen years in the House when I cast the *only* vote on one side of an issue, decided 159 to 1—a unique feeling).

The success of one hospital coalition bred the creation of others, leading to a growing crush of bills, each seeking to modify the system to favor one set of hospitals over others. Meanwhile, Nelson Gifford's Coalition ended its existence in 1986 in deference to the newly established Special Commission whose job was to figure out how to modify the rate setting model to permit more market-based hospital competition and to establish universal coverage. The new commission, like the others before it, proved unable to deliver on either of its key charges and disbanded without a final report in June 1987, with the rate setting structure scheduled to sunset by the end of that September and agreement on a replacement system nowhere in sight.

The Special Commission's work had been thrown off balance in March 1987 when the powerful chairwoman of the State Senate's Committee on Ways and Means, Patricia McGovern, made her own public recommendation to create universal health insurance by requiring all employers to buy health insurance for their workers. Though her plan was sketchy on details, it catapulted the previously obscure issue to front-and-center prominence in the State House. While other legislators had made similar calls in the recent past, none of us had McGovern's clout to move the issue.

During this same time, another development sucked up huge amounts of media and political attention: the growing prospects for Governor Michael Dukakis as a candidate for the Democratic nomination for U.S. president. Dukakis lost his first bid for reelection in 1978 but came roaring back in 1982, and since then had presided over an extraordinarily prosperous state economy that had been dubbed "the Massachusetts Miracle" and had earned him a national reputation for innovative public management. While his directive to his appointee on the Health Care Special Commission was to agree to no initiatives that would require new taxes or additional spending, Dukakis began to reassess that position in the summer of 1987, after the Special Commission had disbanded. With one eye on his need to develop positions that would distinguish his presidential run, Dukakis announced in August 1987 his own plan for "universal health care" in Massachusetts, specifically requiring all employers to provide health coverage for their workers. Dukakis filed his plan as part of legislation to extend the hospital rate setting system for four more years, a system facing an imminent sunset at the end of September. To mollify hospital critics of the rate setting system, Dukakis proposed to permit all hospitals to increase their charges annually by medical inflation *plus* 1 percent (changing the formula in existence since 1982 that permitted increases at the rate of medical inflation *minus* 1 percent). If this concession was needed to win hospital support for universal access legislation, I thought at the time, so be it.

To me, a second-term legislator, it was tremendously exciting to see this issue attain such prominence. I, along with other legislators and friends at Health Care for All, a health access advocacy group in Boston, had been urging Governor Dukakis and his key aides to adopt health care reform as a signal issue for his campaign and as a legislative initiative, and we now felt our urgings had made a difference and fundamental, nationally significant reform was at hand. Hospital leaders, however, responded to his plan by bringing about 10,000 of their workers to the Boston Common in September to denounce the proposed rate setting limits as too stringent. Meanwhile, small business leaders began to organize vigorously to oppose the employer mandate at the heart of the Dukakis plan. HMO leaders opposed a new tax on their premiums that was part of the financing scheme, while other health insurance industry leaders opposed elements that would permit state government to sell rival insurance policies to their customers.

While Senator McGovern gathered significant support in the State Senate for the Dukakis plan, House leaders were openly skeptical of its viability and only moved it forward to the full House of Representatives in early October 1987 out of a sense of duty to their home-state presidential candidate. On the floor of the House, the Dukakis plan suffered a legislative "near-death experience" when it was hustled back to the Committee on Ways and Means rather than face an overwhelming and embarrassing defeat. Several weeks later, the House passed and sent to the Senate a limited bill that merely extended the life of the hospital rate setting system for one additional year. Some thought the matter was dead at that point.

But McGovern took the narrow House bill and used it as a vehicle to reassemble the key parties that had been part of the rate setting negotiation process from the late 1970s. In a long and arduous series of meetings during November and December, she traded and engineered concessions that permitted big business, labor, hospital, insurance, and consumer interests to endorse her new bill in late December 1987. The principal group she wooed was the hospital industry, by offering major financial concessions that transformed its members from entrenched opponents to avid proponents, including an across-the-board rate increase of medical inflation plus 3 percent, as well as other add-ons that allowed huge increases, effectively wiping out all of the cost containment progress made by the rate setting system during the previous ten years. The final "universal health care" package barely passed a reluctant House of Representatives by a mere 77-to-75 margin in April 1988 and the Senate by a more comfortable margin. The changes to the hospital rate setting system took effect immediately, while the universal health care employer mandate—celebrated in an elaborate signing ceremony on the State House steps with balloons, bands, and banners—was not effective until 1992, a concession intended to mollify a furious and rapidly mobilizing small business community.

The delay in implementation of the employer mandate did not ease small business objections but only gave opponents a long lead time to organize and to wait for other events to overtake it. Two key events interceded. First, a severe recession took over the state's economy in 1989 and 1990 and caused budget crises, unemployment and business failure surges, and a deep sense of unease. Legislators were now unwilling to implement the health care employer mandate for fear it could exacerbate the economic distress. Second, Democratic Governor Dukakis, whose reputation as a skillful manager was shredded by the recession, was replaced by Republican William Weld who was as determined to repeal the mandate as Dukakis had been to implement it. (The ultimate fate of the employer mandate is described in chapter 7.)

While the economic recession drove away jobs and drained state revenues, hospitals and the entire health care sector boomed. The 1988 rate setting and "universal health care" law, known officially as Chapter 23, allowed hospitals to increase their charges by such large amounts that most institutions could not even take full advantage of them within their legally permitted revenue limits. These years coincided with a period of huge national health care inflation, with annual insurance premium growth of 20 percent and more. Businesses, large and small, screamed about increasing costs and their inability to stop them; workers lost health insurance coverage in record numbers; and government at all levels saw double-digit increases in the cost of their health programs as their overall revenue collections decreased. While much of these increases would have occurred—and did occur in other states—in the absence of hospital rate setting, Chapter 23 provided hospitals with a legally sanctioned excuse for their exorbitant rate hikes. Those of us committed to universal coverage and cost control had made a Faustian bargain in 1988, agreeing to a period of substantial hospital rate increases in order to achieve passage and implementation of the universal health care law. Now we saw the mandate losing support while the rate increases destabilized the entire regulatory system.

Just about everyone could agree that the system wasn't working—but what change could win majority support and fix the system?

THE ROAD TO CHANGE

The late 1980s and early 1990s were challenging and frustrating years for health policy nationally and in Massachusetts. Nothing seemed to work to slow down the relentless cost growth in the system. Regulation was increasingly viewed as a failure (except in the anomalous state of Maryland whose rate setting system continued to drive down the rate of growth in hospital costs). Market competition through managed care and HMOs was also regarded as ineffective. Meanwhile, the growth in numbers of the uninsured, about one million a year, caused increasing and serious alarm. Even major corporate and industry leaders began to talk openly of the need for a more radical solution, and discussion of the Cana-

dian-style single-payer financing scheme—under which most system revenues were generated through federal and provincial taxation and coverage was universal—attracted respectful and vigorous debate and consideration. Since entering the legislature in 1985, I had viewed the
single-payer concept with interest but dismissed its realistic prospects,
federal or state, as fantasy. Yet while no state government had approved
its own single-payer plan during this period, in several states such as New
York and Washington, one legislative chamber actually found a majority of votes to approve single-payer legislation. Maybe, I began to think,
the health system crisis was opening reform possibilities that would have
been unimaginable a few short years before.

As a member of the legislature's Joint Committee on Health Care during these years between 1988 and 1991, I became increasingly frustrated
defending a dysfunctional rate setting system as well as the controversial "universal health care" employer mandate that was full of loopholes.
Researchers such as Ken Thorpe, then at the Harvard School of Public
Health, showed us that the Massachusetts health care mandate—because
of design exceptions, such as exempting all employers with six or fewer
full-time workers from the requirement—would cover less than half the
state's uninsured population even if fully implemented.

Together with my allies at the Massachusetts consumer health organization Health Care for All, chiefly Rob Restuccia and Michael Miller,
I started working in the spring of 1990 on a proposal to create a Massachusetts single-payer system and called it the "Family Health Plan." Unlike most single-payer proposals, which were consciously designed to re-
semble Canada's fee-for-service structure, the FHP would be built on a
managed-care model. Consumers would be allowed to select a health plan
from a choice of HMOs in order to hold down costs and could opt for
a fee-for-service option at a higher cost. The system would be financed
through new employer payroll taxes that would replace existing employer
and employee health insurance premiums; the state would pay managed-
care organizations a lump sum for each resident they enrolled. Coverage would be universal, benefits would be uniform, and costs would be
held down by the dual pressure from managed-care utilization controls
and a systemwide "global budget." Knowing that the Chapter 23 rate
setting scheme was set to expire at the end of September 1991, we introduced the FHP at the start of the 1991 session as a proposed replacement system. Whatever else would happen during the course of
1991—and with a new governor, who could tell?—we wanted discussion of a single-payer option to be part of the mix.

We knew FHP was a "radical" proposal by any standard. But who knew how great the public's appetite for reform really was? Who knew how bad the twin problems of cost and access would become? Who had a better idea? Nonetheless, in the actual bill, we fudged on critically important questions: for example, how big a tax would be required to replace the private revenue generated by health insurance premiums? We knew that number would be our Achilles' heel, and so we left important decisions up to the proposed Health Care Authority which would manage the new system.

Also during 1990, I convinced legislative leaders to establish yet another special commission to bring key parties together to begin discussing what should happen to the Massachusetts rate setting system when it reached its sunset date at the end of September 1991. The Special Commission on Health Care Finance and Delivery Reform was created in mid-1990 and included all the usual suspects: the Massachusetts Hospital Association, Blue Cross of Massachusetts, the Life Insurance Association of Massachusetts, the Massachusetts Association of HMOs, the Massachusetts AFL-CIO, Associated Industries of Massachusetts, the Massachusetts League of Community Health Centers, Health Care for All, as well as a representative of the Dukakis administration and several legislators. I cochaired the group with Senator Edward Burke, who was the Senate chair of the legislature's Health Care Committee, and Representative Sherwood Guernsey, who was also a vice chairman of the Health Care Committee.

In the past, the processes involved in legislating hospital rate setting statutes had resembled elaborate poker games, with few players willing to show their cards until the latest possible moment in the game. I was one of the willing ones: Chapter 23 had been a dismal failure; we needed either to scrap the entire system in favor of a single-payer model such as the Family Health Plan or to modify the rate regulation system along the lines of the successful Maryland structure, which was more tightly controlled. Senator Burke, a liberal Democrat whom I had long admired, stunned me by advocating complete deregulation. He was frustrated by the continuous gaming and complexity, and he was joined by Bob Hughes, the aggressive head of the state's HMO association. Hughes feared that either a single-payer plan or a Maryland-type approach, such as the ones I advocated, would cause HMOs to lose their exemption from the rate setting system, something that had given them an enormous competitive advantage over Blue Cross and commercial insurers. While commercial plans and Blue Cross were required to pay hospitals on the basis of their state-approved charges, HMOs were free to negotiate lower rates of payment that allowed them to offer substantially lower premiums to their customers. This exclusion had not mattered much in 1982 when HMOs were a tiny part of the Massachusetts market, but it became a serious discrepancy in 1990 when they covered more than 25 percent of the privately insured market. Blue Cross, which was facing a major financial crisis and loss of enrollment at the time, wanted either of two scenarios: HMOs placed within the regulatory system on a par with all other plans or the system deregulated, permitting all plans to negotiate market-based rates of payment. Either way, change was essential for Blue Cross's future competitive position.

The hospital industry, an incessant critic of the rate setting system for years, surprised nearly everyone in December 1990 by announcing its organization's support for continued rate regulation and opposing a surge into competition and market-based contracting. Its position was especially surprising because one month before, in November 1990, William F. Weld became the first Republican to be elected governor in twenty years. A fierce market proponent, he had made no statements on the future of hospital rate regulation during his tough campaign, except to remark that "profit should not be a dirty word in health care." Had the hospitals wanted to move to competition, they would have enjoyed an immediate ally in the governor-elect. Their reluctance to do so suggested they had, in reality, benefited from the rate setting system and they knew it.

As happened with all health care special commissions since the 1970s, this one also could not reach agreement. There was no point in pushing the commission on a single-payer option, because it could not have received more than one-third of the votes. So we held back on that option. With Senator Burke and Bob Hughes dissenting, on the last day of December 1990 the commission endorsed a general statement in favor of continued but modified hospital rate regulation, pointing to the Maryland system as an example. With the state's economy still stuck in a serious recession, and with the public awaiting the inauguration of a new administration that promised radical change from business as usual, the commission's milquetoast recommendations went largely unnoticed.

POWER STRUGGLES

The executive branch was not the only part of state government anticipating major change in early 1991. The Speaker of the House of Representatives, George Keverian, was also stepping down. Keverian had assumed the Speaker's chair in 1985 after a bruising political brawl with his predecessor, Tommy McGee, a former Marine from the working-class city of Lynn. McGee had served longer than any Speaker in the history of the Massachusetts House but broke the promise he had made to Keverian to step down after the 1984 elections. When McGee announced in the fall of 1983 his changed intentions to run for reelection and to hold onto the Speaker's chair in 1985, his majority leader, Keverian, assumed the leadership of a rules reform revolt against his former boss.

Keverian could not have been more unlike the former Speaker. Eschewing the iron hand for a velvet glove, he gracefully overlooked the unruly and outlandish activities of members who regularly thumbed their noses at his requests for votes and loyalty. As a new rank-and-file member in 1985 who supported the revolt against McGee, I received enormous support from Keverian to carry out my agenda; in return, he always had my gratitude and support. Many members regularly complained of the Speaker's unwillingness to set a clear course and to lead, but then ran away from supporting him at every possible turn when the fiscal crisis hit with full force in 1989. He had agreed in 1985 to stay no more than eight years as Speaker, a stretch that would be up at the end of 1992. He thus took advantage of the 1990 state elections to run for the position of state treasurer. The support he counted on from members did not materialize; he lost the Democratic primary and gave up the Speaker's gavel in late December 1990, embittered and alone.

Keverian's successor as Speaker was never in doubt. Charles Flaherty of Cambridge was a smart, working-class liberal who voted progressive but liked to hang out with his conservative pals who had not abandoned Tommy McGee. Flaherty had played the critical role engineering Keverian's 1985 triumph and waited six more years as majority leader for his long-desired chance to lead. "Charlie," as he was universally known, had a talent for convincing nearly everyone that he was their close friend. His ascension to the Speaker's chair in early January 1991 was eagerly anticipated and unanimously approved.

During my first six years in the House, between 1985 and the end of 1990, I had served as a rank-and-file member of the Joint Committee on Health Care under the chairmanship of Malden's Representative John McNeil, who rivaled Keverian for an obesity problem but pursued the darker side of human character as opposed to the Speaker's warmer manner. Over the years, he opposed Keverian and Flaherty on numerous critical votes and lost their confidence as both looked to me and Sherwood Guernsey for advice on health care matters. McNeil had little interest in health policy, instead pursuing other passions: collecting antique cars, Coca Cola paraphernalia, and campaign donations.

It was considered certain that Flaherty would not reappoint McNeil as House chairman of the Joint Committee on Health Care in January 1991, and many considered it nearly as certain that I would be appointed in his place. I had spent six years working on a wide variety of health care issues, including finance, access, lead poisoning, AIDS, Medicaid, immunizations, and more. I knew that the future of the rate setting law would be a major priority and was eager to take it on. The only member who had spent as much time as I on health policy had been Sherwood Guernsey, who gave up his seat in 1990 to make an unsuccessful run for the State Senate. As did everyone else, I felt I had a strong, positive relationship with Flaherty and that he looked to me for advice on health policy issues. During the early days of the 1989–90 fiscal crisis when I rebelled against Ways and Means Chairman Richard Voke's budget-cutting approach, I frequently sought and received advice and direction from Flaherty. In late December 1990, a *Boston Globe* medical writer and friend, Richard Knox, had written that I was "widely considered to be the next health care committee chairman," a comment I feared would jinx my chances.

A colleague who entered the House with me in 1985, Carmen Buell from western Massachusetts, was also seeking a chairmanship in 1991. Smart, savvy, and hardworking, she also saw Flaherty's ascension as her opportunity to move up. But her work had been focused on nonhealth human service issues, and the human services committee was certain to be chaired by the well-respected and well-liked Paul Kollios. Buell and I had worked together in 1990 on a special Ways and Means Committee task force on Medicaid, and we got along well. My State House sources began to tell me in early January that she was pushing hard for Flaherty to name her as a committee chair and that the health care post was her most likely prospect.

In Massachusetts, the choice of committee chairs is made by the Speaker, who sends his nominations to the House Democratic caucus, which dutifully ratifies his choices in a secret ballot where all ballots are destroyed immediately after voting, sight unseen except by a few of the Speaker's handpicked loyalists. To revolt against this model and fail would guarantee political oblivion, so no one does. The Speaker waits until the third week in January to announce his choices, one week after the House debates adoption of rules for the coming two years. Regardless of who is Speaker, the message is always clear: make a fuss in the rules debate and watch any prospects of a chairmanship or favorable committee assignments sink like a stone the following week.

On schedule, Speaker Flaherty made his picks known and chose Carmen Buell to be his new Health Care Committee chair. On one level I was not surprised, and on another I was devastated. While I knew that Carmen was a solid choice, I felt my own career path in the House was suddenly dead-ended. I got in to see Charlie in his wood-paneled Speaker's office the following week and sputtered to get an answer out of him. What had I done wrong? How could I have done it differently? He looked at me somewhat surprised and perplexed, saying, "You just don't understand—you didn't fit into my plan."

THE NEW ORDER

The new Weld administration took power in early January 1991 facing continuing budget crises brought on by an economic recession that wouldn't quit. It engaged in early and heated combat with the newly energized House of Representatives led by Flaherty and his new team, including a fiscally conservative, sharp-tongued, and tough-minded chairman of Ways and Means, Tommy Finneran from Dorchester. The progressive-liberal community—within and outside the legislature—had high hopes that Flaherty would use his considerable political skills to hold back a conservative assault on state government. Indeed, several early and high-profile battles seemed to presage years of intense executive-legislative conflict. But the need to convince Wall Street bond houses that the Commonwealth's political as well as fiscal house was in order led the leaders of each branch by springtime to set aside their differences and to apply negotiation and collaboration—not confrontation—as their characteristic techniques.

Interest in the fate of the hospital rate setting system during these early months was restricted to a small circle. State Senator Ed Burke, who remained the Senate chairman of the Joint Committee on Health Care, invited Buell and me to accompany him in February 1991 on a trip to Maryland to meet with hospital representatives, state regulators, and others who had made their hospital rate setting system the envy of the nation. Buell turned down the request, and so Burke, a Senate aide, and I spent a Friday in early February talking with a variety of players, all of whom extolled the system's ability to hold down costs and to maintain the political support of key parties, including the hospitals. (When Maryland began its rate setting system in the mid-1970s, its inpatient hospital costs were about 25 percent above the national average; by 1990, they had dropped to about 10 percent *below* the national average.) At the end of the day, the three of us had some extra time and used it to walk around the stunning new Aquarium on the Baltimore waterfront and couldn't resist comparing the various fish with parties in the rate setting pool—hospitals were the sharks, we all agreed. Burke seemed as impressed with the Maryland system as I, and as we flew back to Boston, I felt convinced that even if my single-payer Family Health Plan was not winnable, at least a Maryland-style regulatory model might win his key support.

Though it was painful and awkward for me, I tried hard to be a supportive and loyal committee member to Buell as she took control of the Health Care Committee along with Burke. I briefed her early about the history of the rate setting system and the work of the special commission that ended unsuccessfully the previous January. Her early comments indicated agreement with my position that rate regulation could be made to work again if structured appropriately and that the evidence for the capacity of a competitive health care market to perform better was non-existent. In July, when the Health Care Committee held its major public hearing on the administration's proposal to deregulate within three years, Burke disappointed me by returning to his position in favor of market competition and deregulation. Buell gave me encouragement with her public statement, "There is no evidence that competition works."

But the lineup at the July 17 public hearing did not give me confidence that her view would prevail. Governor Weld's point person at the hearing and on the issue was Charles Baker who, like Speaker Flaherty, was always called "Charlie." Baker had been the director of a right-tilting Massachusetts think tank called the Pioneer Institute and had used that spot to criticize the universal health care employer mandate. Weld named him undersecretary of health and human services, with a clear mandate to lead health policy development for the new administration. Unlike the consensus style that characterized policymaking during the Dukakis years, Baker employed a more directed leadership style that made him, in the words of one industry leader, "the center of gravity." During Weld's transition period the previous December, Baker asked the governor-elect whether he wanted to delay the rate setting debate for a year by simply passing a bill to extend rate setting for an additional year, or preferred to move right away for deregulation.

"No. You should be thinking a lot between January and February about where people are and what's important to them, because we really want to fix this right after we get the budget done," Weld told Baker.

Hospital rate setting had never been an issue that stirred the masses. While the stakes were huge and the passions of the inside players erupted easily, no one expected to see any more 10,000-person rallies on the Boston Common over this matter. The July public hearing attracted several hundred hospital, business, insurance, and labor figures and was the largest public event in the 1991 process. Baker spent considerable time during his first few months talking with affected parties about the future prospects for the system. While the Massachusetts Hospital Association had taken an organizational position in favor of continued regulation the previous December, many individual hospital leaders were fed up with the system and thought they would do better under a freer, open market. With Baker's encouragement, they became more forthright and confident in speaking to legislators in support of junking the system. Leaders of Blue Cross, recognizing that more extensive regulatory controls implicit in the Maryland model were not part of the new administration's thinking, also began to embrace the logic of deregulation, hoping to achieve it before their financial fortunes worsened further. Significant segments of the business community, organized around new regional health purchasing networks, had already decided that promotion of competition was in their interest, which was to reduce their employee health costs. Some of the leading business groups, chiefly the Associated Industries of Massachusetts, expressed concern that the removal of rate regulation would lead to short-term explosive increases in hospital costs, but their rank-and-file members muted those concerns. Many of them were already engaged in negotiations with hospitals over rates of payment and found that they held substantial negotiating leverage.

The hearing was the first public demonstration of an essential component of the punctuated equilibrium model: the emergence of an alternative organizing idea. After years of support for regulation as the only realistic option to hold down the rate of growth in hospital costs, business leaders, insurers, hospital officials, and key administration leaders now began to talk openly of the value of competitive, market-based contracting as a replacement organizing idea for the system. The lobbyist for commercial insurance companies, which were not ready to break with regulation, recognized the significance of the shift at the hearing: "It was the first public manifestation that this was an idea that had come of age; it was clear that the idea had arrived." An essential dynamic of the punctuated equilibrium model is for change advocates to create a new "policy image" of the status quo and of their new proposed structure. In this case, they performed that role expertly.

The forces at the hearing opposed to deregulation were less clear. My consumer allies at Health Care for All argued for the single-payer Family Health Plan as an alternative system, an alternative organizing idea, though without broad-based support. Labor unions argued against a retreat from regulation because of the feared impact on health care and hospital workers, though some of the construction trades unions complained bitterly about the inability of the rate setting system to hold down hospital costs during the preceding four years. Academics from area universities suggested that competition as a device to control spending had no support in the research literature. On that point they were correct. But health purchasers from business groups answered back that they were seeing benefits of competition for nonhospital services every day in their own operations. The world of health care and hospital finance was changing in ways that the research community had not yet been able to verify empirically. But it was happening nonetheless.

Carmen Buell struggled with the issue from July through September. She had me, along with consumer groups, labor unions, and academics, warning her against competition. She had hospital leaders, Blue Cross and the state's HMOs, business groups, Senator Burke, and Charlie Baker urging her to embrace the market. She began to work with a group of academics organized at a policy center at Brandeis University to devise a middle route: gradual deregulation over three years, with a vague, global budget cap imposed on overall hospital spending. Her position delighted competition supporters who felt that problems with the proposed legislation—particularly the global budget caps—could be ironed out as it worked its way through the legislative process. Buell and Burke called an executive session of the seventeen-member Health Care Committee on September 19 to vote out a bill. At the session, many of the panel's members spoke at length on their positions. I was one of a few to argue against the proposed bill and had my name listed as a "dissenter." The most memorable comment, though, came from Burke, speaking in favor of competition among hospitals: "I favor putting the scorpions in the same bottle and letting them fight it out."

Rank-and-file legislators typically follow their party leadership unless a compelling reason pushes them in a different direction. The rank and file followed their leaders in the 1970s and 1980s when told that rate setting regulation was needed, and I knew at the outset most would support deregulation if that was the judgment of their leaders. In the heavily Democratic-dominated Massachusetts legislature, the proponents of competition could now count on overwhelming Republican and sizable Democratic support. I found myself in the uncomfortable posture of the dissenter, the critic trying to disrupt the growing consensus in favor of market-based competition. From the Joint Health Care Committee, the deregulation legislation moved first to the House of Representatives, where its first stop was the House Committee on Ways and Means, the committee that considered all legislation that had any impact on the Commonwealth's finances. As the dissenter, I felt I had two advantages over Buell: first, that I was a member of the Ways and Means Committee, and second, that I had enjoyed a friendly relationship with the chairman, Tommy Finneran, who frequently asked for my advice on health policy issues.

Finneran's selection as Ways and Means chairman the previous January was a surprise to many. Much more conservative than the liberal Speaker Flaherty, he had an intense style and voracious appetite for work. While he would invite representatives of various points of view to his office to meet, decision making was reserved to himself and his key aide, Joe Trainor. He listened respectfully as I advocated a Maryland-style regulatory overhaul and Buell urged a careful, three-year deregulation path with global budget caps to guarantee price stability. Instead, he and Trainor wrote a new bill that moved immediately to rate deregulation, with only one year of very loose and ineffectual price controls. "We couldn't reconcile the public and explicit embrace of a free market, and yet being just a little timid to say it and do it," Finneran told me. He called an unusual Saturday afternoon executive session of the House Ways and Means Committee in mid-November to vote out the bill. I spoke at length and to no avail against the bill. Deregulation was heading to the House floor on the Monday of Thanksgiving week.

What to do when the bill reached the House floor? Option 1 was to let it go. I had said my piece in the Health Care and Ways and Means Committees and attracted no substantial support. It was considered bad form to oppose one's own leadership on the floor, and I had been trying to act as a team player. Option 2 was to simply oppose the bill and urge members to vote against it. Option 3 was to propose an alternative regulatory model based on Maryland's successful rate setting program. But recognizing that no more than five members of the institution even understood what the existing system was about, it seemed far fetched that they would bother to develop an understanding of the workings of a more complex system from another state. Option 4 was to use the occasion of debate to present a genuinely radical alternative, the single-payer Family Health Plan.

Throughout 1991, my allies at Health Care for All and I had continued to educate, speak, and mobilize in behalf of our newly developed plan. In the process, we had attracted interest, generated some compelling debates, and demonstrated little broad-based support. Numerous health care leaders applauded the innovative and detailed ideas but doubted the plan's practical potential to win support. Even traditional single-payer advocates withheld their backing because the Family Health Plan incorporated managed care as the delivery structure instead of the Canadian fee-for-service model. But three other states—New York, Vermont, and Washington—had developed substantial support for single-payer programs that actually won approval in one or the other legislative branch. Even if we couldn't win in 1991, perhaps putting it forward would gain credibility for the notion when the consequences of market-based competition became fully apparent to people. Even if we couldn't win on Monday, we could plant seeds that might bear fruit in the future. Option 4 was our choice.

My allies at Health Care for All, some labor unions, and some academics had done as much as we could to warn legislators of the risks of an unregulated health care market. Alan Sager from the Boston University School of Public Health held a press conference at the State House and identified hospitals that would be most at risk in a competitive market. Local 285 of the Service Employees Union, representing health care workers across the state, released a report on how the growing corporate involvement in hospitals was undermining patient care. I sent a steady stream of articles and information to my colleagues to warn them that competition could damage one of their most important local institutions and employers.

When debate on the floor of the House began, only the size of the margin of our defeat was in doubt. For two days, members debated the respective merits and demerits of competition versus regulation in health care. But the debate lacked any sense of intensity or urgency as most members went about their daily business while a few of us staged a last stand on the floor. At this point in 1991, most health care consumers who belonged to health maintenance organizations or other forms of managed care had opted voluntarily for this choice. The consumer and provider backlash against HMOs that developed with such intensity in the mid-1990s was not yet visible. On the floor of the House in November 1991, advocates of deregulation and the competitive model repeatedly extolled the virtues of managed care. I could not argue against that approach as even my Family Health Plan amendment incorporated managed care, albeit in a different framework.

In the House of Representatives, members are permitted to speak for up to one half hour at a time. On the first day of debate, I used up my full thirty minutes, something I had never before done, in order to detail the threat of market competition to the value and integrity of our health system. Buell spoke of the failures of the current system and the values that industry leaders and employers were finding in a prudent purchaser-contracting approach that enabled businesses to cut their own best deals for price and quality. On the second day, I presented my amendment to substitute the Family Health Plan for the entire deregulation bill. Buell did not bother to counter my debate, sending her vice chairman to respond to my arguments. The moment of truth came in a recorded roll call. My amendment was voted down, 120 to 29. Not long thereafter, the deregulation bill was approved by a vote of 119 to 27.

Moral victory is not something in which I have ever found much value. Being in the majority, an overwhelming majority at that, had permitted me to realize numerous legislative victories during my six years in the House. Most of the time, there is a need for someone to stand up and to present a minority position, even if it has no chance of passage, if only to ensure serious consideration and debate by the membership. In this case, the Democratic majority and the Republican minority were completely in sync, and it was left to Democratic progressives to forge a minority position. However one may rationalize the necessity of the role, it is lonely and frustrating.

In the State Senate, where the legislation went next, not a single member opposed the deregulation initiative, for which Finneran's framework now served as the vehicle. As with any large piece of legislation, many members sought to add various riders to benefit their favored projects. A substantial part of this legislative package also included plans to reorganize the commercial health insurance market for small businesses with one to twenty-five workers, something happening in many other states during this period. Also, the deregulation plan required changes in the structure of the Commonwealth's uncompensated care hospital pool which provided a means to pay for hospital services to the growing population of uninsured individuals. Through Buell's initiative, the legislation also created a "Healthy Kids" program to provide primary-care services to a limited number of uninsured children through age six. The significant number of complex details slowed the pace of the legislation during the holiday season.

It was about 4 A.M. on December 20 when the final version of the deregulation statute came to the House for approval of the conference committee report. The legislature was wrapping up its work for the year in one of its late-night, marathon sessions when some members take naps in their seats or in the lounge, others sit around telling jokes and stories, and a few others work feverishly to get their priority bills through the process before the session concludes. I had been one of the nappers until I heard the deregulation bill would be coming up soon for approval. After this vote, the bill would go to the governor's desk. It seemed to me to be my final opportunity to warn legislators and the public about the dangers of the market-based health care financing approach on which we were about to embark. I thought it one of my more eloquent moments as a member of the chamber, a speech I had been mulling since the November defeat:

> Nineteen ninety-one will be a landmark year for health care, not because of anything we do here. This year poliomyletis will be eradicated from the Western Hemisphere, and we are on target for global eradication by 2000. This follows the eradication of smallpox in 1978, an astonishing story of how doctors tracked and eliminated this disease from humankind. When we talk about health care and what's important, these achievements are what counts—victories of planning and coordination. It's no surprise that in the past decade with the emergence of competition and the market, we have seen the resurgence of measles, tuberculosis and other forgotten diseases. The imperatives of the market do not coincide in any way with the imperatives of health. . . . This legislation takes a health system which should be our chariot of the sun and reduces it to a market cart which will result in the degradation of the health of the people of this state and which will be traced to this bill. No member will rue a vote against this bill—we will all regret the forces this will set in motion.

Before the end of the year, Governor Weld signed the bill into law at a press conference with all the key supporters smiling their approval.

AFTERMATH

My late-night speech included some nice words, and years later I still wholeheartedly agreed with the sentiments and general principles regarding the role of for-profit medicine in our health care system. But on the particular matter of the disposition of the ill-fated Massachusetts hospital rate setting system, I was dead wrong. The September 1987 hospital rally on the Boston Common signified that the consensus to hold down hospital costs under a governmentally mediated system had collapsed. We were entering an epoch of everyone for themselves.

I didn't see it coming. For six years, I had so totally absorbed myself in the regulatory minutiae of an impossibly complex and bureaucratic system that I knew more about its intricacies and details than the combined knowledge of the other 199 senators and representatives. I knew so much detail that I had lost perspective and the ability to ask the larger and more important questions concerning its performance and value—the precise questions that legislators need to address. Tom Finneran and Carmen Buell, among others, were able to look at the system with fresh eyes, unencumbered by the detailed baggage I carried. Better than I could, they saw that heavy-handed government sector price regulation represented an idea whose time had come and gone. In the 1960s and 1970s, there was no better way to bring discipline to an out-of-control health and hospital sector, but the world of health care had changed since then in two important ways.

First, Massachusetts government had lost the ability to manage its hospital regulatory system with discipline and integrity. Every participant in the system—most especially, legislators, the executive branch, and the hospitals—had acted in ways that made continuation of the system counterproductive. Senator Ed Burke had often described the statutes authorizing the system to be "like Sanskrit, completely incomprehensible." While that characterization would fit many statutes and government regulations, his language helped to symbolize how the system had become obscure and indecipherable even to those most deeply involved and responsible, whose participation and support were indispensable to its effective operation.

The incomprehensibility led everyone to believe other players were getting something special from the system. Like prison detainees in the classic "prisoner's dilemma" where neither participant can predict what the other prisoner will confess about their joint crime, each hospital and group of hospitals sensed they were getting gypped by other, more savvy players, and they needed their own lobbyists, coalitions, and legislative proposals to claim their share of the pie. Legislators, unable to comprehend the intricacies of the system, valiantly sought to look like hometown heroes to their local institutions. The result became less a prisoner's dilemma and more a regulatory "tragedy of the commons" where everyone grazed cattle herds on the same land at greater and greater intensity until there was nothing left.

Consistent with the requirements of the punctuated equilibrium model, rate setting had its own "policy monopoly" that guarded and directed the system for years. But the gang was breaking up. The hospitals were divided, with many favoring an approach permitting them to determine their own fates. Blue Cross, facing its own financial disaster, wanted out. Many business voices echoed the belief that competition and contracting could, at last, work. Added to these critical participants in the coalition were the Weld administration and the new legislative leadership who refused to adhere to a regulatory formula just because it had been there for a long time. Their confidence in the potential for change epitomized the second major development in the Commonwealth's health care system.

The second major difference was that the health system had reached a point where hospitals were no longer the undisputed center of the system. The hospital at the center of the system was a critical feature of the rate setting idea. But by the early 1990s, health plans, allied with their employer clients, had achieved a level of sophistication and bargaining power enabling them to cut better deals than could be obtained through joint industry-government negotiations. They were doing it every day at multiple levels within the system and were confident in their ability to do it with hospitals as well.

I questioned deregulation supporters repeatedly: where is any evidence that market-based contracting, competition, and managed care can work? I possessed dozens of empirically based studies documenting that rate setting had reduced the rate of growth in hospital costs relative to unregulated systems and an equal number of studies showing that managed care and HMOs made no difference. No one disputed my research or offered counterevidence of any consequence. Only later did I recognize a critical point I had missed: the most recent research available was based on data collected before 1985 because it takes years for reliable numbers to become available, used, and disseminated by the research community. The business and insurer voices were talking about what was happening on the ground to them in 1990 and 1991, and it turned out to be more useful than a mountain of empirical research based on data from 1975 to 1985.

The punctuated equilibrium model suggests something important and heartening to those looking for hope in the policy and political process: ideas matter in the policy arena. The deregulation process in Massachusetts in 1991 affirms this view. Hospital rate setting was based on an idea, namely, that the health sector was a dramatic example of market failure and government-directed regulation was necessary to correct it. This idea was maintained and defended for about fifteen years by a wide array of interests. It was toppled in Massachusetts in 1991 (and in other states in other years) because major participants no longer believed in that idea and because an alternative idea emerged that made more sense to key policymakers. The new idea was that market-based contracting, organized around managed care, could correct the worst aspects of market failure, not perfectly but far better than regulation.

This idea was powerfully embraced by elements of the business community that purchased health care services for their employees. But it was just as powerfully embraced by government sector purchasers, chiefly the state's Medicaid program. Under rate setting, Medicaid had a terrific paper advantage: while most private purchasers were required to pay between 92 and 100 percent of hospital charges, Medicaid had to pay only about 80 percent of those charges. But the structure left the program vulnerable to manipulation of charges by hospitals to meet predetermined revenue targets. Massachusetts Medicaid Commissioner Bruce Bullen said that payers "had no way to know whether the hospital was going to gouge them or not. Deregulation was a shift of control to let the payers set the terms." It was not coincidental that deregulation occurred during the end of an intense fiscal crisis that saw huge Medicaid budget increases while the state's overall revenues were dropping. Hospital rate setting had been initiated during the previous state fiscal crisis of the mid-1970s as a strategy to control Medicaid spending. It was discontinued at the end of another fiscal crisis, again as a different strategy to control Medicaid costs.

With the institutionalization of the new idea—market competition and managed care as cost control strategies—a new policy monopoly formed to defend it from future threats. The new policy monopoly involved the Weld administration (especially Baker, who was later promoted to secretary of health and human services and still later to secretary of administration and finance, often called "deputy governor"), the business community, the HMO industry, Blue Cross, and various legislative leaders including Tommy Finneran, later elected Speaker of the House of Representatives in 1996. Provider groups such as hospitals and physicians no longer found themselves comfortably on the inside and were often found banging on the door from the outside to get attention. In the prior days of regulation-driven health care, consumer groups often found themselves aligned with business groups seeking to hold down price increases, and even with HMOs, the new players in the system who sought to hold down costs and emphasize prevention. In the new competitive era, consumers often found themselves aligned with provider groups seeking to impose mandates and other requirements on health plans to protect both consumers and providers.

This new dynamic has played out across the nation and Massachusetts since the early 1990s. Particularly with the demise of national health care reform in 1994, the growth of managed care rapidly accelerated. While HMO penetration in Massachusetts had been among the nation's highest since the early 1980s, it has become dominant in all segments of the health financing system since 1991 with the exception of the Medicare population. Consistent with national trends, the rate of growth in health insurance premiums moderated substantially in Massachusetts after 1993, slowing the growth in state Medicaid spending to a crawl as well (until 1998 and 1999 when premiums began rising again at rates far faster than overall inflation). The moderation in the growth of health spending removed health care costs as an issue of public concern and left room for consideration of other issues affecting consumers in the new health care environment.

Since 1994, nearly all states have passed a substantial number of new laws to protect consumers and providers in managed-care plans. Consumers have won rights to grievance procedures and appeals of service denials, while providers won measures designed to enhance their contractual rights and bargaining leverage with HMOs. Massachusetts was among the earliest states to enact a series of discrete legal protections, including regulation of maternity lengths of stays in acute hospitals and prohibition of so-called gag clauses in HMO-physician contracts, but was distinctly slower in addressing more comprehensive legislation. In a "Kuhnian" sense, the question arises: does the managed-care backlash represent incremental or fundamental change? Clearly, the new round of regulation is incremental, in that it seeks to modify, not overturn, the managed-care paradigm now governing the system. Consumers and providers unite to press for changes and negotiate with the managed-care/purchaser interests representing the new governing policy monopoly.

For Massachusetts hospitals, the 1990s were tumultuous times. Many institutions closed, merged, or affiliated with stronger ones. But as an industry, they saw their healthiest financial margins in many years until federal Medicare cutbacks damaged their bottom lines in the latter part of the decade. Nonetheless, deregulation was actually a healthy event for most of them. During the era of rate setting intrigue, hospitals reflexively looked to the State House whenever they got into trouble. Whatever went bad within an institution could be reflexively blamed on politicians and rate setting regulators. Immense amounts of time, money, and energy went into efforts by hospital executives to tweak the system to their own advantage. Deregulation changed that dynamic completely. After 1991, when a hospital got into trouble, it was on its own and had no one to blame but itself.

After 1991, I quickly realized that I did not miss the games and manipulations of the rate setting madness. In fact, it was a great relief. Its absence allowed me to focus more on my issue of greatest concern: access for the uninsured and underinsured. In promoting deregulation, Governor Weld and his allies suggested that the measure would lead to lower numbers of uninsured as the market worked to lower health care costs. I knew this claim was laughable, but no one ever took it seriously enough to make a retort worth the effort—and besides, how could one disprove it ahead of time? In fact, year after year in the early 1990s, the numbers of uninsured in Massachusetts swelled dramatically. Economic improvement did not at all abate their growing numbers.

For several years after deregulation's enactment, I continued working with my Health Care for All allies to promote the Family Health Plan, our single-payer proposal. We saw the November 1991 vote as a benchmark and expected to see improvements in our level of support year after year as the worst aspects of deregulation and a competitive market became apparent. For the 1992 legislative session, we worked hard to gather sponsors and actually convinced about sixty-five senators and representatives to sign onto the bill. But in truth, most of them did not understand the nature and intricacies of the plan, and we never succeeded in gaining sufficient support to bring it up for a vote in the Health Care Committee, which politely killed the measure year after year by placing it in a "study," a convenient term for the legislative graveyard.

In 1993 and 1994, most discussion of state-based health care reform came to a halt while the nation debated the merits of President Clinton's Health Security Plan. The president's proposal was an elaborate scheme based on an untested model called *managed competition* that sought a balance between universal coverage and managed care, using both public regulatory pressures and private markets. In truth, it was close to the concepts and structures that formed the Family Health Plan. But the mind-bending complexity of the president's plan enabled its insurance and small business opponents to instill fear in the minds of enough Americans to guarantee its demise in September 1994 without a vote in either the U.S. Senate or the U.S. House of Representatives.

Many of the proponents of a national single-payer plan derided the Clinton plan as a sellout and suggested that had the president pushed a more courageous single-payer proposal, he would have catalyzed a wave of political support that would have dwarfed opposition and forced approval from both houses of Congress—in other words, that single payer was the missed political opportunity of 1993–94. Indeed, about 100 members of the U.S. House, led by Washington Congressman James Mc-Dermott, a psychiatrist, actively promoted a single-payer plan during the entire reform period.

It was left to voters in California to demonstrate that single payer was not the missed opportunity of 1993 and 1994. Health care activists, displeased with the direction of Clinton-style reform, gathered sufficient signatures to place on the November 1994 California ballot an initiative proposal to establish a single-payer plan in their state. For their efforts, reformers were handed a staggering defeat by a margin of 73 to 27 percent, even less than the 33 percent of the public that usually indicates support for single payer in public opinion surveys. The plan's advocates were quick to point out that they were outspent by the insurance industry by $10 million to about $3 million in campaign spending, suggesting this imbalance accounted for the defeat.

But the initiative's opponents offered a different and revealing interpretation. The perspective of insurance industry leaders was that they did not begin to spend the amount of money to defeat the question they were prepared to commit had it been necessary. Republican political consultant and pollster William McInturff reported that his telephone poll takers had gauged support for the single-payer plan by reading the proponents' own description to prospective voters and found that support dropped precipitously with the addition of each successive sentence. In 1988, the California insurance industry spent more than $60 million in an unsuccessful effort to defeat a ballot initiative aimed at controlling auto insurance premiums. In 1994, in its leaders' view, the industry didn't break sweat in swatting down the single-payer health plan. In the process, California voters demonstrated conclusively that single payer was *not* the missed opportunity of 1994.

In 1995, I stopped filing the Family Health Plan bill in the Massachusetts legislature.

·   ·   ·

The deregulation of hospital rate setting in Massachusetts in 1991 is another demonstration that big changes do happen in American politics and policy. They happen when the existing framework in a policy venue no longer satisfies the needs of enough key decision makers and power sources. But change only happens when a replacement idea exists and is ready to take its place. The new idea does not have to be better in everyone's mind, but it does need to appear better to enough of those with the power and responsibility to act.

In the late 1980s and early 1990s, numerous reports and analyses showed how the growth in health system spending was out of control, dangerously threatening the national economy and other important societal needs. Some suggested that by 2000, health spending would consume nearly 20 percent of the gross domestic product, up from about 12 percent in 1990—if current trends continued. Analysts with more faith in markets suggested that the economy and society would not stand for this rate of growth. They were right, and the doom analysts were wrong. Had the results been reversed, the Family Health Plan—and other plans like it—might well be on their way to enactment and implementation in many states. As it stands now, single payer has vanished as a viable political option.

Managed care and the market are now dominant throughout the system. Their hold is thorough and tight. But the constant attacks on them from providers and consumers suggest—as was true during the heyday of government regulatory controls—that their hold is by no means secure. The punctuated equilibrium model shows us that they will remain in place, weakened or not, facing only incremental alterations, until an attractive and politically viable replacement idea emerges to challenge them.

You can't beat something with nothing.

CHAPTER SEVEN

Agendas and Children's Health Care

... chance favours only the prepared mind.
Louis Pasteur

It was a gorgeous spring day, with luxuriant blossoms dressing the trees that lined the Hooker entrance to the State House. Imperturbably guarding the entrance is the equestrian statue of Joseph Hooker, the Civil War general who briefly commanded the Army of the Potomac in 1863. It was my first year in the House, 1985, and I wasn't paying much attention to the surroundings, thinking instead of the hell-on-wheels week just past. It seemed I could do nothing right. Issues kept popping up that threw me off balance, and everyone in sight was angry or disappointed in me for one reason or another. As I stood on the steps, the legendary Senate President William Bulger happened to walk by, wearing his familiar grin suggesting nothing got him down. "Boy, this is tougher than I thought," I said in response to his polite, "How's it goin' kid?" "Listen," he said, lowering his voice, "you get so wrapped up in the day-to-day issues around here, and you think if you don't do things the way people want, they'll never speak to you again. And you're always wrong, because they always come back for more."

His words were comforting relief I remember to this day. Nonetheless, the odd, unpredictable, and chaotic way that issues popped up on the public's and the legislature's radar screens was puzzling and troubling to me. It seemed too random and out of control to be real, not just in Massachusetts but everywhere I looked. Some issues, such as welfare and immigration reform, suddenly reach the center stage of public attention, become incessant topics of controversy in governmental corridors, newspaper columns, and policy discussions, and then result in the enactment of new laws. Other issues, such as universal health care and comprehensive national tobacco control, may reach the public agenda, generate substantial attention, and then collapse before enactment or implementation of any new policy or law. Still other issues that may reflect major public problems, such as homelessness, can languish offstage for many years with no significant public concern.

Is this just random luck of the draw? While it often seems that way from afar, the appearance of randomness is an illusion. Throughout many layers of society, all the time, individuals and groups inside and outside of government are hard at work setting up their next opportunities to create change. Those who understand the dynamics of a process called agenda setting and who operate according to its principles have a valuable advantage over those who do not. There is, indeed, an element of luck involved in this process. But, as Pasteur suggests, luck most often happens to those who prepare for it.

This chapter describes the dynamics of agenda setting, relying on a model developed by John Kingdon. In explaining his model, I use President Bill Clinton's ill-fated national health reform plan of 1993–94 to illustrate how the framework can be used retrospectively to analyze a successful or unsuccessful legislative campaign. I then describe how I used Kingdon's model prospectively to plan and promote major health care access legislation in Massachusetts in 1996.

AGENDA SETTING

Kingdon developed a simple and elegant model in the early 1980s to explain the emergence and recession of issues from the policy agenda.[1] I have found this framework genuinely useful in real life and one that people can easily understand. Because politics is both science and art, no model can explain everything. Rather, good models work like helpful tools—a hammer, a saw, a screwdriver—that can be used by most of us to perform a necessary job. Of course, there is always more to a successful job, such as the skill of the craftsperson, the quality of the materials. But the tools can also help a lot.

Kingdon's model was adapted from organizational theory that describes decision making in firms, whether for profit or not, governmental or nongovernmental. The model's basic premise is that leaders and managers in organizations and in politics are at the receiving end of a constant stream of disconnected, random, and chaotic information and

Open Window of Opportunity

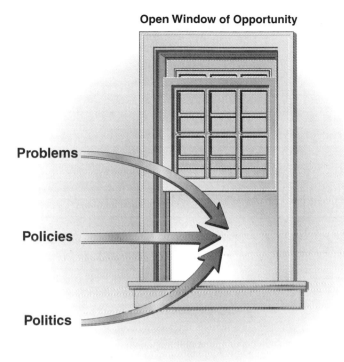

Problems

Policies

Politics

The Agenda Setting Model

feedback, flowing together in a form that makes little sense on its own. Creating some degree of order from all this varied input, finding a path through it, and then crafting an agenda for action are the essential challenges facing leaders both in organizations and in politics.

According to Kingdon's model, change can only happen when a "window of opportunity" for that change opens up—no open window, no change. For the window to open, three streams or dynamic processes must be moving at roughly the same time. The first stream is the _problem_ stream, the sense among _those with the power to act_ that a legitimate problem exists that deserves to be addressed. No genuine sense of a problem most often equals no action. Who are those with the power to act? That depends entirely on the forum in which the issue is being pursued. Changing a state insurance policy may require acceptance of legitimacy by the insurance commissioner and his or her appointing authority. Changing a university policy may require belief in the legitimacy of the issue by the president, the dean, and the board of trustees. If the issue requires action in a legislative body, then key legislative leaders and committee chairs are the ones who must recognize the legitimacy of the problem. Change in the regulatory structure governing managed care was a major issue in the Massachusetts legislature in 1997 and 1998 (as in many other states), with many bills and lots of interested organizations involved in the fray. Ultimately, nothing happened, largely because the Speaker of the House, in his gut, did not believe that the dispute represented a genuine problem and thus used his power to delay any consideration until very late in the session. In this example, the political and policy streams were moving well, while the problem stream was halted by a critical person with the power to act.

The second stream is the *political* stream, the sense among those with the power to act that the timing for action is right in relation to public sentiment and consistency with other policy objectives. This stream combines the mood of the electorate, election results (who has been put into positions of power), the process by which groups are mobilized, and more. Promoting a major public spending proposal during a recession when budgets are being cut and pushing a major antiabortion bill in a state with high levels of pro-choice support are two examples where there may be an implementable policy and even officials who strongly support it. But progress will be held back by the political stream.

The third stream is the *policy* stream, the existence of an implementable policy that fits the scope of the problem, is understandable to those who need to understand it, and can attain sufficient support. At all times, so-called *policy networks* in every conceivable area and microarea of public policy are at work developing, refining, and promoting policy ideas and proposals. These networks are composed of government officials, academics, industry leaders, consultants, journalists, and more. They argue and test out ideas with each other, hungrily anticipating the moment when a problem will emerge to which their favored solution or policy can be applied. Indeed, policy solutions often precede the emergence of problems; effective *policy entrepreneurs* work hard to spot emerging problems to which their new policy ideas can be applied.

When all three streams are flowing at a sufficient pace, the window of opportunity opens, creating the possibility for substantive policy change. Implicit in the model are several important caveats. First, having only one or two of the three streams in motion is usually insufficient, particularly on matters that generate substantial controversy and attention. Retrospective analyses of failed attempts to change policy can usually reveal deficiencies in one or more of the streams. Second, just as surely as windows of opportunity open, they close, making it important for advocates to move before an opening vanishes. Timing is not everything, but often it will be pretty close. Third, all window openings are not the same size. A policy proposal can easily be of a scale too large to fit through the size of the open window, either because the policy addresses far more than the perceived problem or because political limitations cannot permit a solution of the scale proposed.

President Bill Clinton's ill-fated national health reform proposal in 1993 and 1994 is a strong example of how Kingdon's model can be used retrospectively to analyze a failed policy initiative.[2] At the time of Clinton's presidential inauguration in January 1993, the problem stream was moving with terrific force. Throughout the 1980s, analysts in numerous health policy networks had demonstrated that out-of-control health spending and rapidly increasing numbers of uninsured Americans were symptoms of a growing systemic crisis. Throughout the decade, the cost of health insurance, public and private, rose at a rate far greater than general inflation or the growth of the overall economy. Health spending rose from less than 10 percent of the gross national product in 1980 to more than 14 percent in the early 1990s, with projections that spending would rise as high as 20 percent by the year 2000 if trends continued (the rate stabilized around 14 percent through the middle and later 1990s). Business and labor leaders, consumer groups, state and federal lawmakers, and media voices concurred that health spending was out of control with no end in sight. During this same period, the numbers of Americans with no health insurance coverage at all began to increase by about a million persons per year, from twenty-five million uninsured in 1980 to more than thirty-eight million by 1993 (and forty-four million by 1999). As both sets of numbers worsened, health policy researchers began paying closer attention to various dimensions of the problem, media began publishing stories describing the human aspects, and state and federal commissions, such as the Pepper Commission chaired by U.S. Senator Jay Rockefeller, further documented the problems and the needs.

Kingdon points out that there are many unfortunate conditions in life that are not recognized as public policy problems. "Conditions become defined as problems when we come to believe that we should do something about them," he observes.[3] By the end of 1992 no credible voice anywhere in the nation doubted the existence of a serious problem in our nation's health system.

Policymakers' sense that the political stream was moving adequately to justify action had evolved over several years. In 1988, Democratic pres-

idential candidate and Massachusetts Governor Michael Dukakis used
health care concerns as a central policy plank in his national campaign.
He had established his credentials on the issue with the signing of a so-
called universal health care law in his own state in April of that year, a
law that included a mandate for most employers to cover their workers
and that was scheduled for implementation in 1992. While the Dukakis
campaign floundered badly in the late summer and early fall in the face
of an aggressive and negative campaign by then Vice President George
Bush, it was widely agreed in campaign postmortems that the health issue had given Dukakis a late campaign lift, though not enough to overcome other weaknesses. The health care issue would increase in prominence in future presidential campaigns, several analysts wrote, though
probably not until 1996.

The event that changed policymakers' perceptions about the political
stream occurred in Pennsylvania in November 1991. Republican U.S. Senator John Heinz had been killed in an air crash in April of that year.
Richard Thornburgh, the sitting U.S. attorney general at the time, resigned his cabinet position to run for Heinz's seat and began the campaign more than forty points ahead of his little-known rival, Democrat
Harris Wofford, who had been appointed to the seat until a special election could be held. While Thornburgh publicly dismissed the notion that
the health system was in crisis, Wofford made health reform his major
issue, running television ads proclaiming, "If criminals have the right to
a lawyer, I think working Americans should have the right to a doctor."
When Wofford won the nationally watched contest, political observers
widely agreed that health care was the issue that turned the election in
his favor, even though his reform prescription was thoroughly undefined.

Democratic presidential candidate Bill Clinton made health cost control and access expansion central parts of his campaign, though once
again in an undefined form embracing an untested, ambiguous concept
called *managed competition*. After his victory, health reform was viewed
as an electoral mandate issue, a point he emphasized repeatedly during
his transition, most prominently at an economic summit he hosted in
Little Rock, in December 1992. By inauguration day, 1993, with Democrats in control of the presidency and both houses of Congress, few
doubted that the political stream was moving strongly in the direction
of comprehensive, national health system reform.

But two streams are not enough to make change, especially big
change, happen. It was the third stream, the existence of an implementable and understandable policy, that created the nascent adminis-

tration's greatest challenge. Deborah Stone discusses how broad labels such as "liberty," "security," "efficiency," and "equity" can be used to mask gaping differences in real policy preferences. By January 1993, the time for discussion of broad and abstract concepts—managed competition, health care reform, universal coverage—had passed. Instead, it was time to talk turkey.

Kingdon's model suggests that early 1993 was the time to take a policy off the shelf and move it through Congress while the problem and political streams were optimal. Instead, President Clinton appointed the much-maligned Health Care Task Force, headed by First Lady Hillary Rodham Clinton, that quickly ballooned to about 500 participants whose job was to figure out what his policy should be. It was not until late September 1993 that the president announced his Health Security Plan to Congress (not delivering an actual bill until late October), after deciding that the plan would follow consideration of his budget package, narrowly approved in August, and ratification of the North American Free Trade Agreement, approved later in the fall.

By the time Congress readied itself for serious deliberation, the size of the open window of opportunity was already narrowing. An improving economy reduced the public's sense of a health care crisis as many Americans regained health benefits when they found new jobs. Enemies of the president's plan in the insurance industry, small business, and the Republican Party took advantage of the delay to find a better footing for their opposition. In January 1994 the public heard a curious and remarkable open conversation over whether the U.S. health system was experiencing a "crisis" (a position espoused by Clinton plan backers) or a "problem" (a position promoted with increasing confidence by Clinton plan opponents). While the crisis advocates won the short-term rhetorical battle, reciting citizen horror stories to the media in droves, opponents succeeded in driving home the point that more than 80 percent of Americans were satisfied with their own coverage, however they might feel about larger systemic issues. The problem stream's flow was beginning to diminish.

The force of the political stream faced a similar depletion. While in January 1993, the U.S. Chamber of Commerce and other national business groups had publicly supported a national employer mandate, by early 1994 other small business voices had organized to force the chamber to reverse its position and to oppose any mandates. The combined weight of the small business community and the commercial health insurance industry, represented by the Health Insurance Association of America

(HIAA), had alternately emboldened and frightened members of Congress to oppose or remain neutral to the president's plan. The sheer complexity and breadth of the plan left many confused and open to negative impressions about its potential impact. Even Clinton's secretary of labor, Robert Reich, who traveled across the nation to speak for the plan, confessed in his memoir, *Locked in the Cabinet,* that he didn't really understand it:

> The health plan plays into its opponents' hands. It's unwieldy. I still don't understand it. I've been to dozens of meetings, defended it on countless radio and TV programs, debated its merits publicly and privately, but I still don't comprehend the whole. In the public arena, nothing is more vulnerable to organized opposition than a huge and complex idea.[4]

The Kingdon model helps to explain the nature of the Health Plan fiasco. An extraordinary opportunity in terms of public recognition of a problem, and political momentum for significant change, was lost because of the failure to develop a coherent, understandable policy and to move it in a timely way. Success with only two of the three streams is not enough to create major public policy change. Missing the moment by not moving forward when the time was most auspicious in January 1993 was a grave mistake. Overestimating the size of the open window of opportunity by proposing a policy change that went far beyond the public's sense of the problem was the other.

Hindsight, of course, is much easier than looking ahead. Like many state health policy leaders in 1993, I supported and worked for passage of the Clinton plan and would have been happy to see a plan that went even further. Understanding the nature of that failure by using the Kingdon model helps us to imagine how the result could have been different. Kingdon's model suggests a successful outcome would have required a less comprehensive plan that would not have nurtured the opposition coalition that formed. For example, had the president moved forward in January 1993 either with a straightforward plan to establish a national employer mandate to require most employers to cover their workers or with a national program to cover all uninsured children, he might have achieved a substantial victory that would have placed the nation's health system in a very different position in the late 1990s. In early 1993, many major business groups were on record in support of an employer mandate. Others groups such as the insurance industry's HIAA that were so highly effective in their opposition to the president's plan also supported an employer mandate and would not have moved forward with their highly publicized and effective "Harry and Louise" television ads against such a requirement absent the other controversial elements of his proposal.

Perhaps this alternative scenario also would have been unsuccessful. I don't think so, but that's actually beside my point, which is to illustrate the usefulness of this model in analyzing highly charged public policy battles. The Clinton Health Security Plan fiasco was, above all, a failure to devise a policy that fit the public perception of the problem and the existing political opportunity. The use of the Kingdon model does just what one would hope: it enables users to see critical facets of a situation that would not be as apparent without applying the framework.

One final aspect of the Kingdon model is helpful to understand. There is a tendency in politics to play the "blame game" when something goes wrong, to point fingers in any direction except at ourselves. Thus, the common reaction of Clinton plan supporters is that the 1993–94 failure was the result of insurance industry–small business–Republican Party opposition. But nothing done by this trio should have been at all surprising. When a legislative proposal seeks to put a substantial professional group out of business (as the Clinton plan would have done to many commercial insurers and insurance agents), it should not be surprising that these forces will fight like hell against the plan. Engaging in critical self-examination in the face of policy failure is a painful experience but also an empowering one. It suggests that the power to make change happen lies significantly within and begins with understanding the true nature of an open window of opportunity.

All this discussion, however, is used retrospectively to analyze a past event. In 1995 and 1996, I had an opportunity to use the Kingdon model in a prospective fashion: to plan and execute a campaign for major health care access reform in Massachusetts. The following case story shows how it happened.

HEALTH CARE ACCESS REFORM, 1995–96

It was the morning of Wednesday, April 3, 1996, as I walked up the marble State House staircase to the Senate Reading Room (where little if any reading ever occurs). I recalled the words of Nick Littlefield, longtime trusted aide to Senator Edward Kennedy, who had told me a few months before, "Nothing big ever happens without someone who gets just passionately crazy about it, and who keeps at it no matter what happens until it gets done." In this situation, that seemed to describe me, the crazy. The main question, though, was whether this exercise would result in tangible accomplishment or simply be one more round of frustration and deadlock.

I was anxious as I walked into the Senate Reading Room, located across an elegantly carpeted corridor from the chamber of the State Senate on the third floor of the State House. Senators use the Reading Room for off-the-record chats and meetings with important guests who are invariably impressed with its ornate ceiling, thick rugs, and high plush curtains. Surrounding the room are imposing portraits of former leaders of the body, including U.S. President Calvin Coolidge who presided over the State Senate during the First World War, Horace Mann, known as the father of American public education, and Kevin Harrington, a dominating six-foot-six leader from the 1970s whose long and imposing cigar is only one of his portrait's distinguishing features.

Large meetings in the Reading Room are rare, and only for those with solid connections. No one doubted that this meeting of fifty or so members of the Success By 6 Coalition met the test. Organized in 1994 by Marian Heard, the dynamic and engaging president of the United Way of Massachusetts Bay, Success By 6 was a coalition of Greater Boston's most powerful and influential business and civic leaders to promote public policy change on behalf of kids up to age six, especially in health care and early education. Members included Chad Gifford, head of the Bank of Boston, Paul O'Brien, former chief of the telephone giant NYNEX, Leo Breitman, the boss of Fleet Bank, Paul LaCamera, the president of Channel Five, and Carol Goldberg of the Stop & Shop grocery store chain. Thrown in for good measure were people like Hubie Jones, former dean of the Boston University School of Social Work, and Dr. Barry Zuckerman, head of pediatrics at Boston Medical Center. Marian displayed extraordinary savvy in leading the group, especially in hiring a skilled political organizer, Margaret Blood, as the group's director. Margaret knew the State House cold and as head of the legislature's Children's Caucus had worked with Representative Carmen Buell in 1991 to establish a small health program for uninsured children.

My study of thirty years of health policymaking in Massachusetts had convinced me of one critical fact: no major health care financing initiative had ever won State House approval without some significant and visible business support. On that April 3 morning, I had none and there were fewer than four months remaining in the legislative session that would end on July 31 to get a bill through both branches and to the governor's desk. My strenuous efforts in 1995 and 1996 to find a meaningful alternative to the health care employer mandate signed into law by Governor Michael Dukakis in 1988 but never implemented had been woefully unsuccessful. The 1988 universal health care mandate was scheduled to take effect on August 1, 1996, but unless I could broker an alternative plan, the legislature had promised to simply repeal the statute and put nothing else in its place. The week before, I had succeeded in getting a controversial access bill voted favorably by the Joint Health Care Committee, which I cochaired, but only by the narrowest of margins, with several members reserving their rights as a favor to me. The broad array of Massachusetts business groups that focused on health issues made clear their opposition to my plan. The prospects of that bill making it through the process and then surviving a certain veto from Governor William Weld were nil. At the same time, the only bill that the governor would sign was unacceptable to me and to other key groups. Success By 6 seemed the most likely business group to win over, but they hated any kind of employer mandate, opposed new taxes, badly wanted to avoid any kind of public confrontation with the governor, whom they personally regarded as their pal and a good guy, and were principally interested in covering kids through age six, not up to eighteen as my plan proposed.

It was time to make a deal. . . .

THE MANDATE

Path dependent is a term that describes the real nature of policymaking. It means that potential actions have to be related in some logical way to whatever has gone before. There may be many potential paths to address any given policy problem, but the list of viable alternatives is sharply narrowed by what has come before. If I am driving down Route 2, I can't just wish myself onto the Massachusetts Turnpike. I have to take myself there, exit by exit, road by road. The health policy debate that came to a head in 1996 in Massachusetts represented the convergence of two paths. The first path involved the 1988 universal health care employer mandate. The other involved the Weld administration's 1994 request for a so-called Medicaid 1115 waiver from the federal government.

In 1988, by extremely narrow margins, the Massachusetts House and Senate approved what was called a "universal health care law" by the public and "Chapter 23" by the health care cognoscenti, referring to its designation as the twenty-third statute signed into law that year. Governor Michael Dukakis, then running for U.S. president, trumpeted the new law as a model for the nation in an elaborate signing ceremony in front of the State House replete with colored balloons, a music band, and banners. While the Dukakis presidential campaign helped to convince a reluctant House of Representatives (I and only a few other reps were enthusiastic backers) to enact the mandate, support in the State Senate was more solid because of determined advocacy on the part of the powerful chair of the Senate Committee on Ways and Means, Patricia McGovern. While Chapter 23 had many complex provisions, the most controversial required all employers with more than six employees either to provide family health coverage for their workers, with employers paying at least 80 percent of the cost, or to pay a $1,680 per worker annual tax to the Commonwealth that the state would then use to finance coverage for the worker and family. In an unsuccessful attempt to mollify small business groups that opposed the mandate, implementation was held off until January 1, 1992.

Two important developments occurred in the four years between 1988 and 1992. First, the Commonwealth plunged into its worst economic recession since the 1930s, with major layoffs, business closings, and financial distress for most public and private employers. This recession greatly exacerbated concerns about the mandate's potential impact on small business. Second, in January 1991 Democratic Governor Dukakis, who was firmly committed to implementation of the employer mandate, was replaced by Republican William Weld, who was as adamantly committed to repealing the requirement and quickly filed legislation to achieve that objective. Weld's key health adviser, Charles Baker, publicly talked of how much he "hated" the mandate and said he would resign his job rather than implement the requirement.

In 1991, the political situation within the Senate and House had also changed. The 1990 election that elevated Weld to the corner office also increased the number of Republicans in the forty-member Senate from eight to sixteen, more than enough to sustain gubernatorial vetoes and—combined with conservative, antimandate Democrats—more than sufficient to repeal most of Chapter 23. McGovern personally warned me in a late-1990 telephone call that "it's up to the House now to keep the employer mandate alive. I can't protect it over here any more."

On the House side, the sentiment of members was clear. If the choice was between implementing or repealing the mandate, repeal would pass overwhelmingly; but if the choice was to repeal or delay implementation, delay had a shot. The new Speaker, Charles Flaherty, was criticized by many progressives and the *Boston Globe* during 1991 for being overly solicitous of the new governor, but he was determined not to lose the opportunity for health reform presented by the mandate. He concurred with the recommendation by his new Health Care Committee chair, Carmen Buell, and me to move legislation to delay the effective date of the mandate from January 1992 to January 1995. Recognizing that the House would not send him legislation repealing the mandate, Weld signed the delay into law. Not coincidentally, 1995 was beyond Weld's current term of office, signaling our hope that a new governor after Weld would view the mandate differently.

But Weld coasted to a massive reelection margin in November 1994, trouncing his Democratic opponent, Mark Roosevelt, who made no campaign issue of health care or the employer mandate. Prospects for ever implementing the 1988 mandate in the wake of President Clinton's own health reform fiasco—which included a national employer mandate—were nil. Carmen Buell and I, however, were determined not to see the mandate repealed without winning some significant health care access expansion as the price for repeal. Again we prevailed upon Flaherty to postpone the mandate's implementation date for one additional year until January 1996 to give us time to work on an alternative health care access plan with the Weld administration. For a second time, in late 1994, the legislature agreed to postpone the mandate's implementation and Weld signed the delay.

By late 1995, Carmen Buell had resigned her seat in the legislature to move to North Carolina where her husband had been named head of the state university, and I had succeeded her as the House chairman of the Joint Committee on Health Care. We had made some progress with the Weld administration in agreeing to a health care reform package but still had a long way to go. Reluctantly, I successfully pleaded with my colleagues for one, final ("I promise!") delay of the mandate, from January 1, 1996, to August 1, 1996, and committed on the floor of the House that if we could not find an acceptable, alternative plan by then, I would personally bring to the floor and support a simple repeal bill. Though I did not know in late 1995 what that final alternative package would include, the selection of August 1 as the drop-dead date was to ensure that sometime before the end of our session on July 31, 1996, the House and Senate would be compelled to address health reform, one way or another. We purposefully put a gun to our own heads.

THE WAIVER

For a laid-back person, Bill Weld is one ambitious guy. Harvard under-grad, Harvard law, Rhodes scholar, with family roots tracing back to the *Mayflower,* the tall, red-haired, red-faced governor had become im-mensely popular with the Commonwealth's voters. He mixed a hard-edged libertarian message of no-new-taxes, pro–death penalty, and tough on welfare recipients with progressive stances in favor of abortion and gay rights, all the while maintaining a goofy, self-effacing personal style that included proposing that all the state's flags be lowered to half-mast in recognition of the death of Grateful Dead guitarist Jerry Garcia. Since the 1950s, Republican voter strength in Massachusetts had been in steady and heavy decline, requiring Weld to stitch together a base that included heavy doses of independent and Democratic voters. Part of his strategy to win the governor's office in 1990 included convincing mod-erate-to-liberal Republican State Senator Paul Cellucci to abandon his own gubernatorial ambitions and to run for lieutenant governor on a ticket with Weld. In gratitude for this gracious move, Weld wanted to do everything possible to get out of the way to give Cellucci a clear path to the corner office by 1998.

In 1993, Weld and his key lieutenants had two related ideas. The first was that Weld might be a viable contender for the Republican presiden-tial nomination in 1996 to challenge incumbent Bill Clinton. Failing that, there would be a potential challenge to U.S. Senator John Kerry, the state's second-term junior senator. The second idea was that in order to appear viable, Weld needed his own plan to address the key national issue of the year, health care access. This was the period when the Clinton health plan was still considered viable and many thought some form of national health reform was inevitable. Weld knew he possessed the talent to cre-ate his own plan.

Within his administration, Weld had two key players eager to meet his need. Charles Baker was a hard-driving supply-sider, the son of a high-ranking health official in the Reagan administration, and the former chief of a right-tilting Massachusetts think tank, the Pioneer Institute. As Weld's assistant secretary of health and human services, Baker was a blunt-speaking, conservative thinker who loved health policy and who led the charge in 1991 to close state hospitals and to dismantle a hospi-tal regulatory system in favor of market-driven health care. In his office was a photo of Bill Weld, personally autographed to Baker as "the soul of the Weld Administration." In 1993, he became Weld's second secretary of health and human services, and would move in 1995 to become Weld's third secretary of administration and finance, a position often called "the deputy governor."

Close to Baker was Bruce Bullen, the low-key but intense commissioner of medical assistance, who ran the state's behemoth Medicaid program, labeled the leading "budget buster" during the heated recession days when the program's costs were rising by more than 20 percent while the overall state budget was hemorrhaging red ink. Despite working for a Republican administration, Bullen came from a Democratic background, having served as budget director to Patricia McGovern at Senate Ways and Means and later moving to Medicaid during the final years of the Dukakis administration in 1989. Baker had admired Bullen's work and kept him on to lead the transformation of the Medicaid program from a passive payer of provider bills to an aggressive health purchaser. Bullen had watched as the state of Tennessee implemented in 1993 an ambitious "TennCare" program that used savings from the implementation of Medicaid managed care to expand coverage to large numbers of uninsured persons. He and Baker thought Massachusetts could do the same thing, and do it better.

In the spring of 1994, the Weld administration filed a request with the federal Health Care Financing Administration (HCFA) for a so-called Section 1115 waiver to permit the state to redesign its Medicaid program in experimental ways. The federal government, through HCFA, pays between 50 and 80 percent of Medicaid expenses in states (50 percent in Massachusetts) and requires conformance to numerous standards related to benefit design, service delivery, and more. States can deviate from these standards only by obtaining at least one of several waivers from the administering agency, HCFA, which runs Medicaid and Medicare within the U.S. Department of Health and Human Services. While the 1115 waiver option provides states with the greatest amount of flexibility to expand access to otherwise ineligible persons, it also includes a "revenue neutrality" requirement so that the federal government will not pay more than it would in the absence of the waiver. From the state's perspective, meeting all the requirements and answering all the questions to obtain the 1115 waiver are major challenges. Governors often complained about the lengthy and burdensome process but sought waivers as the only way to experiment with the program while retaining cherished federal dollars.

The Weld administration 1115 waiver proposal as crafted by Baker and Bullen included several complex and related parts.

First, eligibility for Medicaid coverage would be expanded to all families whose incomes were below 133 percent of the federal poverty line (about $20,000 for a family of four) instead of the traditional standard where coverage was only provided to some poor people, those who fit into specific categories such as Aid to Families with Dependent Children (AFDC) or Supplemental Security Income (SSI).

Second, a new program of tax credits to employers and subsidies to low-wage workers would be provided when the worker had a family income below 200 percent of the federal poverty level (about $32,000 for a family of four) and the employer provided health insurance paying at least half the cost. The employer would get a $400 per year tax credit for providing individual coverage, $800 for spousal coverage, and $1,000 for family coverage. The worker subsidy would be greater, scaled according to income. The administration labeled this proposal the Insurance Reimbursement Program (IRP).

Third, and most controversial, principal funding for the IRP would be obtained by diverting more than $200 million from the state's Uncompensated Care Pool, a $315 million program created in 1985 to assist hospitals in paying the cost of caring for persons in need of hospital services who had no health insurance. From the hospitals' perspective, this was *their* money and it was already insufficient to cover their growing charity care costs.

Fourth, the administration urged the legislature to reform the so-called nongroup insurance market that exists for individuals who cannot obtain group coverage through employers. This coverage is too expensive for most uninsured persons to afford, and many were excluded from useful coverage because of restrictions on persons with preexisting conditions, experience rating, and a variety of other requirements.

Fifth, the administration proposed to the legislature the creation of a state tax break for so-called medical savings accounts that permit individuals to set aside funds in tax-deferred accounts to use for their own medical costs. The concept was highly popular in Republican circles as a means to encourage health consumers to spend money on health needs more prudently and unpopular with Democrats because of the feared and expected negative effect on remaining insured populations.

Sixth, the administration proposed to repeal the 1988 employer mandate.

The first two items required specific approval from HCFA because of the intended use of federal dollars to finance the reforms. The latter four required no federal action but would be part of a legislative package submitted to the House and Senate to implement the waiver once needed federal approvals were obtained.

There are two ways for a governor to win the necessary approvals to implement a Medicaid waiver. One is to get agreement and approval from the legislature first and then seek federal approval. The risk is that HCFA may require modifications requiring another round of legislative approval, something most governors prefer to avoid. The second route is to obtain federal permission and then seek ratification of the arrangement from the state legislature. The risk here is that the legislature may not agree with the structure of the waiver as negotiated by the administration, requiring further approvals from the feds. Governor Weld and Lieutenant Governor Cellucci decided to follow the second route, filing their plan for an 1115 waiver with HCFA with fanfare in April 1994. "Universal coverage without an employer mandate" was their tagline, claiming that more than 400,000 of the Commonwealth's 500,000 uninsured residents would be covered if the plan were fully implemented.

Later detailed examination of the administration's claims would reveal that at most 150,000 of 700,000 uninsured would be covered, and only if *everything* went precisely according to plan. No one publicly challenged the administration's estimates at the time, thus allowing Weld to boast that he had found the route to universal health care without the harsh medicine of an employer mandate. Aside from exaggerated estimates, the Weld plan had several other looming problems, chief among them opposition from the hospital industry at the prospect of more than $200 million being diverted from the uncompensated care pool to finance the IRP tax credits and subsidies at a time when hospitals were feeling financially pressed by growing competition and growing numbers of uninsured patients.

By the end of 1994, Governor Weld had been reelected with a historic margin, the drive for national health reform had ended in ignominious defeat, the 1115 waiver was still pending before HCFA, and the Dukakis employer mandate was scheduled to become effective in January. The legislation approved at the end of 1994 to delay implementation of the mandate until January 1996 anticipated that the waiver would be approved in some form by federal officials and thus directed the governor to establish a special commission to review the waiver and to report to the legislature its recommendations for implementation. The expectation was that this work could be completed by the end of 1995, permitting a final resolution to the fate of the mandate.

On December 24, 1994, the Weld administration suspended any further admissions into a small state program called the Children's Medical Security Plan that had been set up in 1991 through the advocacy of Representative Carmen Buell, Margaret Blood, and others to provide a basic package of primary and preventive care services to uninsured children. Budget limits kept most kids out of the program, but advocates had been informing more and more parents of the option and were outraged and mobilized by the freeze. Two days after the freeze, a Children's Health Coalition formed, made up of the advocacy group Health Care for All, the Massachusetts Medical Society, the Massachusetts Academy of Pediatrics, and the Massachusetts Teachers Association. It was an unusual coalition, and MTA President Bob Murphy declared at its start, "Our goal is that no child in Massachusetts will go without needed health care."

In late April 1995, the federal government approved the Weld administration's 1115 waiver request, with some modifications and pending review and approval by the state legislature. Only a handful of the 200 senators and representatives had any sense at all of what the administration's plans contained. To decide the next move, eyes turned toward the newly formed special commission.

THE COMMISSION

Legislatures like to create special commissions to examine complex and controversial problems. Legislators tend to be generalists: even the most expert lawmakers are usually not as up-to-date as outside experts and constituency leaders. When outsiders can be brought together in a way that leads to consensus, the route to legislative approval can be considerably smoothed. One key challenge is composition. Stacking a commission with people who agree with the appointing authority's point of view gets the report he or she may prefer, but it then enjoys less credibility; constructing a diverse and conflicting membership may lead to no recommendations at all, setting back the process considerably.

Despite their regular use, special commissions in Massachusetts on complex health matters had generally followed the second pattern and had been uniformly unsuccessful. Special commissions in 1981, 1987, and 1990 all failed to reach agreement on reforming critical elements of the Commonwealth's health care financing laws. Health care providers and insurers simply had too much at stake to make their deals at the commission stage, which preceded normal legislative considerations. Final deals usually were cut much later in quieter rooms where the brokers were Ways and Means chairs, House Speakers, or Senate Presidents.

Carmen Buell, the House chair of the Health Care Committee, was the point person for health care reform in 1994 and 1995. Smart, progressive, and politically savvy, she entered the House in the same class as I did in 1985 and beat me in a competition for Health Care chair in January 1991. Flaherty named me House chair of the Joint Committee on Insurance in January 1995, giving me a stronger role in health policy discussions. Buell and I shared a strong commitment to finding a way to expand access to growing numbers of uninsured. Buell was Speaker Charlie Flaherty's key leader on this issue, and I worked with and supported her.

Buell and the Senate Health chair, Marc Pacheco, agreed on a plan for the composition of the commission that was included in its enabling legislation: three senators and four representatives (one Republican from each branch); Weld's secretary of health and human services (this would be a new player, Gerald Whitburn, brought in from Wisconsin by the Weld administration because of his reputation for aggressive welfare restructuring—he readily admitted to knowing little about health care); Weld's commissioner of insurance; and "six members appointed by the governor, two [of whom] shall be consumers representing diverse cultural backgrounds and geographic regions, three [of whom] shall be members of the business community who represent different size employers and geographic regions, and one [of whom] shall be nominated by the Massachusetts AFL-CIO." To Buell's calculation, the five Democratic legislators and two consumer reps and one labor union rep would give our side eight votes, with Whitburn, Weld's insurance commissioner, two Republican legislators, and the three business seats giving their side seven votes—if it came down to a voting, instead of a consensus, situation.

Though establishment of the commission was authorized in January 1995, Governor Weld waited until May 1995—after HCFA gave its initial approval of the 1115 waiver—to make his appointments, giving the commission little more than four months to complete the review by its September 30 legislatively mandated deadline. Rather than appoint a mix of two consumer and three business representatives, Weld appointed five business group leaders, two men and three women, all white, to the panel. This move gave Weld's allies a nine-to-six voting majority for their positions. Buell and Pacheco, who became the commission cochairs, seeking to move the commission forward as rapidly as possible to meet a tight deadline, decided not to contest the governor's clear violation of legislative intent regarding the composition of the nongovernmental appointees. The governor's appointees liked to refer to the panel as the "Blue Ribbon Commission." I loathed the term and refused to use it. It made me feel like a judge of the prize pig contest at the State Fair. The official and statutory title of the panel was a "special commission established for the purpose of making an investigation and study of methods for achieving universal health coverage for residents of the commonwealth."

Shortly after the start of the commission's work, Buell announced that she would be resigning from her legislative seat in July to move to North Carolina with her husband, Michael Hooker, who had just been named head of the University of North Carolina at Chapel Hill. With her departure, House Speaker Flaherty moved me from chairmanship of the Insurance Committee to the Health Care Committee, and the Special Commission members chose me to assume Buell's cochairmanship of that group as well. Prior to Buell's departure, I had deferred to her lead, having my own load of issues (nongroup health insurance market reform, homeowner insurance redlining discrimination, long-term care insurance reform) to carry as chairman of the Insurance Committee. Now, finally, in July 1995, ten and a half years after entering the House, working with my Senate chair, Marc Pacheco, I was in charge.

In discussions with Weld's point person on the commission, Secretary Whitburn, it became clear that the governor was in no mood to make any significant concessions on health reform. The political climate in the summer and fall of 1995 was markedly different from the atmosphere prevailing in the heady health reform days of 1993 and 1994. With Newt Gingrich as the new Speaker of the U.S. House of Representatives and triumphant Republican majorities in both houses of Congress looking confidently to revolutionize the Medicaid program—seeking to create block grants to give near–carte blanche authority to states to run the programs as we saw fit—the relevance of the 1115 waiver seemed questionable. According to Whitburn, the governor would consider no compromise on repeal of the employer mandate, no new state revenues to finance additional health expansions, and no major changes to his plan. In fact, it was apparent that Weld didn't care very much whether we moved on the waiver at all. Since late 1994, he had aggressively pursued a tough-on-crime, no-new-taxes, and tough-on-welfare-recipients agenda. Health care was off the list. Take it or leave it was the message. It was also clear that Whitburn commanded a majority on the commission, nine for him and six for us.

In the process of the commission's work during the summer, the governor's appointees emphasized their enthusiastic support for their sponsor's plans, especially for the tax credits and subsidies to businesses that insured workers with family incomes below 200 percent of poverty (the so-called IRP), repeal of the employer mandate, individual market insurance reform, and creation of medical savings accounts. It became increasingly apparent to those of us not with the governor that many of the numbers behind his plan were cooked. Most important in this regard was the IRP portion of the plan that would provide tax credits to eligible employers and employees, including employers who were already covering their workers. It was obvious to us that most firms currently providing health benefits would claim the credit, but what percent of firms not offering coverage would start doing so because of the IRP? This was crucial in order to judge how effective the approach would be. The administration's confidently stated answer was "70 percent." I was suspicious, knowing that similar tax credits in other states attracted no more than 15 percent of eligible employers. I kept asking them, "Where did you get 70 percent?" When they realized that I wouldn't stop asking, one of the administration's operatives told me privately, "It was a guess."

In September, after a series of public hearings, meetings and working groups, Pacheco and I decided to euthanize the commission as quickly and quietly as possible. The next stage after the commission would be at the legislature's Joint Committee on Health Care, which we solidly controlled. We permitted Whitburn to write most of the language that he wanted in the final report, and we included our dissenting opinions wherever we chose. The final report, which all members signed, included useful information on the background of the reform issues facing the Commonwealth but confirmed that the commission members had been unable to reach agreement on the most controversial and important matters. As Pacheco and I had intended, the issuing of the commission's final report was a nonevent.

When it suited our purposes, we would speak about the broad areas of agreement that commission members had found—but those areas were minuscule in comparison with the disagreements. Pacheco and I used that language of consensus to convince the House and Senate in November to postpone implementation of the employer mandate to August 1, 1996. We both committed publicly on the floors of our respective chambers that we would not ask for any more extensions after this. One way or another, we would resolve the issues behind the employer mandate and the waiver before the end of formal sessions on July 31, 1996. Now we just had to figure out what to do. . . .

THE STREAMS

It was September 1995, and everything seemed a mess. The employer mandate had minuscule support at best and nowhere to go. The administration's waiver plan was full of holes. The public clamor for health care reform was nowhere. Congress seemed on the verge of dismantling the basic structure of Medicaid as President Clinton began to move in the Republicans' direction. The Massachusetts House was experiencing growing tension as a federal criminal investigation of Speaker Charles Flaherty gathered steam with an incessant stream of newspaper leaks; meanwhile, Flaherty's majority leader, Richard Voke, and his Ways and Means chairman, Tom Finneran, had begun sub-rosa but intense and bitter campaigns to line up votes should the Speaker's chair become vacant. On the personal front, I had only eight months to write and complete my doctoral dissertation or else violate the terms of a federal grant I had received to help me write it.

In midsummer, shortly after becoming Health Care chair, I picked up my copy of John Kingdon's book *Agendas, Alternatives, and Public Policies*. I recalled the intuitive simplicity and elegance of the Kingdon model, the three streams and the window of opportunity that I recently learned in doctoral studies at the University of Michigan from John Tierney of Boston College. I thought, "What about trying to use this model to plan a campaign prospectively instead of just using it to analyze a political effort after the fact? Hey, do I have a better idea? What do I have to lose?" Without telling anyone, several times a month I would sit down and evaluate progress and plan next steps according to the three streams. . . .

Problems.   Kingdon's framework suggests that *those with the power to decide* must be convinced that a genuine and significant problem exists in order for this first stream to move. In 1995, the challenge was to convince not only key lawmakers but also the media and the public. Support for expansion of access to health care services seemed to have disappeared during the first year of the Republican revolution in Washington and in the aftermath of the Clinton health plan fiasco. Discussions concerning health care "reform" focused overwhelmingly on Republican plans to reduce substantially the rate of Medicare spending growth and to transform the Medicaid program into flexible block grants to states that also would lessen federal expenditures. In October of that year, I attended a joint National Governor's Association–National Conference of State Legislatures session in Washington, D.C., where speaker after speaker advised us to get ready for the brave, new, and inevitable world of Medicaid block grants.

At one session, my friend and then Michigan Medicaid director, Vern Smith, posed a vivid metaphor to describe our state of mind in anticipating block grants and the removal of federal regulatory authority. His son had taken up sky diving and recalled looking out the doorway of the flying plane, holding onto a bar above his head. He looked down at the earth below and froze. He looked up, closed his eyes, and then "just let go," enjoying a liberating and energizing experience. "And, friends, that's what we have to prepare ourselves to do," said Smith. "We have to have the confidence in ourselves to *just let go.*"

The time for comments came, and I couldn't resist. My days when I would flame out at the drop of a hat had passed but rushed back to me. "As we anticipate the brave new world of block grants and just letting go, I'd like to speak on behalf of all the folks out there without parachutes. I can recall coming to meetings like this in the 1980s when we would discuss how to meet the challenge to provide health coverage for all Americans. Today, we have millions more uninsured Americans and all we're talking about is how to cut back. We have a moral imperative to meet their needs." Scattered applause. More than a few scowls. A senator from Wyoming got up to say that all his people wanted was to get Washington off their backs. I thought of myself as Donald Sutherland in the remake of the movie *Invasion of the Body Snatchers.* Who *were* all these people? Would we ever be able to change the topic of conversation back to the uninsured?

One way to refocus attention on the problem was to develop evidence of its scope and to create awareness—according to Deborah Stone's approach—of a number. Back in 1988, our best estimates indicated that about 600,000 of six million Massachusetts residents lacked any health insurance. By 1990, because of access expansions in the 1988 universal health care law, data indicated that the number of uninsured had dropped to about 450,000. By 1994, Carmen Buell and I believed that the number had risen substantially to perhaps as high as 700,000 because of anecdotal reports from health care providers and growing demands on the hospital uncompensated care pool. Weld administration officials openly suggested their belief that the number had actually declined to between 200,000 to 300,000. Buell had the foresight to push for and win a budget appropriation directing the administration to contract for a professional research study to estimate the actual number of residents without coverage in 1995.

The Weld administration contracted with three respected health research professionals from the Harvard School of Public Health, Robert Blendon, Katherine Swartz, and Karen Donelan, who used the Lou Harris polling firm to conduct a telephone survey of Massachusetts households during late May 1995. The results indicated that the number of residents without coverage had risen from 455,000 in 1989 to 683,000 in 1995, while the number of uninsured children had risen from 90,000 to 160,000 during the same time frame. The researchers informally gave me the results in July. Because the researchers had a contract giving the administration control over release of the data, I held onto the results until Weld officials chose to release them.

Government and media relations specialists know there are good times and bad times to release information, depending on one's desire for extensive or limited media coverage. Weld administration officials waited until the second Friday in August, in the afternoon, to release the results of the Harvard study. The timing of the release ensured that coverage of the story would appear in the Saturday newspapers, the least-read edition of the week, during one of the least-noticed weekends of the year. Good news from the Weld administration gets announced in Room 157 in the State House, with its deep-blue carpet and sky-blue walls, prefabricated speaking platform and stage, and elevated back platform for the cameras. Good news, the kind of news the administration wanted to get out, would be announced by Bill Weld himself or at a minimum, his lieutenant governor, Paul Cellucci. On August 11, the news about the new number of uninsured in Massachusetts, a huge 50 percent increase, was announced by Weld's secretary of health and human services, Gerald Whitburn. The news was not announced in the State House but rather in Whitburn's office on the eleventh floor of the John McCormack State Office Building.

"At least our numbers are still below the national average," offered Whitburn in a vain attempt to find a silver lining in the report's clouds. The next day's story appeared on page 23 of the Saturday, August 12, *Boston Globe*. The Weld administration's efforts to keep the issue of the uninsured away from central public attention, to manage the public agenda by minimizing the public's sense of the problem, had seemed to succeed.

The Harvard team's contract with the Weld administration lasted until the end of September. Before then, they were contractually unable to speak out or testify on the results of their study without Whitburn's prior approval, and all comments and testimony had to be approved beforehand as well. Beginning on October 1, they would be free agents. On September 25, the Special Commission issued its final report and dissolved, unmourned except for the five business representatives who frequently asked Pacheco and me to file legislation to extend the panel's life. "That would be very difficult," I said. "We have a long way to go through the legislative process, and need to get moving." Privately, I thought, "in your dreams."

But the release of the commission's final report gave Pacheco and me a plausible rationale to call a public hearing of the Health Care Committee during October. Instead of placing the commission's report at the top of the hearing agenda, when the TV cameras and press paid the most attention, we asked Blendon, Schwartz, and Donelan to lay out the details of their findings on the growth in the Commonwealth's uninsured population. The rest of the hearing was uneventful. A decent amount of press coverage gave the numbers of uninsured the attention we had wanted. From that point onward, every speech, presentation, discussion, interview, article, comment from me included mention of two numbers: nearly 700,000 uninsured residents and 160,000 uninsured children. We distributed the commission report only to those who asked; we distributed the Blendon report everywhere.

Deborah Stone's work on discourse theory emphasizes that numbers are both tools and weapons in politics, never complete unto themselves, always used in a specific context with a political purpose in mind. I was clear about my purpose in using numbers: to nurture a sense that the problem of uninsurance was serious, unacceptable, growing, and in need of a significant public response by government. My tool of choice in the fall of 1995 was a number, 700,000. When Speaker Flaherty and I made our first public proposal in January 1996, Karen Van Kooy of my staff prepared a large poster board with the oversized figures "700,000 uninsured residents."

Later in 1996, when it became clear we would not be able to address the needs of the broader population of uninsured and instead chose to focus on uninsured children, we switched to talking exhaustively about "160,000 uninsured kids." In March, U.S. Senator John Kerry began a series of nine vitriolic and bitter debates with his formidable challenger,

Bill Weld. In every one of those debates, at some point, Kerry hurled "160,000 uninsured kids in Massachusetts" at Weld. Kerry's reference was not coincidental; a handful of influential Kerry backers and I worked aggressively beginning in December 1995 to convince Kerry to help us carry this issue into his U.S. Senate fight. By the time the debates actually occurred on the floor of the Massachusetts House of Representatives in June and on the floor of the Senate in early July, awareness of the number, 160,000, had spread widely across the state.

Creating awareness of the problem through recognition of a number was clearly insufficient to move major policy change through the legislature. But it was an essential prerequisite that placed our opponents in a defensive and awkward position, forcing them to preface each statement in opposition with some variant of the phrase, "I agree that we need to do something about the problem of so many uninsured kids, but . . ." Increasingly, the second clause of the sentence would be irrelevant.

Policies.   From the beginning of efforts to achieve universal health coverage, finding a meaningful, implementable, and politically viable policy had been the hardest challenge. While most people easily agree with the statement "Everyone should have health insurance," how does one accomplish this goal? In the fall of 1995, I spent lots of time thinking about this dilemma throughout the day, whatever else I was doing at the time: cleaning my house, driving the car, fixing up my yard—an intense mental distraction. On one weekday in October I was sitting on one of the high-topped, stiff black leather chairs at the front of the House chamber mulling this quandary, while the rest of the House membership was engaged in spirited debate over legislation to raise the state's minimum wage by one dollar. In spite of the Republican ascendancy in Washington, D.C., Democrats in the Massachusetts House and Senate remained firmly and lopsidedly in control of our respective chambers. Raising the minimum wage from $4.15 to $4.65 in January 1996 and to $5.15 in January 1997 was a plan vigorously opposed by most Republicans in both chambers and by Governor Weld, who promised a veto. Our reply was vintage Clint Eastwood: "Make our day!" Weld did, and we overrode his veto with pleasure and ease.

My mind turned back and forth between the one-dollar minimum wage hike and the 1988 employer mandate that would have required employers to provide health coverage to their workers or pay a $1,680 per worker tax for use by the Commonwealth to buy coverage for the worker. A one-dollar-per-hour increase in the minimum wage comes to about 40 dollars per week for a full-time worker. I took out my pen and scratched on the white back of my copy of the daily House calendar:

$$\begin{array}{r} 40 \ \text{dollars per week} \\ \times \ 52 \ \text{weeks} \\ \hline 80 \ \ \ \ \ \ \ \ \ \ \ \ \ \ \ \ \\ 200 \ \ \ \ \ \ \ \ \ \ \ \ \ \ \\ \hline = 2{,}080 \ \text{dollars per year} \end{array}$$

Why, I wondered, was it so difficult to sell my colleagues on a $1,680 employer health tax and so easy to sell these same legislators on a $2,080 mandatory wage increase on many of these same employers? Was there a lesson here? Gradually, I came to the conclusion the problem was part packaging and part substance. The 1988 requirement was perceived as Cadillac health coverage for workers, requiring employers to kick in the equivalent (in 1988 dollars) of 80 percent of the cost for full family coverage. What if, instead, we devised an alternative requirement that worked more like the minimum wage? What if, instead of setting a "maximum" mandate that would require new costs and compliance by most employers, we looked at mandated coverage as a minimum, a floor below which employers couldn't go? All workers should be offered—at a minimum—individual coverage by their employers, I thought, and those employers should agree to pay at least half the cost.

OK, but what about the low-wage, marginal employers for whom even a minimalist mandate could spell disaster? For low-wage employers, we could agree to implement Governor Weld's Insurance Reimbursement Program, which would assist vulnerable employers with tax credits and workers with subsidies to pay their share of the cost. We could even call the plan "the Health Care Minimum Wage." I disliked Weld's IRP because it gave no assurance that employers who didn't cover their workers would actually do so. But an IRP linked to a minimum health care mandate made a lot of sense to me.

I immediately went to work on the idea with my committee research director, Brian Rosman. Several months earlier, having just assumed the Health Care Committee chairmanship, I hired Brian as my research director. He was low-key and intensely effective, an attorney who had worked previously for a member of Congress and for former Senate Ways and Means Chair Patricia McGovern. Having just returned from two years in Israel with his wife, a rabbi, he was eager to reengage in serious policy work. Over several weeks in October, we developed the substance of the proposal to establish the health care minimum wage.

Other elements of a legislative package also began to come together. Senior citizen advocates had been pushing unsuccessfully for about eight years to establish and fund a program to help lower-income seniors to purchase prescription drugs. I had known Manny Weiner, president of the Massachusetts Senior Action Council, since my days as an organizer for the Amalgamated Clothing and Textile Workers Union and his days as the president of a steelworkers' union local in Everett, north of Boston. Manny was now in his early eighties, slowing down and a little cranky but earnest and determined. He asked me to include a $30 million senior drug program in whatever health access bill we reported out. I was derisive. "I've got one bottom line, brick wall requirement from House leadership," I told Manny and his companions. "The bill has to be revenue neutral in terms of a hit on the state budget. Where the hell do you think I can come up with 30 million bucks? Get real! Who are you kidding?"

Here was one of my worst flaws. Other politicians learn to listen, nod, smile, shake hands, and then, after visitors depart, shake their heads. I've never been good at playing poker or keeping a straight face. Manny sent me a handwritten personal note the next day: "I have never been so disgusted at the treatment I received from any politician. . . . We're just trying to help people in need and you ought to be ashamed of yourself!"

I told the story to several House colleagues, one of whom gave me an important piece of information. The House chairman of Ways and Means, conservative and tight-fisted Tommy Finneran from Dorchester, who had personally beaten aside previous attempts by legislators and elderly groups to pass a senior prescription drug program, had recently appeared before the legislative senior caucus, a gathering place for legislators and advocates interested in issues affecting the elderly. Asked about his long-standing opposition to the establishment of the program, Finneran replied: "I have no objection to the program in principle. I agree with the need. If we could find a reasonable way to fund it, I would like to see it established."

Hmmm. In working with Rosman to craft the package, I had wanted to find a way to finance a major expansion of the Children's Medical Security Plan for uninsured kids. The governor's proposal would cover all kids in families with incomes below 133 percent of the federal poverty line (about $20,000 for a family of four) through expansion of the Medicaid program, but that left out well more than half of the state's uninsured kids who fell above that income line. The CMSP had been started as a small pilot program in 1991 by Carmen Buell (initially called "Healthy Kids") to provide a basic package of primary and preventive care services to uninsured kids under age six. While the package was limited (no inpatient hospitalization, no dental, vision, or hearing services, very limited drug and mental health coverage), it was a heck of a lot better than being completely uncovered. In 1994, eligibility had been increased to age twelve, but enrollment had topped off at about 15,000 kids due to funding restrictions; meanwhile, data showed about 160,000 uninsured kids. Wouldn't it be good if we could come up with a way to expand CMSP to kids up to age eighteen and provide sufficient additional funding so that every uninsured kid in the state could get in?

Conventional State House wisdom was that raising taxes was impossible during the Weld years. But my mind increasingly turned to tobacco taxes as a new and viable funding source. In the late 1980s and early 1990s, I had tried on several occasions to hike the cigarette tax to fund public health programs. In 1991, in the midst of our deep and damaging recession, I proposed during the House budget debate a four-cent cigarette tax increase that would have raised about $16 million to be used to avert serious cuts in public health programs. Flaherty and Finneran toyed with the idea and abandoned it. I moved the amendment on the floor anyway and lost by 115 to 41.

I knew that the public, though, had a different feeling about tobacco taxes. In 1992, the state branches of the American Cancer Society and the American Lung Association formed a coalition to promote a state ballot initiative to raise the cigarette tax by twenty-five cents, directing the funds toward smoking prevention and other public health purposes. Though the coalition started its campaign with over 70 percent public support in the polls, by election day it won its initiative by a margin of 54 to 46 percent, surviving a heavily financed opposition campaign by the tobacco industry. Clearly, the public had far less antipathy toward tobacco taxes than did the legislature.

A new twenty-five-cent cigarette tax increase would generate about $100 million a year over five years, according to our best estimates. If we gave $30 million to a senior pharmacy program, that would leave about $70 million for a kids' health expansion and other parts of our plan. Even if our cigarette tax estimates proved to be high, there would be a ton of money for the program. I tested the waters with Speaker Flaherty who was willing to see if the tax could fly and with Ways and Means

Chairman Finneran who had no problem with tobacco taxes and always appreciated legislators who proposed new spending programs that also included new revenues to pay for them.

By late October, the form of a legislative package began to take shape:

1.   The Health Care Minimum Wage, requiring all employers to offer individual coverage to their workers, with employers paying at least half the cost;

2.   To address business concerns about the cost of the new mandate, a proposed decrease in the recently approved increase in the state's minimum wage in January 1997—from $5.15 to $5.05;

3.   The governor's proposed Insurance Reimbursement Program to assist employers in complying with the HCMW, funded from the Hospital Uncompensated Care Pool, as proposed by the governor;

4.   Repeal of the 1988 universal health care employer mandate;

5.   The restructuring of Medicaid envisioned in the administration's 1115 waiver to open eligibility to all families—adults and children—with incomes below 133 percent of the federal poverty line;

6.   Major expansion of the Children's Medical Security Plan to cover all other uninsured kids, funded at $70 million;

7.   The Senior Pharmacy Program, funded at $30 million;

8.   A twenty-five-cent increase in the cigarette tax to finance the expansions (with the additional benefit of discouraging teenage smoking); and

9.   Creation of a formal study commission to examine ways to restructure the financing of the hospital Uncompensated Care Pool, addressing concerns expressed by the hospital industry.

By early November, it was time to start testing the waters. My longtime personal aide, Liz Malia, bought a four-by-eight-foot, white, secondhand writing board that fit perfectly on one large wall in my Health Committee office. As I met with groups and individuals in November and December, I didn't want to give anyone anything on paper, knowing that it might immediately get out to the media before I was ready. And so, during those two months, on about fifty separate occasions, I wrote out the plan on the board, step by step, throwing in lots of numbers and arrows and other scribblings to explain the complex package to anyone who wanted to listen.

The reactions varied widely: physicians from the Massachusetts Medical Society—"great, we love it"; leaders from the Massachusetts Hospital Association—"intriguing, challenging, but we think our members have grave concerns about using the hospital pool to finance the IRP"; consumers and their advocates—"we love it!"; business groups—"thank you for presenting this to us and we'll have to take this back to our members, but you know that we can't support any kind of health care mandate"; nurses from the Massachusetts Nurses Association—"we're with you!"; commercial insurers and Blue Cross—"very positive, we can work with this"; senior groups—"yes!"; health maintenance organizations—"we can support this direction"; children's groups—"this is very exciting to us!"; Weld administration officials—"no mandates and no new taxes; except for that, we can talk"; Health Care Committee members—"this looks promising, let's see how it goes"; Marc Pacheco, my Senate cochair—"we'll get killed if we propose new taxes, and killed on any kind of mandate."

Health Care for All and the Massachusetts Medical Society, two groups that in earlier times had been antagonists, joined together to form the Coalition to Improve Health Care Access to establish a broad support network for the plan. Rob Restuccia led HCFA's involvement, and lobbyist Mike Kelly coordinated for the MMS. They told me they were finding interest among a number of organizations that wanted to participate in the coalition in order to have better access to me. I thought that was great.

The reaction from the important labor community, though, was more mixed. Union leaders were very positive in their support for an employer mandate but were extremely anxious about giving away any piece—even a dime—of the minimum wage increase they had recently won. At their request, in early December, I attended a meeting of the Massachusetts AFL-CIO executive board at the Boston Teacher's Union Hall in Dorchester. I sat there while fifty of the state's most powerful union leaders argued with each other about the merits of this one element of the plan. Knowing how difficult it would be to sell any kind of mandate, I had put the 10-cent decrease in my plan to mollify business complaints and to demonstrate our serious intent. After about an hour of intense and bitter debate, I threw in the towel on that element of the plan—the first (and not the last) to go. I needed strong and united labor backing to have a chance and could not risk an early rift with them.

By the end of December, I had tested the outlines of the plan enough to know it was time to go public. On our side we had: consumers, physicians, nurses, community health centers, labor, seniors, and, most important to me, Speaker Flaherty. Likely against us: the Weld administration, tobacco interests, and business. Somewhere in the middle: insurers and HMOs, the hospitals, most of the members of the Health Care Committee, and, importantly, my Senate cochairman, Marc Pacheco. Flaherty agreed that early January was the right time to put a plan out for public discussion. I gave him a choice: "If you want to announce this as your plan, I'm with you all the way. If you want me to go out on the plank, and you watch how it goes, that's fine with me, too." The two of us held a well-attended press conference on the morning of January 11, 1996, in Nurses' Hall on the second floor of the State House where a large bronze statue to Civil War nurses stands at the bottom of two marble staircases, one leading to the governor's office and the other to the State Senate chamber.

In order to get maximum coverage for the press conference, especially from the TV stations, which were getting harder and harder to attract because of their ratings wars, I leaked the details of the access plan and proposed legislation ahead of time to Richard Knox, the respected medical editor of the *Boston Globe,* who had been covering health issues in the state for more than twenty years, and to Connie Paige, State House reporter for the *Boston Herald.* Both papers gave our plan top-of-the-front-page coverage that day, thus guaranteeing good media coverage of the event. "Democrats Push Health Coverage, New Proposal Applies to All Mass. Workers," headlined the *Globe.* "Let's make the minimal provision of health care benefits part of the minimum wage, and see how it sells," I was quoted as saying. "Maybe it won't, but we're going to give it a try." Weld, asked on camera for his reaction, smirked and said, "Mandates and taxes! What is this, bring back Dukakis week?" An effective retort, I had to admit. The next day, the *Globe,* which was especially generous to my plan, titled its lead editorial of the day, "Rep. McDonough's Sound Health Plan."

The press conference, which came off without a hitch, represented the beginning of an external sales strategy. After two months of off-the-record, nothing-in-writing discussions in my Health Committee office, I spent the next three months moving all over the state, meeting with business, consumer, physician, senior, and other groups, making presentations to newspaper editors and reporters, using the same pitch and the same lines five to fifteen times per day. On Tuesday, January 16, five days after the press conference, the Health Care Committee held a daylong hearing on the new plan, with U.S. Senator Edward Kennedy, Boston

Mayor Tom Menino, and Attorney General Scott Harshbarger as my leadoff witnesses in support of the plan. On Martin Luther King Day, I appeared on a public radio talk show, *The Connection,* bracing myself for whatever. Talk radio is not for the meek but for those who can take it; the experience is enormously energizing as the calls come from all directions. Much to my surprise, out of about a dozen calls during the hour, only one was distinctly negative.

Much to their surprise, I went out of my way to meet with business groups across the state, making my pitch, hearing their comments and concerns, answering their questions as best I could. They genuinely appreciated my approach but respectfully disagreed. I recall meeting in late March with members of the Neponset Valley Chamber of Commerce. Sitting quietly through my presentation was the owner of a Domino's Pizza Shop, wearing his uniform of various shades of blue. "You just don't understand," he finally said. "I compete against pizza stores that pay everything and everyone under the table. I pay unemployment, workers comp, FICA, you name it, and you want to add one more thing that I have to dig up while my competitors pay none of those things? Come on. . . ." To lots of critics and questioners, I had ready answers. But to Mr. Domino's, I had to admit that his point cut through.

The noted political scientist Charles Lindblom suggests that the pluralist explanation of how politics works—that it's open season, and anyone can join the game to shape the outcome—misses the trump card the corporate community gets to play: business most always brings a larger degree of influence in political contests than other groups do. It's an observation that makes intuitive sense: politicians usually do better in good economic times than bad ones, and our fates are most closely tied to the fate of our district's and state's businesses. That dynamic was certainly in evidence in this situation and conformed to my own awareness of the heavy influence of business views in Massachusetts health policy discussions for more than thirty years. After three months of heavy outreach between January and March, a large amount of media coverage and favorable publicity, promising poll numbers, and the beginnings of an effective lobbying effort inside the State House by consumer, senior, and labor groups, I had moved nowhere in influencing the business community and, by extension, the legislators who listened to it. Those reps and senators who opposed the 1988 employer mandate had already heard from their local business groups and had no inclination to view my Health Care Minimum Wage plan in a more favorable light.

On March 27, in order to move the issue forward, I convinced a ma-

jority of the seventeen Health Care Committee members to allow the
bill to be reported from the committee favorably. I had far less than a
real majority of votes, but most members, including my new Senate
cochair, Mark Montigny of New Bedford, "reserved their rights" out
of respect for the work I had done (Marc Pacheco supported the losing candidate in a battle for the Senate presidency in late 1995 and had
been removed as Senate Health Care chairman in January 1996 as a
result). I knew there was zero chance for this bill to become law but
wanted the Health Committee, which I chaired, to go on record in support of the kind of reform really needed to address the needs of the
uninsured.

At the end of the afternoon executive session, Rob Restuccia, the executive director of Health Care for All and my ideological twin and ally
in countless health access battles, pulled me aside. "We can get a lot of
good things done now," he said. "But holding out for the mandate will
kill it all. I've supported it as long and hard as you have, but it's time to
let it go." He felt momentum building for an expansion of children's coverage in particular through the work of the Children's Access Coalition.
He had a much clearer perspective on emerging events than I did, and
he was right. We had an open window of opportunity to win some important health care access expansions, but a package that included any
kind of employer mandate would be too large to fit. We were already
thinking of what the new bill should include. Our original bill was now
moving on to the House Committee on Ways and Means, and we would
need to recommend a modified bill for its consideration.

The mandates, new and old, had to go. The governor's IRP, with its
phony estimates and its elaborate tax credits and subsidies taken from
the Hospital Uncompensated Care Pool, was also out. The package Brian
Rosman and I put together included the following key elements:

1. Restructuring of the Medicaid program along the lines envisioned
in the original Weld 1115 waiver, making all families with incomes below 133 percent of the federal poverty line eligible for Medicaid;

2. Expanding children's eligibility for Medicaid further to all kids
in families with incomes below 200 percent of the federal poverty line
($32,000 versus $20,000 for a family of four at 133) to be phased in;

3. Providing sufficient funding to open the Children's Medical Security Plan to all other uninsured kids who would not be eligible for
Medicaid;

4. Establishing the Senior Pharmacy Assistance Program, funded at $30 million;

5. Raising the cigarette tax by twenty-five cents to seventy-six cents to finance the senior and children's health expansions;

6. Creating a Special Commission to develop a new way to finance the hospital Uncompensated Care Pool; and

7. Repealing the 1988 universal health care employer mandate.

By early April, we had our final package assembled. We had created a genuine sense of a compelling public problem in need of resolution. We finally had developed a viable, implementable, road-tested, and funded policy proposal. From here until the end of July, it would be all about one thing . . .

Politics. Moving the political stream in a favorable direction, and keeping it going that way, was a formidable challenge—on numerous fronts. Some of the challenges included: instability in both the Senate and the House because of resignations by the presiding officer in both chambers, the President (in January 1996) and the Speaker (in April 1996), respectively; the need to develop and demonstrate support among the public; the need to counter an expected avalanche of opposition generated by the tobacco industry; the urgent need to develop an effective support coalition that could lobby inside the State House and generate public support on the outside; the dilemma of how to work with and move the business community; and, of course, the puzzle of how to deal with his excellency, the governor, who had other things on his mind.

In November 1995, Governor William F. Weld ended months of speculation by announcing that he would challenge two-term incumbent U.S. Senator John Kerry in the November 1996 general election. In his announcement, Weld stressed that his campaign would focus on three issues: crime, welfare, and taxes, and he began immediately to emphasize differences between himself and Kerry on these matters. It was widely recognized that this would be a bare-knuckle brawl between two experienced public figures. Knowing Weld's long-standing commitment to help his lieutenant governor, Paul Cellucci, become the next governor, and Weld's love for the national scene, I had felt for some time he would enter the race. My immediate thought, though, was how this race would affect our chances to pass the nascent health bill, still in development at the time of Weld's announcement. Many smart people advised me it was now foolish to entertain any thoughts of a health bill that included new taxes. Weld could never afford to violate his no-new-taxes pledge, repeated firmly and directly in his Senate-run announcement. He would surely be able to use the visibility provided by the race to scare legislators away from voting for a new tax on cigarettes and certainly would be able to scare up enough votes to sustain a veto in either the House or Senate. Maybe, I thought, and maybe not, wondering to myself if I was being naïve and foolhardy.

One way to gauge our chances was to ask the public. Lou DiNatale is a tough, Democratic street fighter, a political operator who had retreated from the field of campaign battles to the more serene atmosphere of the John McCormack Public Policy Institute at the University of Massachusetts in Boston. In the past, he had offered me the free services of a polling operation available through the institute. Together, we devised two questions for a February 22, 1996, poll. The first was on the health care minimum wage: "A 'health care minimum wage'proposal would require employers to pay half their employees' health insurance premiums, give employers a tax credit, and provide subsidies to employees who don't earn enough to pay half their premiums. Would you support or oppose this plan?" The second dealt with the other elements in the plan: "A proposal has been made in the State House to raise cigarette taxes by 25 cents to fund health insurance for children who don't have it and help buy prescription drugs for elders who can't afford such coverage. Would you support or oppose such a plan?"

We had the survey numbers by late February. Over 65 percent supported the health care minimum wage plan (77 percent of Democrats and 44 percent of Republicans), about the same proportion that had always supported the 1988 mandate. They were nice numbers, but not high enough to move anyone inside the State House. The results on the second question were much better: 77 percent agreed, while only 19 percent opposed; importantly, even 73 percent of *Republican* voters agreed with our plan. We waited until the end of March to release the poll results at the same time as the Joint Health Care Committee reported the health care minimum wage bill favorably. From then on, we constantly reminded all 160 representatives and 40 senators about the numbers for the second question. "Even 73 percent of *Republican* voters," we would say.

We knew the tobacco industry would spare no expense in opposing a cigarette tax hike, having demonstrated its willingness to invest millions to defeat legislative and ballot initiatives everywhere in the nation.

(The industry had spent $7 million in an unsuccessful effort to defeat the 1992 ballot question, versus $1 million spent by proponents.) We expected, and saw, what's referred to as "astroturf lobbying." Gathering thousands of names from promotions, coupons, and other public relations devices, the industry breaks the names down by state legislative district. Paid phone callers reach the individuals, ask if they would oppose a cigarette tax hike, and then directly connect the individual to his or her legislator's office. Warning legislators ahead of time to expect this ploy was one effective countermeasure, but the more vital one was building a huge support coalition of our own.

At the epicenter was the consumer advocacy group Health Care for All. Formed in 1985 to advocate the health needs of low-income people, its focus broadened as health system problems affected larger segments of the population. Executive Director Rob Restuccia, bearded, articulate, and fortyish, rejected more doctrinaire forms of advocacy in favor of "what we can get." He became accustomed to hits from more ideological health advocates who wanted a Canadian-style, tax-financed, single-payer health system, and nothing else. (One single payer advocate wrote: "The McDonough bill is so watered down, it resembles homeopathy.") Joining him in the newly formed Campaign for Children were leaders and operatives from a broad array of forces: provider groups, consumer and advocacy organizations, senior citizen groups, and health insurers. Key supporters included the Massachusetts Medical Society, Children's Hospital, Harvard Pilgrim Health Care, the Massachusetts Teachers Association, Blue Cross, and smoking prevention groups such as the American Cancer Society—all of whom backed up their verbal support with significant dollar commitments to enable this grassroots campaign to function at a skilled, professional level. At various points, one or another group would suggest to me adding something to the legislation that would invariably alienate one or another part of the coalition. For example, the Medical Society, which abhorred managed care, suggested adding a tax on health maintenance organizations to finance additional expansions. My answer was, "No. We need to keep as big a tent as possible to beat the tobacco industry and Bill Weld. I want the HMOs with us, not against us." It was the same answer I gave to every group—with the exception of the senior citizens. Adding the senior pharmacy program to the bill gave us an enormous political boost with senior groups and virtually no loss in support from anyone else.

The coalition raised over $300,000 in three months, organized itself into fund-raising, lobbying, and grassroots organizing committees, ran four telephone banks, and sent out over 30,000 legislative alerts bulletins. Blue Cross contributed funds that enabled the coalition to hire a senior public relations professional, Geri Denterlein, who generated newspaper and television stories across the Commonwealth.

One major health interest (which to this day prefers anonymity) bought us the lobbying services of Judy Meredith, a fiftyish, hard-boiled pro who cut her lobbying teeth in the 1970s as a naïve suburban mom advocating reform of adoption laws. She caught the lobbying bug and quickly became a respected and skillful operator within the State House. Meredith billed herself "the poor people's lobbyist," and she and I had worked closely together in the early 1980s lobbying for tenant protection laws. Each of the major groups participating in the coalition sent their own lobbyist to coalition strategy meetings where Judy carried the bullwhip. As the chair of a key legislative committee whose ear they all needed, I would occasionally show up to remind the thirty or so lobbyists that Judy reported to me every day who was carrying out their assignments—and who was not.

One major group we were unable to attract to the coalition was business. Adamantly opposed to the 1988 employer mandate and the health care minimum wage proposal, business was poised to block whatever it didn't like. This was a change. Back in 1988, two major business groups, Associated Industries of Massachusetts and the Massachusetts Business Roundtable, stood on the stage in front of the State House applauding as Governor Michael Dukakis signed the universal health care bill into law. By 1994, under pressure from small business groups and in the context of the national health reform disaster, both groups had withdrawn their support. Now, about thirty business groups, including AIM and MBR, met together on a regular basis to plot common strategy on health care issues.

The most likely break in the business chain appeared in the form of the Success By 6 Coalition, the business-backed group formed by the United Way to promote better health care and child care for kids through age six. With some of the most powerful business leaders in the state in the group, and some influential allies of mine among them, this was the first group to move if any movement on new taxes was possible within the business community.

On the morning of Wednesday, April 3, more than fifty Success By 6 leaders held a meeting in the Senate Reading Room. I made my offer to the group: we would repeal the 1988 employer mandate and not propose the health care minimum wage—or any other requirement—in its place; but we would raise tobacco taxes by twenty-five cents and raise Medicaid eligibility for uninsured kids up to 200 percent of poverty, expanding the Children's Medical Security Plan to cover the rest of the kids; we wanted to cover all kids, not just kids up to age six. And we would set up the program to help seniors buy prescription drugs. I asked for their support.

Paul O'Brien, the former head of NYNEX, a powerful and respected business leader in the state for many years, stood first and addressed me. "To us," he said, "employer mandates are mortal sins. Cigarette taxes are more in the category of venial sins. I think we can all live with that kind of sin."

Shortly after my part, Senate President Thomas Birmingham walked in to address the gathering. Working-class from the streets of Chelsea, Harvard- and Oxford-educated, Birmingham had prevailed in a bruising fight to become Senate President the preceding January by effectively using his power over the budget as chairman of Senate Ways and Means. Once in power, he removed Mark Pacheco, who had backed his opponent, as Senate Health Care chair and installed New Bedford's Mark Montigny in his place. Birmingham had issued mildly sympathetic responses to my January proposal but on other occasions had clearly stated that no new taxes would be considered by the Senate in 1996. Standing before the Success By 6 group, Birmingham was visibly taken aback to hear O'Brien, a business voice, ask if he would support a cigarette tax hike to finance health coverage for kids. A chain smoker, Birmingham hesitatingly replied, "That would be very difficult to pass especially in an election year."

After Birmingham departed and the meeting ended, some of the group's leaders approached me in the back of the room to express their disappointment at his response. I was delighted. "What he means is, 'Show me the support is there, and we'll see what we can do.' It's just what he should say, and it's *great* news."

During this same period, the political situation in the House of Representatives became wildly unstable. Back in December 1992, a group of legislators led by House Speaker Charles Flaherty traveled to Puerto Rico for the expressed purpose of attending the winter meeting of the Council of State Governments but instead made their way to a luxury resort on the other side of the island, accompanied by a select group of high-powered lobbyists and unbeknownst to them, the *Boston Globe*. A front-page exposé appeared in May 1993 with a full-color picture of the Speaker in his bathing suit. That series convinced the U.S. attorney's office in Boston to begin an extraordinarily intensive series of investigations designed to bring Flaherty down. While other legislators and lobbyists were fined and embarrassed by the Puerto Rico affair, nothing was found illegal on the Speaker's part. Instead, investigators focused on a house on Cape Cod at which the Speaker had stayed with a friend for a vacation in the early 1990s, a house owned by a parking lot operator with an interest in various legislative matters. By March 1996, leaks and rumors had reached a feverish pitch, suggesting Flaherty would plead guilty to a minor violation, pay fines, and relinquish the Speaker's gavel.

As early as mid-1995, two highly placed Democrats began quietly lining up votes to succeed Flaherty. The moderate liberal majority leader, Richard Voke, held the position which normally precedes that of Speaker and used his years of favors and service to line up a solid majority of votes—including mine—in the House Democratic caucus. Ordinarily, the winner in the caucus proceeds to election in the full House with the backing of most or all Democrats, as the Republicans support their own leader in a final predictable piece of theatre. But Voke was challenged by the moderate conservative House Ways and Means chairman, Tom Finneran, who used his intense, aggressive style and ability to hand out budget favors to build a team of committed loyalists. Despite his challenge, Finneran could not shake Voke's solid lock on control of the caucus.

Just hours after the Success By 6 meeting on April 3, Flaherty announced to a stunned House Democratic caucus that he would plead guilty to a minor tax violation and step down as Speaker on June 30. Pressure built immediately from the media and public for him to step down at once, and he agreed to do so. On Monday, April 8, Finneran held a press conference to announce a lock on 82 of the 160 votes to be elected Speaker. With quiet support from Weld, he convinced every one of the 32 House Republicans to commit to voting for him and not one of their own. Combining these with his solid 50 Democratic votes, he successfully employed an end run around the Democratic caucus and was elected Speaker of a bitterly divided House.

I felt a unique perspective on these events: would the bitter, ugly division within the House and the inevitable leadership changes derail what were becoming increasingly promising prospects for passage of major health reform? This was my primary concern—everything else was secondary. Shortly after announcing his vote lock on the Speakership, Finneran told reporters the names of several Voke-supporting committee chairs whom he intended to put on his new leadership team, with my name mentioned first on the list. I read his words carefully and knew his word would be good for the rest of 1996 but implied no commitment after January 1997 when he would once again reorganize his leadership team at the start of a new term. He waited until May 21 to call a Democratic caucus to ratify his recommendations for leadership changes. Every member who supported Voke was either left in his or her current position or demoted, about half and half; nearly all Finneran backers were promoted, with a few left in place. A hard core of the Voke faction—very good friends of mine—became the active opposition within the House, challenging Finneran's control at many turns, mostly losing. To attain more than two-thirds support of the House membership for my health bill, I desperately needed strong support from both sides of this divide. I shut my mouth, bit my tongue, and felt like dirt.

In terms of the legislative process, I saw one major thing that could go wrong, something I had worried silently about for months. According to the rules of the institution, anything, *anything,* can be proposed as an amendment to an "appropriations" (or budget) bill: death penalty, agency reorganization, gay rights, you name it. Floor amendments to all other bills had to be "within the scope" of the bill's subject matter; but in a budget bill, everything and anything was "within the scope." We were scheduled to debate the House version of the coming fiscal year 1997 budget during the week of April 8–13, and if Republican members acted true to form, at least one of them would file an amendment to repeal the 1988 employer mandate. Were that to pass, and were the Senate to add a similar item to its version of the budget (and the Senate supported repeal more strongly than did the House), there would be no compelling need for any health bill (much less mine) to reach the governor's desk before July 31, the day before scheduled implementation of the 1988 mandate. This would be fatal. I could plead with members to wait, assuring them that a repeal bill would reach the floor but lose because of many members' unwillingness to be recorded publicly against repeal of the mandate.

To avert this threat, I filed early my own amendment to repeal the mandate and let the Republicans know it. Because they, along with most other House members, were distracted by the leadership struggle and other matters, they neglected to file an amendment of their own. After the deadline for filing amendments had passed, I quietly withdrew my amendment, eliminating any chance for the matter to be inserted into the House budget. After that, even had the Senate added it during their debate, it would have been deleted in the budget conference committee by the Democratic conferees who supported my position.

To me, this was a quiet, unobserved, and yet critically important win in dealing with the business community. Political scientist and game theorist William Riker made the key observation that legislative bodies only process alternatives in a *pairwise* fashion, two at a time. For example, suppose there are three proposed solutions to a given problem with varying degrees of support: option A has 45 percent, option B has 35 percent, and option C has 20 percent. Assume that everybody who supports option C supports option B as a second choice and that option B supporters break half and half for A or C as a second preference. If the choice is between A and C, A wins, 62.5 to 37.5; but if the choice is between A and B, B wins 55 to 45. Thus, the ordering of the presentation of choices can have a decisive impact on the legislative outcome.

The business community—hostile to any new mandate and any new tax, with the exception of Success By 6—saw three health policy choices arrayed before them in April 1996, presented in their order of preference. Option A was simple repeal of the 1988 employer mandate. Option B was my new bill, repeal of the mandate plus the cigarette tax increase that they didn't like. Option C was implementation on August 1 of the 1988 employer mandate, if nothing passed. By ensuring during the House budget debate that the House would not have the option of a simple mandate repeal—option A—I gave the business community a choice only between options B and C. On May 13, Brian Rosman and I met with about thirty of them at the offices of the Greater Boston Chamber of Commerce. Much to their dismay, Success By 6, Associated Industries of Massachusetts, and the Massachusetts Business Roundtable were already with us or moving in our direction. The association representing convenience stores and the groups near New Hampshire (which lured Massachusetts smokers with lower cigarette taxes) were bitterly opposed to our plan and sought every angle to attack my bill. But by early June, shortly before the House of Representatives took up the health access bill, we had won official support from the MBR, AIM, the Greater Boston Chamber of Commerce, and the *Boston Business Journal*. The solid wall of business opposition had broken, and we began letting everyone know it.

With the conclusion of the Special Commission back in September 1995 and the start of Governor Weld's Senate campaign in November, the Weld administration abandoned any pretense of interest in enacting major health reform legislation in 1996. In meetings with Human Services Secretary Whitburn in November 1995 and February 1996, the message was simple and clear: no mandates and no taxes, take it or leave it. They knew that the legislature would not allow the 1988 mandate to become law, figured they could block any new taxes, and thought I was being, in the words of Medicaid Director Bruce Bullen, "excessively ideological." They even seemed to have lost interest in enacting their own proposals that were part of the Medicaid 1115 waiver.

An April 30 *Boston Globe* article gave the administration a severe jolt. A Richard Knox piece, "Weld Trails Pack on Cigarette Tax," reported that

> a high visibility group of business and community leaders that strongly supports raising the state cigarette tax to provide health insurance for children has at least one dissenting member: Gov. William F. Weld, who has vowed to veto the bill. Lt. Gov. Paul Cellucci and Charles D. Baker, the Weld administration's secretary of administration and finance, are also among the 56 members of the Success By 6 Leadership Council, which lobbies for programs benefiting young children. The situation illustrates how the Weld administration is becoming isolated on the health insurance issue, which is attracting support from leaders of both big- and small-business sectors. Opposition is currently expected only from the tobacco industry and convenience store owners who sell cigarettes.

Within days, Baker called reporters into his State House office to announce that the Weld administration was hard at work developing a new alternative health plan—without mandates or new taxes—that would be "more kid friendly."

Key to the emerging Weld strategy was wooing the hospital industry to the governor's side, away from what was now called the "McDonough-Montigny Health Access Bill," by promising an immediate restructuring of the hospital uncompensated care pool. The pool, as originally devised in 1985, had all hospitals kicking in a proportionate share of about $300 million, money which was then diverted to hospitals that provided disproportionately high amounts of care to uninsured persons. Almost half of the funds went to two urban hospitals, Cambridge City and Boston City. Hospitals passed their pool liability onto their customers, similar to a meal or sales tax. But hospital rate deregulation in 1991 ended the inclusion of an explicit "uncompensated care surcharge" as a direct pass-through and instead left it to hospitals on their own to recoup their pool liabilities in rate negotiations with individual payers. By the mid-1990s, the reimbursement environment for hospitals had become perilous, as an overcapacity system left health insurers and businesses who paid the bills in the driver's seat. In the spring of 1996, a forceful coalition of community hospitals, angry at their subsidization of the two public hospi-

tals, broke ranks with the Massachusetts Hospital Association and began to lobby the State Senate for a new $200 million tax on health in-
surers and a reduction in their liability to the pool by the same amount.

In late May, Weld and Cellucci proposed their own alternative to the
McDonough-Montigny Bill, including a new $200 million assessment on
hospital payers. But the administration's hopes that the proposal would
break the hospital community away from support for McDonough-Montigny backfired. First, while the MHA thanked the governor for his recognition of the hospital community's concerns, the association's leaders did
not believe that the governor's alternative would win and did not want
to alienate House and Senate leaders; they refused to withdraw their support for our bill. Second, the governor's plan enraged business and insurer community forces who recognized they were being asked to pick
up what amounted to a new $200 million tax on health insurance pre-
miums. The plan served one useful function for the governor: for about
six weeks, when asked why he opposed the McDonough-Montigny Bill,
Weld replied that he had his own better plan—no mandates, no new taxes,
$200 million in new funds to help hospitals, plenty of coverage for kids.
For the uninitiated, it sounded fine, but why was he so adamant against
a cigarette tax?

"Tax increases are a no-brainer for me," he told the *Globe* in early
June. Later that month, asked if he felt uneasy being in league with cigarette manufacturers, Weld replied, "No, not at all. I don't brake for tax
increases."

To demonstrate that we had viable support to pass the bill over a now-
certain veto, we needed to win initial House approval not just by the necessary 81-vote majority but by at least two-thirds, or 107 votes out of
160. The Children's Access Coalition worked aggressively at getting its
participants to lobby their legislators. While Judy Meredith and her team
of lobbyists had divided up the House and were polling and probing members daily, I kept my own tally based solely on my own one-on-one conversations with colleagues. I ranked them 1 to 5, 1 solidly for, 2 leaning
for, 3 undecided, 4 leaning against, and 5 solidly against. By late May, I
counted nearly 100 "1's" but couldn't move the final batch, who were
waiting for a signal from the new Speaker.

Speaker Finneran put me up before the House Democratic caucus on
Thursday afternoon, June 6. I had been in this position only once before, for the 1994 campaign finance legislation, but felt confident. I could
tell the Speaker had not yet made a final decision on moving forward,
or on the final shape of a bill, and this caucus would be his test. I spent

about ninety minutes explaining the plan, fielding questions, and taking hits from antitax and New Hampshire border reps. One tough line of questioning suggested that we should put the tax increase on the ballot to let the voters decide. Aside from the fact that the state constitution would allow us to make it only advisory and nonbinding, I suggested a more personal motive for members to reject that idea:

> In 1992, the tobacco industry spent about $7 million dollars to defeat the last tax increase. Most of that money was spent trying to convince voters they couldn't and shouldn't trust the Legislature, namely *you*, to use the money appropriately. If you want to give the tobacco industry an invitation to spend another $7 million attacking Y-O-U, be my guest.

That idea soon dropped from sight. Another group started complaining that we should not pick on the tobacco industry and let other societal vices such as alcohol and gambling off scot-free. I remembered an interesting fact from a book I had just finished reading on the history of the tobacco industry, *Ashes to Ashes*.[5] There were two principal reasons, I suggested:

> First, we can generate enough money from tobacco taxes, and quite frankly, opposition from that industry is more than enough for me, thank you. Second, about five to ten percent of alcohol users become problem drinkers, and about the same number of people who gamble become problem gamblers. But there is no known safe level of cigarette smoking. By definition, all smokers are problem smokers. That's a big difference.

On Monday, June 10, after about three hours of debate, the House voted for the access bill 115 to 42, more than enough to override a gubernatorial veto with ease. Finneran's lieutenants had rounded up enough votes in the final days to ensure safe passage. For the Speaker, this had become one of his new Speakership's defining battles, showing that he could promote and pass a big "D" Democratic policy initiative and that he would not knuckle under to the wishes of Governor Weld. Importantly, 11 of the 32 House Republican members deserted Weld and voted for the bill. Without their help, we would not have had sufficient votes to override.

On Tuesday, July 2, after six hours of debate, the State Senate voted to pass the bill by a margin of 31 to 8, comfortably more than the 26 votes needed for an override. After fighting the bill fiercely for hours, six of the chamber's ten Republicans voted for passage, again providing the critical margin needed to override a veto. Many of those six had been personally lobbied by the Success By 6 big business leaders who lived in their well-heeled districts. Mark Montigny, who took over Senate leadership of the Health Care Committee in January in the wake of the Birmingham Senate Presidency election, and who resisted my entreaties to support a version of the Health Care Minimum Wage, had come into his own during this process. At times brash and quick on the trigger, he basked in the attention that came to him by carrying the major legislative initiative of the two-year session and pulling it off flawlessly. At one point, several senators close to the community hospital coalition proposed an amendment to create a new $200 million tax on insurers to refinance the uncompensated care pool. Montigny quickly filed a substitute amendment to create a special study commission on the issue and prevailed. Oftentimes Mark would drive me crazy. But watching him on the TV in my office on the day of the Senate vote, I thought, "God, is he good!" I called him at home that night to leave a sincere congratulatory message on his tape machine.

The rest of July resembled ritualized Kabuki theatre, a play without surprises, where all the moves are well known ahead of time—with one exception. Once we knew we had sufficient votes to override a veto, and the administration knew it would lose, the tension and interest rapidly diminished. The Massachusetts Teachers Association, which had been an active participant in the Children's Access Coalition, began running radio ads ridiculing the governor for his inevitable and increasingly foolish-looking veto. For a brief period of days, Weld's lieutenants lamely suggested that they might use the governor's constitutional prerogatives to delay the final legislative steps so that the House and Senate would be unable to vote to override Weld's veto before the July 31 end of our session, running out the clock. But when the business community heard of this stratagem, they rose in united outrage reminding the governor that this move would trigger implementation of the despised 1988 universal health care mandate. Red-faced, Weld and his aides abruptly retreated. The trap we had laid way back in November 1995 by delaying the mandate's implementation until August 1, 1996, sprang perfectly.

On Friday, July 19, Weld returned the bill—as he is permitted to do once—with amendments that would have made our bill into a new version of his own late May proposal. At a rare Saturday session on July 20, the House and Senate rejected his amendments and returned the bill to him. As promised, he vetoed the bill early the next week, and both branches voted by wide margins to override his veto on Wednesday, July 24. The legislative fight was over.

The Children's Access Coalition organized a sizable celebration that week in front of the State House, the same spot on which Governor Michael Dukakis had celebrated the enactment of the universal health care employer mandate in 1988. Now we were celebrating the new law that included its repeal, an irony that few beyond me and Rob Restuccia recognized. The featured guest was Marian Wright Edelman, head of the national Children's Defense Fund. We were already thinking that our formula—children's health expansion funded by new tobacco taxes—had national implications, and Marian's presence reflected that intent.

A week later, the new law received its official chapter number, given numerically in the order that laws are passed each year. Brian Rosman gave me the news. "It's Chapter 203 of the acts of 1996," he said. "In other words, it's Chapter 23 with a hole in the middle for the employer mandate."

AFTERMATH

Four years later, most of the major elements of Chapter 203 had been implemented, some more successfully than others, but not badly considering the scope and complexity of the programs involved. Mark Montigny, Charlie Baker, and I served as the cochairs of a special commission on hospital uncompensated care and in January 1997 came up with a compromise plan agreed to by the hospitals, business, and insurers that was signed into law in July 1997 in one of Bill Weld's last official acts as the Commonwealth's chief executive.

In November 1996 Governor Weld lost his U.S. senatorial race to incumbent John Kerry who savaged him in voluminous television ads for his veto of the children's health law. In the spring of 1997, President Bill Clinton announced that he would nominate Weld as the new U.S. Ambassador to Mexico, a choice that ran into immediate trouble with Republican U.S. Senator Jesse Helms, chairman of the Senate Foreign Relations Committee. Weld resigned as governor in July to fight for the job and to make way for Paul Cellucci to run for governor in 1998 as an incumbent. In September, Weld withdrew his name from consideration for the ambassador's post.

Right after the November 1996 election, Brian Rosman, Dr. Barry Zuckerman of Boston Medical Center, and I spent several hours with U.S. Senator Edward Kennedy discussing our legislative fight and the extraordinary synergy that we found between the issues of children's health care access and new tobacco taxes. Kennedy told us he was doubtful any kind of cigarette tax would be feasible in Washington, D.C. We didn't argue with him but just gave as much information as we could about our experience. Zuckerman later told me that within several weeks, Senator Kennedy was repeating the same lines we had used with him. In February 1997 Kennedy and Republican U.S. Senator Orrin Hatch announced their own bill to hike federal tobacco taxes by forty-three cents, using most of the money to expand children's health insurance coverage. Their efforts directly led in July 1997 to the passage by Congress of Title XXI, the State Children's Health Insurance Program (SCHIP), which now provides $24 billion to states to provide insurance to uninsured kids.

FINAL COMMENT ON KINGDON

Using Kingdon's model *retrospectively*—how most people use it—gives the impression that the three streams are fixed and not subject to human control or manipulation. If this story does anything, I hope it dispels that erroneous impression. The streams are constantly subject to change and manipulation by self-conscious political actors determined to achieve their objectives. My colleagues and I did it. Using the Kingdon model *prospectively* allows one to appreciate this important dynamic. The model can help to assess one's current status and progress and point to areas most in need of attention and improvement.

The other important element is that while windows of opportunity open, they just as surely close, often quite suddenly, for reasons no one might see coming. It's important to be thoughtful, methodical, and careful in planning and executing political strategy. But it's also foolish to squander opportunity and to waste valuable time. Opportunity and luck will surely come around. The challenge, as Pasteur suggests, is to make oneself ready for when they do.

PART FOUR

Endings

How to wrap up a book that introduces readers to different ways of seeing the political in their lives and seeks to keep them hungry for more? I thought of several ways. First, I present not a model but a duality, a pair of contrasting metaphors that characterize important elements of politics. This final construct, or way of viewing politics, is meant to be easier on the eyes. Second, I relate a dramatic and compelling story that engulfed my final weeks as a member of the Massachusetts House, an unexpected conflict that dominated the agenda like no other issue. Finally, I offer summary and concluding thoughts on the models, legislatures and legislators, U.S. health policy, and our politics in these times.

CHAPTER EIGHT

Conversations, Games, and the Death Penalty

My work is a game, a very serious game.

M. C. Escher

I first heard the news at my father's wake in mid-January 1997. Speaker of the House Thomas Finneran had scheduled a 1 P.M. caucus of House Democrats to announce his new slate of leadership appointments for the 1997–98 session at the exact time of the service for my eighty-seven-year-old father. Finneran had won his position as House Speaker the previous spring after a fierce battle with Majority Leader Richard Voke and had announced publicly at the time that he would retain in their posts a small group of former Speaker Charles Flaherty's committee chairs who had not supported his leadership bid. Without asking, he included my name first on the list. But those of us who retained our chairmanships during that tumultuous spring knew that in January 1997 the Speaker, who by then would have consolidated his tenuous hold on a majority of the House Democratic caucus, would have another chance to remove us from our positions. Lobbyist and longtime friend Judy Meredith, one of the first arrivals at the wake, didn't want to tell me, but I insisted. "All the Voke chairmen, including you, were removed," she said.

My reaction was mixed. Being at my father's wake helped to put the news in perspective, though as word spread through my family, I began to wonder for whom this service was being held. The new Speaker's aloof demeanor since his election had already convinced me removal was more than possible. Moreover, I had experienced this kind of disappointment before, in 1991, when I was bypassed for appointment as Health Committee chair, and had better prepared myself this time. Originally, I had not intended to run for reelection in 1996, feeling it was time to move on. But the challenges connected with being Health chair were too enticing to abandon after only sixteen months in that position, and so I decided to run for one last term. I knew I needed to move on to begin saving money for my kids' college education, something I could never do on the House salary. In many ways, I felt more upset about the demotions of some of my colleagues who had done great jobs and wanted to stay. All in all, it seemed a mixed blessing in disguise.

My initial plan was to complete the 1997–98 term and not run for reelection. After my removal as chair, I made suggestions to the Speaker about roles I could play to help him and his untested new team. He listened politely, said he would get back to me, and—typically—never did. After the invigorating challenges of twelve years in the House, I felt like a crow on the wire watching the world go by. In the summer of 1997, I received several attractive job offers, and in September, I accepted one. I had originally intended to resign at the end of September. The House would be meeting in formal sessions until mid-November, but I could count on one hand the number of times that an important matter was decided by one vote. Still, I wanted to make sure that legislation implementing the new federal Children's Health Insurance Program in Massachusetts was approved before I left. Besides, one could never tell when something might come up where one vote would matter. In late September, I announced my intention to resign at the end of November.

As it turns out, one vote did make all the difference on two separate occasions in late 1997, as described in this chapter. The chapter also proposes one final way of understanding politics by presenting a powerful pair of competing metaphors that elegantly captures its dual nature. The case story provides an illustration of these two metaphors at work.

THE CONVERSATION AND THE GAME

This book's central premise is that there are compelling concepts, models, and structures that can explain politics in ways accessible and helpful to broad audiences. Once I realized useful models were out there, I became a scavenger for them, searching journals and books to find newer and better ones. In 1997, I found a pearl in the journal *PS*, published by the American Political Science Association. Professor Brian Frederking of Syracuse University wrote a brief item about how he makes political science more compelling for his students by presenting politics as two contrasting metaphors, the conversation and the game.[1] His insight grabbed me immediately and became a personal theme for my final months in the House, as well as for this chapter.

POLITICS IS A CONVERSATION

As described in chapter 1, politics is how we decide who gets what in society without resorting to violence. An essential way we pursue our political objectives is through conversation, broadly defined. The conversation can be heard or read in any political controversy. The conversation may occur in many places. In international controversies, it may take place at the United Nations, through the media, or across a negotiating table—often the end of conversation means the beginning of armed conflict. If the issue is legislative, the conversation may reach the floors of the House and Senate, committee hearing rooms where the matter is referred, press conferences, and other staged events by partisans of any viewpoint. Invariably, the conversation spills into the media, and especially into the newspapers—through news stories, analyses, editorials, paid advertisements, op-ed columns, and letters to the editor. If noteworthy, controversies also spread to television and radio, the nightly newscasts, the Sunday morning "talking head" shows, the radio talk and call-in programs, public and cable news channels, and Internet sites. If an issue has "legs," discussion will reach America's coffee shops and office water coolers, lunch and dinner tables, schools and places of worship, and on and on.

Some discussions are short-lived, while others can go on for years, decades, or generations. The formal conversation regarding reform of the U.S. Internal Revenue Service proceeded from start to finish within the span of 1997–98. The formal conversation regarding President Bill Clinton's ill-fated Health Security Plan can be traced from the fall 1992 presidential campaign to its demise in Congress in September 1994, though conversations about establishing a national health insurance system have proceeded since about 1915. Conversations about the U.S. role in the Vietnam War raged intensely from the first major buildup in 1965 until our final withdrawal in 1975, though discussions about our appropriate role began in smaller circles as far back as the late 1940s. (I vividly recall the extended conversations, called "teach-ins," on Vietnam held at my high school and across the nation in 1970–71.) The existence of slavery in the United States provoked conversation lasting more than two hundred years, and finally required not talk but armed conflict to settle.

Though political conversation unfolds in disparate locations and over varying stretches of time, it often moves forward in a surprisingly logical fashion. Each side brings to bear its perceived strongest evidence and assertions, presented in whatever medium is most available and accessible. Parties with competing interests and points of view do their best to dissect and undermine the claims made by the original party. Where their attacks succeed, the first party will tend to abandon losing points, reinforce its stronger assertions, and develop new lines of argument. As the circle of conflict grows, so will the number of competing voices, from widely varying points of view, each seeking to shape the evolving opinions of policymakers and the public. Up close, the conversation can seem like a Tower of Babel, with numerous commentators and writers weighing in, creating more heat than light and more confusion than inspiration. But over time, one can recognize the path and progress of the conversation, the dropping of lines of argument by each side, and the development of new ones.

A vivid example of political conversation occurred in the 1787–88 debates over the adoption of the proposed federal constitution, well before the advent of modern communications. While *The Federalist Papers* are widely judged the best writings in support of the proposed constitution, they were not written in a vacuum or without substantial disagreement. Emery Lee, among others, has shown that the tenth *Federalist,* written by Madison under the name Publius, is best understood as a response to anti-Federalist writings, especially those of the anonymous Brutus whose first essay appeared in New York on October 18, 1787, preceding Publius's tenth by only three weeks.[2] Over time, each side can be observed dropping unsuccessful arguments and trying out new ones. The early addition of the Bill of Rights as the first ten amendments to the new Constitution was a direct result of the criticisms made by anti-Federalists in this compelling national conversation. There are many dynamics at work in politics, but a key one is the conversation. To ignore it is to miss a vital ingredient.

It must be noted that accepting the conversation metaphor does not imply that access to avenues of public discourse is equal or fair. A president or governor can usually gain more attention for his or her comments than can any single legislator. A large corporation generally has more ability to buy exposure for its viewpoints than individual citizens or public interest groups. In E. E. Schattschneider's observation (cited earlier), "The flaw in the pluralist heaven is that the heavenly chorus sings with a strong upper-class accent."[3] But American society is also filled with examples where individuals and groups with diminished access to public media were able to attain their objectives in spite of this disadvantage. Acknowledging inequities in the ability to be heard does not diminish the power of the conversation as an essential way to understand politics.

POLITICS IS A GAME

Many writers have noted the gamelike qualities of political conflict for good reason. Inevitably, most political disputes arrive in a public venue for resolution. Every one of these bodies or forums—legislatures, executive offices, regulatory agencies, courts, ballot initiatives—has a set of rules established prior to the arrival of the dispute that determine how it will be addressed. In most legislative bodies, rules are adopted at the beginning of each newly elected sitting; in other locales, such as courts and regulatory agencies, the rules stay in place and evolve slowly over many years. It is usually difficult to predict how newly adopted rules will affect, positively or negatively, most of the issues that reach the affected public entity, because the shape of those issues has not yet fully formed. Experienced and savvy political players seek to understand and use rules to gain advantage for their own position. They do so fully expecting their adversaries to engage in the same exercise. Paying attention to the impact of rules and using them to create advantages over one's opposition are essential components of any effective political strategy. It is in this respect that political conflict most resembles a game.

Games of one form or another are familiar to most of us: football, baseball, soccer, croquet, chess, tennis, checkers, Monopoly, Scrabble, poker, hearts, blackjack, old maid, charades, Trivial Pursuit, Pictionary, tag, hide and seek, crosswords, Jeopardy, Wheel of Fortune, Powerball, and more. (One of the most publicized and discussed books of 1997, *The Rules*,[4] gave explicit instructions regarding the "game of love" to women seeking marriage.) The first step for any first-time player is to gain some understanding of the rules of the game. Usually, one reads written rules or has a companion explain them. This initial perusal provides the basics, allowing someone to begin to play. Over time, the rules come to life as players encounter unexpected situations requiring referral to and interpretation of the rules. Some games have participants such as umpires or referees whose only role is to interpret and enforce the rules. Legislative bodies have parliamentarians who serve a similar function.

The word *game* has several meanings that can confuse. "[A]n amusement or pastime" and "fun; sport of any kind; joke" are two references that suggest trifles and play. But games can also be deadly serious: "a competitive activity involving skill, chance, or endurance on the part of two or more persons who play according to a set of rules."[5] Parents who lose their tempers at the soccer games of their toddler children show that games are not necessarily fun or funny. It may be only a game, but fierce conflict often may erupt over the interpretation and enforcement of rules in almost any game.

For young people, our culture promotes the value of games as training for life. Teamwork, cooperation, competition, practice, judgment, endurance, tools for managing conflict, and other positive qualities are thought to emerge. Moving into work and professional life, we encounter innumerable processes that involve learning and mastering rules, processes that—while not considered games—often seem game-like. Attorneys and judges must learn the rules of procedure, evidence, cross-examination, and more. Physicians must pay attention to rules required for licensure, certification, and reimbursement. Scholars must master the rules of scientific evidence and the requirements for publishing and promotion. Journalists need to demonstrate mastery of the rules of reporting. Stockbrokers have to adhere to the rules of the various exchanges and the Securities and Exchange Commission. Likewise, legislators and lobbyists must master the rules of the chambers in which they operate. All of these settings are more than games, but all become part of the "game of life."

Several case stories in this book have exemplified the game aspect of political conflict. In chapter 3, senators used their right to "lay matters on the table" to delay consideration of legislation to regulate condominium conversions, and later, tenant advocates used rules in a failed attempt to thwart a ballot initiative on rent control. In chapter 5, I used the legislative rules to prevent consideration of an amendment to the campaign finance legislation that would have prohibited the accumulation of so-called warchests by incumbent officials. In chapter 6, Governor William Weld attempted unsuccessfully to use the limited number of days left at the end of the 1996 session to hold back health care access legislation before the House and Senate could override his veto; cries of "foul" by his business allies quickly forced the governor to back down.

Later, Weld himself became an example of how the failure to understand rules can be fatal. In August 1997, he resigned as governor after President Clinton disclosed his intent to nominate Weld as U.S. Ambassador to Mexico. Initially, the nomination seemed a cinch: a Republican nominated by a Democratic president appeared to have no problem in a U.S. Senate controlled by Republicans. However, Senate Foreign Relations Chairman Jesse Helms of North Carolina announced his opposition to the nomination and his determination to prevent its consideration. Weld waged a public campaign to force Helms to hold a public hearing on the nomination but then was surprised to learn that it is practically impossible under the Senate rules to require any chairman to hold a confirmation hearing. After months of frustration, Weld withdrew his nomination and retired to private life, wiser in the ways of U.S. Senate rules, though not much better for it.

The Weld example illustrates another facet of the game: not only are there formal rules, but often there are informal rules that critically affect outcomes. On the floor of the Massachusetts House, for example, any member has the right in the formal rules to challenge any ruling by the Speaker—"Mr. Speaker, I doubt the ruling of the chair"—and thus bring the matter up for an immediate vote of the entire membership. Freshmen Democratic members learn early never to doubt the ruling of the Speaker and never to vote against leadership on such procedural rulings. Every member understands ahead of time that such a challenge is futile. It's not written anywhere, but it exerts enough peer pressure to appear as though it were an article of the state constitution.

Politics is a game. It is not a joke and is only occasionally funny. But it has the essential qualities of a game. To ignore this dynamic is to miss an essential and compelling fact of political life.

POLITICS IS BOTH A CONVERSATION AND A GAME

Frederking observes that Americans like and respect political conversation and despise political games. In association with the game metaphor, he presents these assumptions: 1. Politics is a game that others play; 2. The object is to win; 3. The players of the game are either winners or losers; 4. Players are constantly worried about who is ahead and who is behind; and 5. The rules are static. In contrast with this, he presents these assumptions behind the conversation metaphor: 1. Politics is a conversation in which we all take part; 2. The object is to solve problems; 3. The participants in the conversation are citizens; 4. Citizens debate the merits of the arguments; and 5. The rules are dynamic. He suggests that emphasizing the conversational aspects of the process can help to diminish disdain for politics and encourage enhanced participation.

I find Frederking's ideas compelling, particularly his suggestion that—

in the game metaphor—politics is about "them," others who are detached from real people's lives. A major challenge for political leaders is to provide multiple opportunities to bring new people into the process, to encourage the uninvolved to participate, and to make politics about "us." The conversation metaphor helps to do that in a useful and compelling way, by demonstrating that political controversies progress and that there are multiple, meaningful ways to become involved.

But a realistic and seasoned sense of politics leads to the recognition that both dynamics, the conversation and the game, are present at all times. To ignore the conversational aspect of politics is to miss a vital component that usually weighs heavily on the final outcome. At the same time, to ignore the game aspect of politics is to miss another vital aspect that frequently means the difference between success and failure. It is not one or the other. It is both.

The final case story provides a real-life example of these two aspects of politics and a vivid illustration of the importance of paying attention to both.

THE DEATH PENALTY DEBATE, 1997

On Wednesday, October 1, 1997, around 3:30 P.M., ten-year-old Jeffrey Curley of Cambridge washed his dog, then wandered away from his grandmother's house, telling her that he had something to do and would be right back. Down the street he climbed into the Cadillac of two young men who had promised to replace his stolen bike. At a parking lot in Newton, one of the men suffocated Jeffrey in the back seat with a gasoline-soaked rag, later sexually abused his body in a New Hampshire apartment, stuffed him into a plastic container filled with lime, and threw the container with the body into a river in Maine. Arrested for the crime within two days were Charles Jayne, twenty-two, a 250-pound auto detailer who had seventy-five outstanding criminal warrants, and Salvatore Sicari, twenty-one, a mechanic with a history of violence; they were discovered by police to be lovers with ample supplies of pornography of men and boys. During the first two days of frantic searching for young Jeffrey, both had participated in the search. Jeffrey's body was found beneath the surface of the Great Works River in Maine on October 7.

Though Jeffrey's funeral was not held until Saturday, October 11, the political implications of the horrific tragedy became apparent on October 8 when his father, Robert, told reporters that the state legislature "has to take a stand. . . . We need a death penalty to protect us from lowlifes who prey on working-class families where both parents have to be out working." Curley's own state representative, Timothy Toomey, who had always opposed the death penalty prior to Jeffrey's murder, was the first legislator to announce his change of heart. "This whole thing has completely stunned me and the city is devastated. This crime is so horrific, I think we have to step back and say something. . . ."[6] No capital punishment statute would affect Jeffrey's killers or bring him back, but an intense conversation about death penalty restoration had begun.

I remember thinking about Jeffrey's funeral, about my eleven-year-old son, and about the death penalty as I cleaned my house on that Saturday. While I had always reflexively opposed the restoration of capital punishment, this situation forced me to reexamine my beliefs. I had been a member of the House during several emotional death penalty debates over the years, but the outcome had never been in doubt, and I always took a back seat as others jumped headlong into the fight. I had no political consequences to fear, knowing that I would be out of the House in two months, never to seek election again. What did I care if these two despicable individuals were put to death? Isn't that what I would want if it happened to a member of my family? I wondered if others of my colleagues were having similar thoughts. I quietly decided that I just might vote for the death penalty in the unlikely event that it came up before my departure at the end of November. And then I wondered, what the heck was going on with the capital punishment bill anyway?

·   ·   ·

The story of the death penalty in Massachusetts traces back to a 1641 colonial document called *The Body of Liberties,* which spelled out offenses punishable by death: idolatry, witchcraft, blasphemy, murder, bestiality, sodomy, adultery, man-stealing, false witness in capital cases, and conspiracy. Over the next 140 years, other offenses added to the list included: rape, cursing or smiting of a natural parent by a child sixteen or over, being a rebellious son sixteen or over, a third offense of burglary ("three strikes and you're out" has a *long* history), a third offense of highway robbery, denying Scripture, the return of a Jesuit after banishment, the return of a Quaker after banishment, piracy, mutiny, military service with the enemy, treason, concealment of the death of a bastard child, incest, polygamy, Romish priest escaping from prison, sleeping of sentinels at their posts, killing by dueling, and more. With the establishment

of the Commonwealth of Massachusetts in 1780, the scope of capital offenses for which death could be imposed was reduced to arson (if at
night), highway robbery, willful murder, burglary at night, and treason.
By 1852, the death penalty was reduced to punishment for the crime of
murder in the first degree, willful and premeditated. In 1952, the legislature amended the death penalty statute to eliminate the mandatory
death penalty, requiring a jury recommendation of capital punishment
except in cases of murder committed in connection with rape.[7]

Throughout more than 300 years, Massachusetts used the death penalty.
Resting serenely on the front lawn of the Massachusetts State House is a
statue of Quaker Mary Dyer, hanged on the Boston Common in 1660 for
attending the wrong church. Other recipients include nineteen persons from
the Salem area executed in the early 1690s as witches. Two Italian anar-
chists, Nicola Sacco and Bartolomeo Vanzetti, executed in 1927 for a
fiercely disputed murder-robbery conviction, had their sentences posthu-
mously pardoned by Governor Michael Dukakis in 1987. The last official
executions in the state, on May 9, 1947, were those of Edward Gertsen
and Philip Bellino for the murder of an acquaintance in Lynn.

In 1972, the United States Supreme Court declared unconstitutional
a Georgia death penalty statute that closely resembled the Massachusetts law. The Court held in *Furman v. Georgia* (408 U.S. 238, 1972)
that "imposition and carrying out of the death penalty in these cases con-
stitutes cruel and unusual punishment in violation of the Eighth and 14th
Amendments." The decision threw into disarray death penalty statutes
across the nation, including the one in Massachusetts. In two 1975 decisions, *Commonwealth v. Harrington* (367 Mass. 13, 1975) and *Commonwealth v. O'Neal* (367 Mass. 440, 1975), the Massachusetts Supreme
Judicial Court declared that the state's death penalty statute violated certain provisions of the Massachusetts constitution as well. In his written
opinion, Chief Justice Joseph Tauro noted, "I would not intend to fore-
close the commonwealth from enacting any statute authorizing the
death penalty. However, if such a statute should be enacted, the burden
would be on the commonwealth to establish that such use of the death
penalty is the least restrictive means for furtherance of a compelling State
interest. . . ." The Massachusetts legislature went to work to devise a new
statute that could meet the requirements of the federal and state consti-
tutions. In 1977, in an advisory opinion to the legislature (*Opinion of
the Justices,* 372 Mass. 912, 1977), the justices stated that the new proposal, while meeting the requirements of the U.S. Constitution (the U.S.
Supreme Court relaxed its 1972 prohibition in 1976), violated Article

26 of the Declaration of Rights of the state constitution against cruel or unusual punishment.

In 1978, Democrat Edward J. King stunned the Commonwealth with an upset victory in the September Democratic gubernatorial primary against incumbent Michael Dukakis. Dukakis had been severely wounded in 1975, his first year in office, when he signed a major tax increase in the face of a severe economic recession, after making a "lead pipe cinch" guarantee in his 1974 campaign that he would not raise taxes. Since then, many observers believed he had repaired his political damage, and he had soared in popularity after a severe winter blizzard in February 1978 when he uncharacteristically appeared on television wearing a sweater. But King was a surprisingly strong and relentless opponent who made restoration of the death penalty his number one campaign issue against Dukakis, a solid and outspoken opponent of capital punishment.

In 1979, the legislature delivered to the new governor a capital punishment statute that he proudly signed as Chapter 488 of the acts of 1979. It attempted to meet all the objections raised by the Supreme Judicial Court in its 1977 opinion and included a preamble declaring the utility of capital punishment as a deterrent to crime. In its 1980 ruling (*District Attorney for the Suffolk District v. James Watson*, 381 Mass. 648, 1980), the SJC again declared the statute in violation of the state constitution's Article 26. "Certainly," the justices stated, "at the time of its adoption, art. 26 was not intended to prohibit capital punishment. Capital punishment was common both before and after its adoption. However, art. 26 . . . must draw its meaning from evolving standards of decency that mark the progress of a maturing society . . . and it is our responsibility to declare it invalid."

In response to this state constitutional roadblock, the legislature began the arduous process of amending the constitution. To accomplish this, the House and Senate must meet jointly in a constitutional convention. The identical proposal must be approved by two successive sittings of the constitutional convention; the first was done in 1980, and the second in 1982. Having passed this threshold, a proposed amendment is then placed on a statewide ballot for the judgment of the Massachusetts electorate. On November 2, 1982, Massachusetts voters approved the addition of two sentences to Article 26 of the state constitution:

> No provisions of the Constitution, however, shall be construed as prohibiting the imposition of the punishment of death. The general court may, for the purpose of protecting the general welfare of the citizens, authorize the impo-

sition of the punishment of death by the courts of law having the jurisdiction of crimes subject to the punishment of death.

During the course of this lengthy process, though, politics had taken another peculiar turn. Michael Dukakis reemerged from political oblivion to challenge Governor King to a "rematch" in the September 1982 Democratic gubernatorial primary and handily defeated him. The pro–death penalty legislature was thus anxious to adopt a new death penalty statute before Dukakis reclaimed the governor's office in January 1983. Under the provisions of the newly approved constitutional amendment, it adopted a new capital punishment statute that was signed in December by the lame-duck governor as Chapter 554 of the acts of 1982 for cases of murder in the first degree. Apparently, the legislature had accomplished a death penalty statute—just before the window of opportunity closed.

It took until 1984 for a capital case to emerge that triggered a constitutional challenge to the new law. The case was *Commonwealth v. Colon-Cruz* (393 Mass. 150, 1984) and involved three defendants accused of murdering a state trooper. This time, the SJC ruled that the death penalty statute violated not Article 26 but Article 12 of the Declaration of Rights of the state constitution. Article 12 addresses an accused person's right against self-incrimination and right to a jury trial. Because Chapter 554 can result in the imposition of death only after a trial by jury, a defendant who pleads guilty under the new statute cannot be put to death. "The inevitable consequence is that defendants are discouraged from asserting their right not to plead guilty and their right to demand a trial by jury," concluded the SJC. "The legislature [m]ay not authorize the imposition of the death penalty in a way that needlessly chills defendants' art. 12 rights."

The 1984 ruling took the wind from death penalty proponents' sails. While the legislature could attempt to write a new statute in conformity with the SJC ruling, the balance of power in the State Senate now favored opponents. Even if sufficient votes could be found for passage, it was inconceivable that two-thirds of the House and Senate would vote to override a certain veto from Governor Dukakis. Bills were filed each year by legislators but never moved far in the legislative process as leaders in both chambers sought to avoid divisive and futile debates.

A significant shift in the constellation of support occurred as a result of the 1990 state elections. Republican William Weld, an outspoken death penalty supporter, was elected governor along with a new State Senate solidly in the pro–capital punishment camp. But at the same time, the political stance of the House of Representatives shifted for the first time from support to opposition with the election of a new Speaker, Charles Flaherty of Cambridge, a working-class liberal with a deep and visceral antagonism to the death penalty. I remember sitting in his office in 1995 and picking up an anti–death penalty book sitting on his desk that had been sent to him by his daughter, with written words of encouragement to "keep up the fight, dad." In his legislative committee appointments, Flaherty made sure that every relevant chairmanship and committee roster had a solid majority of death penalty opponents. Between 1991 and 1994, the restoration of fiscal stability—and the urgent need for collaboration between the executive and legislative branches—kept death penalty restoration off the political agenda: no debates, no votes.

In 1995, Governor Weld began his second term with renewed confidence from a record-shattering electoral victory margin, a desire to satisfy frustrated Republican activists, and an eye on future electoral possibilities that included the U.S. Senate seat held by John Kerry. He worked with House Republican leaders to force a reluctant Speaker Flaherty to bring a death penalty bill up for debate before the full House. Flaherty eventually agreed and worked intensely to line up votes to defeat the proposal by a convincing margin. He developed a friendship with Sister Helen Prejean, the Catholic nun whose book *Dead Man Walking* was made into a successful Hollywood film. Sister Prejean joined Flaherty in personally lobbying members. In July 1995 the measure was defeated in the House, 83 to 74, not a landslide margin but large enough to convince observers that a shift in the House position was unlikely.

In April 1996, Flaherty resigned as House Speaker, conceding to a federal tax violation after an intensive, three-year investigation by the U.S. attorney's office. While his departure was certain to have numerous consequences, a change in the stance of the House relative to the death penalty was not considered among them. His successor, moderate conservative Tom Finneran from the Dorchester section of Boston, had once supported restoration but now summed up his opposition in three words: "Bobby Joe Leaster." Leaster, an African American, served fifteen and a half years of a life sentence in a Massachusetts prison after being wrongly convicted at age nineteen of a 1970 slaying of a shopkeeper. At his trial, the judge specifically instructed the jury that it could consider the death penalty. The father and son attorneys Robert and Christopher Muse worked ten years to prove Leaster's innocence and won his release the day after Christmas, 1986. Finneran also worked relentlessly for years to provide Commonwealth compensation for Leaster, now a city of Boston youth counselor who visits schools to talk about the criminal justice system. At one dramatic legislative hearing on restoration in 1994, as Governor Weld spoke in favor of the death penalty, the House chairman of the committee, Joe McIntyre from New Bedford, signaled Leaster to come forward and stand next to the governor. Weld's lieutenant governor, Paul Cellucci, earlier had suggested that the execution of innocent persons under a death penalty statute was "an acceptable price to pay" in order to have the punishment. McIntyre used this moment to challenge both of them: "Governor, can you look this man in the eye and tell him why making a mistake that would sacrifice his life is an acceptable price to pay?" The normally voluble Weld stumbled a forgettable response. Enthusiasm for the capital punishment issue waned considerably after the decisive negative House vote in 1995.

Thus, the prospects for death penalty restoration did not appear strong as the 1997 legislative session got under way. It was understood that the Senate would most likely pass a restoration statute that subsequently would be defeated or unaddressed by the House. One important difference between Flaherty and Finneran, however, was in their committee appointments: the latter appointed chairs and committee members to the relevant committees without consideration of their death penalty sympathies. As it turned out, Finneran's chairmen of the Committee on Criminal Justice and the Committee on Ways and Means were both committed death penalty proponents as were the majorities of their respective committees.

While the death penalty bill moved forward, it was hard to argue that restoration was on the fast track in the session. In late June 1997 the Committee on Criminal Justice reported favorably to the Senate a capital punishment restoration bill whose consideration was promptly delayed until September. When the matter was brought up in the early fall, Senate opponents began using the familiar stalling tactics of moving "to lay the matter on the table" and filing amendments that would delay consideration until each subsequent formal session. On Tuesday, September 30, a motion to lay on the table was "negatived," while further debate was postponed pending the printing of a new amendment, another familiar Senate stalling procedure.

The next day, ten-year-old Jeffrey Curley was kidnapped and murdered.

·   ·   ·

Massachusetts is one of only twelve states that does not permit capital punishment as a criminal justice option. New York had been the principal holdout during the twelve-year administration of Democratic Governor Mario Cuomo, a passionate opponent, but passed its own death penalty statute in 1995 during the first year of his successor, Republican George Pataki. Discussion of a political-legislative issue might have seemed inappropriate to some during the period of mourning for Jeffrey Curley, but not after his father, Robert, publicly indicated his desire to see death penalty restoration as a memorial for his lost son two days before he was laid to rest. Immediately, the conversation exploded forth in headlines, news articles, editorials, columns, letters, cartoons, radio call-ins, TV panels, daily and unending, fiercely argued from both perspectives, and each side hurling emotional charges at the other.

I devoured as much information, analysis, and opinion as I could, with the intent of establishing a defensible rationale for changing my long-standing position. But I couldn't do it. There was no single article or comment that turned me. Instead, the intensity of venom on the pro-restoration side convinced me the sole rationale for the death penalty was retribution, nothing more. I was disturbed to learn that Jeffrey's killers both had long criminal histories and that one continued to walk free despite more than seventy outstanding criminal warrants. Criminal attorneys I trusted told me how death penalty cases become "black holes" in the judicial system, devouring the time, resources, and talents of the best attorneys, prosecutors, judges, and staff and diminishing everything else. In my needy, "crime-ridden" district, I had worked hard with community leaders and others to address urgent public safety issues and had labored to establish "community policing" programs at the city and state level focused on prevention—programs that received budget vetoes from Governor Weld in our early years. Our efforts were successful and making a real difference. I asked key legislative death penalty proponents if they had any estimates of how much restoration would cost and from where the money and resources would come. Despite numerous reports from across the nation suggesting that the costs were considerable, the answer I received was always the same: "There are so many competing estimates, it's impossible to make any useful prediction." I thought to myself, if I ever said that about one of my proposals, I'd get laughed out of the room. Why is it that "fiscal conservatives" can get away with this? Over several weeks, I moved back to firm and open opposition.

On the day of Jeffrey's funeral, the house minority leader, Republican David Peters of Charlton, called on Speaker Finneran to bring the death penalty matter before the House before the end of the legislative session in mid-November or else Republican members would use any legislative vehicle to force debate. At that time, the Senate had not yet even acted; on October 7, in respect for Jeffrey, senators voted to postpone debate until October 21. Robert Curley began a series of appearances on local news and public affairs programs to argue in favor of death penalty restoration. On October 18, more than 15,000 signatures on petitions calling for death penalty restoration were delivered to the State House. Huge numbers of people now were joining in the public conversation.

Meanwhile, news about another horrific murder burst onto the front pages of local newspapers. Elaine Donahue, an outgoing obstetrics nurse and mother of four who lived in the suburban town of Reading, had been missing since mid-September. Intense searches by hundreds, led by her husband, Edward, had been fruitless. On October 19, police discovered her body wrapped in plastic and stuffed inside a fifty-gallon plastic container in a Lynnfield storage locker. She had been murdered by her husband, an unemployed accountant with a gambling addiction and numerous debts, and left in the basement for weeks. Edward apparently got the idea for the plastic container by reading accounts of the Jeffrey Curley killing. How much worse could things get? Several days later, a woman in the city of Lawrence was shot to death by her boyfriend at a school bus stop in front of her child.

On October 21, after lengthy debate and consideration of many amendments, the State Senate adopted its version of death penalty legislation by a vote of 22 to 14. All the parliamentary delaying tactics employed by opponents prior to Jeffrey's murder were now laid aside. The key issue in the debate was not whether to restore capital punishment but how broadly to apply it. The original bill sent to the Senate in June by the Criminal Justice Committee would have restored capital punishment only in the case of the first-degree murder of police officers. Proponents had wanted this narrow range to create the strongest possible pressure on the House to approve the legislation. But the dynamics now had changed, and senators debated a plethora of amendments to apply capital punishment in other situations such as Jeffrey's. The Senate approved legislation creating twelve capital punishment–eligible offenses, including the murder of children under age fourteen who are kidnapped and sexually assaulted, first-degree murders involving torture and extreme cruelty, the murder of judges and multiple victims, and murders related to bombings and drug trafficking. Reinstatement proponents, whose numbers included Jeffrey's father and mother, wore yellow ribbons as they watched the proceedings from the Senate gallery.

Prior to the Senate action, on October 19 and 20, House Speaker Thomas Finneran made clear his intention to hold off House consideration of the death penalty matter until the spring of 1998, saying that legislators needed a period of "calm reflection" before deciding on such an emotional issue. "I don't think it is inappropriate or harmful to have a period of time to reflect," he stated. In the eighteen months since his ascension to the Speaker's chair, Finneran's will had not been altered by anyone, legislator or citizen. I assumed my vote would not matter because I was leaving at the end of November and focused on other matters. But flooded with calls from outraged citizens, Finneran uncharacteristically reversed his posture on October 22, announcing that he would schedule a vote within two weeks: "It was my assessment over the next two to three weeks that this was going to dominate to the point of eclipsing any other legislative proposal that we hoped to bring to bear," he announced.[8] His about-face was an example of the impact of the *conversation,* as the Speaker clearly heard and responded to the voices of citizens demanding swifter action by the House of Representatives. But it was also an example of the *game,* as House Republican leaders made clear their intention to block the passage of other important legislation unless the death penalty was also addressed.

Finneran also signaled his intention to handle this debate differently from his predecessor, Charlie Flaherty. "I have not done any head count," he declared, "nor will I do any arm twisting." While members of his top leadership did actively lobby against restoration, Finneran's key chairmen of the Committees on Criminal Justice and Ways and Means were leaders on the other side. The Ways and Means chairman, Paul Haley, brought before his committee on Monday, October 27, a bill that expanded to fifteen the number of offenses that could trigger the death penalty. Added to the list were murders in violation of domestic violence restraining orders, murders committed as part of a pattern of terroristic physical abuse, and murders committed in the presence of an immediate family member. As a member of the committee, I pressed Haley in the public session on whether his committee staff—responsible for the budgetary impact of legislation—had developed cost estimates for the bill.

"We haven't looked at that," he replied.

Even more aggressive than House advocates, however, was the acting governor, Argeo Paul Cellucci, who had taken charge in August when Governor William Weld resigned in his ill-fated pursuit of an ambassadorship to Mexico. Cellucci had been a moderate liberal Republican state representative and senator in the 1970s and 1980s who had always voted against capital punishment. In 1989, he abruptly switched sides, shortly before declaring his intention to run for governor in 1990. In the fall of 1989, he agreed to run for lieutenant governor on a ticket with Weld and subsequently formed a successful governing team. Now he was gearing up for a 1998 run at the top office as the "acting" incumbent and was blunt about his determination to use the death penalty as a cornerstone of his campaign—either trumpeting his success at reinstatement or arguing that his reelection was essential to win the issue. Unlike Weld, Cellucci eagerly engaged in personal, one-on-one lobbying of legislators. He organized a State House rally with crime victims and law enforcement officials. He officially declared October 28—the day of the House vote—to be "Jeffrey Curley and Victims of Murder Memorial Day." He publicly threatened death penalty–opposing legislators that he would campaign in their districts against them on this issue in 1998.

Slow and timid at first, death penalty opponents eventually joined the conversation. A letter of opposition was signed and released by eighteen Cambridge clergy, including the pastor of Jeffrey Curley's Catholic Church. Press conferences, vigils, and rallies were organized by opponents. The four Roman Catholic bishops sent a letter to all legislators and to all the state's parishes to be read at Sunday services on October 26. Families of other homicide victims, organized as the National Coalition of Survivors for Violence Prevention, began their own lobbying; one of them, South Boston's Michael MacDonald, spoke of his reactions to the furor: "You know that feeling as you watch the Curleys and these other families; you know that face; you can empathize with the way they're feeling. But it doesn't do a damn thing. The Revenge Fantasy doesn't work." Boston's Roman Catholic leader Bernard Cardinal Law wrote: ". . . support for capital punishment is not a litmus test for revulsion at Jeffrey Curley's murder."[9]

Nonetheless, it was evident that the ten-vote margin that had defeated capital punishment in the House in 1995 was eroding. "I came to realize that there are some sick animals out there," said Haverhill's Representative Brian Dempsey, explaining his change of heart. Finneran scheduled debate for Tuesday, October 28, hoping to avoid further desertions. It didn't help. After twelve hours of emotional and intense debate (with each side pointing to its own synecdoche: Jeffrey Curley versus Bobby Joe Leaster) the House of Representatives voted 81 to 79 to pass the bill—an 80–80 tie would have killed it. Eight members who voted against the death penalty in 1995 changed their positions, and none changed in the other direction. Death penalty supporters on the floor whooped and cheered when the numbers appeared on the roll call board. In the House gallery, Jeffrey's uncle, John, stood up and shouted, "Thank you for saving our children!" Those of us who worked against the bill looked at each other blankly and silently, feeling depleted and worn out. It appeared the fight was over. After all the strenuous lobbying and debate, it seemed inconceivable that any member would now change, much less in our direction. There were still other legislative steps and procedures to be followed, but they seemed only like "endgame."

The next day, Speaker Finneran publicly promised not to stop the bill from reaching acting Governor Cellucci's desk. Because the Senate and House versions were not identical—for example, the Senate version included twelve categories of murder eligible for capital punishment while the House version had fifteen—senators had to decide whether to "concur" with the House version or to "non-concur," thus requiring the creation of a committee of conference. Republican senators and some Democrats, fearing a glitch, argued that the Senate should simply concur but were defeated on Thursday, October 30, in that motion, 10 to 27. As a matter of institutional pride, the Senate would never simply accept the House version of such a controversial matter.

Three senators and three representatives compose a committee of conference in the Massachusetts General Court, two Democrats and one Republican from each chamber. Though the individual appointments are made by the Senate President and House Speaker, only members who voted in favor of the bill are permitted to be conferees, minimizing the chance for in-conference mischief. Indeed, all six appointees were strong death penalty backers, determined to construct a compromise bill (or "conference report") that would hold onto all eighty-one House votes and do it as rapidly as possible. The conference report would need to be approved by a majority of members in each chamber, after which a final, up-or-down "enactment" vote is required, again in each chamber, before the bill is sent to the governor's desk. If a conference report is not accepted by a majority of "yes" votes in either the House or the Senate, the leaders in both chambers are then required to appoint a new conference committee to attempt to devise a new conference report which can win majority support on both sides.

After recovering from the shock of defeat on Tuesday, October 28, death penalty opponents took several days to regroup. On Wednesday, November 5, members of the Progressive Legislators Group (PLG) met in room 167, a plain conference room in a far corner of the State House, to discuss potential strategies. When we examined our realistic prospects, the situation appeared even more dim. First, we needed to find a representative who would switch. But even if we could pull off that unexpected miracle, rejection of the conference report on the House floor would only trigger the creation of a new conference committee. That new conference committee then would hold onto the bill until January when two death penalty opponents (Representative David Cohen who had been elected mayor of Newton the previous day and I) would have resigned our seats. The second conference committee could then report out the death penalty bill again and win by a vote of 80 to 78. Switching a vote would subject the switcher to enormous personal vilification by death penalty backers and prove to be only a Pyrrhic victory for us.

As we talked, we could imagine only one scenario to avert this dilemma. If we could get the House members to approve acceptance of the conference report as a pro forma vote—perhaps even having it accepted on a voice vote—and then conduct the full debate at the next stage when the House would later vote on enactment, a vote in our favor would not trigger a new conference committee but would instead defeat the bill for the entire two-year legislative session, not just for 1997 but for 1998 as well. "How could we ever get the death penalty backers to go along with that?" asked one member incredulously. In truth, none of us believed that we could pull this off. But at least we had some kind of a strategy, and that was more than we had started the conversation with.

As we discussed legislative strategy, other forces opposing the death penalty kept talking to members, probing for representatives who might reconsider their positions. I recall talking with one rep, a decent, hardworking, committed young guy. We had been friends through a couple of tough fights. I looked him in the eye and said: "You really don't believe in this bill, do you?"

"No," he replied. "But the truth is I'm scared shit of what would happen to me if I switched now. I'd be humiliated and get killed."

On that Wednesday, though, one member was having an unexpected change of heart. A thirty-nine-year-old attorney in his second term, Jack Slattery from Peabody, who had run for the House in 1994 on a platform that included death penalty restoration, who had voted for restoration in 1995, and who debated on the House floor in support of restoration on October 28, silently made up his mind that night to switch. Other attorneys active in the Coalition Against the Death Penalty had spent hours talking with him about their experiences with the flaws of the judicial system. Since the October 28 House vote, a jury in Middlesex County in Massachusetts voted on Thursday, October 30, to convict an English au pair, Louise Woodward, of second-degree murder in the shaking death of her baby charge, igniting an international uproar over the follies and frailties of the criminal justice system in Massachusetts. Slattery decided to change his vote because of the doubts implanted in his mind by the Woodward verdict and because the final draft issued by the conference committee eliminated protections for juveniles and minorities that had been included in prior versions. Early Thursday afternoon, he went to the office of House Majority Leader Bill Nagle, who had been coordinating the anti–death penalty efforts for the Speaker, and told him of his intention to switch.

Several hours after Slattery's visit to Nagle, the conference committee report was brought before the full House. Rumors were spreading on our side of the floor that there might be a switch and it might be Slattery. Representative Jim Marzilli, a smart, staunch progressive from Arlington and a good friend, had been communicating with House leaders on behalf of the PLG on the strategic issues should there be a switch. Shortly before debate on acceptance of the conference report was to start, Speaker Finneran called Marzilli and House Minority Leader Dave Peters to the ornate rostrum, five steps above the floor of the House, to discuss procedure. Few in the chamber noticed what was happening, though I spotted it right away and anxiously watched from the back row of the House. Marzilli was talking to Finneran and Peters, gesturing politely with his hands. I couldn't hear, but I knew exactly what he was saying: "Let's approve the conference report on a voice vote and have the final debate on enactment so we don't have to go through it twice and keep members here too late." Finneran said something, and then he and Marzilli looked at Peters. I couldn't hear, but I could recognize what Peters was saying: "That sounds OK to me; we can skip the debate 'til later; but I still want to have a roll call on accepting the conference report." Back and forth they went several times. All three heads nodded. Marzilli and Peters left the rostrum.

Marzilli immediately caucused with several of us. "We agreed to move right away to a conference committee vote and save debate for enactment. But he insisted on a roll call on acceptance of the conference report, and I had no way to make him back down." Alarm! If the conference report was voted down by a tie vote, the Speaker would then be compelled to name another conference committee which would wait until the votes were there. How could we avoid this?

Speaker Finneran started: "The House will come to order. Question comes on acceptance of the report of the committee on conference. Those in favor of acceptance will vote yes, those opposed will vote no. The roll call machine is now open and will remain open for five minutes."

One of us, I don't remember who, said: "Let's get as many of us as we can to vote 'yes' or else to not vote at all to confuse the other side and to make sure that the report is approved." We spread quickly to all corners of the floor to talk with strong death penalty opponents, asking them to vote green or to not vote. Most of them looked at us as though we had lost our minds.

I remember pausing several seconds right before I pressed the green "yes" button on my desk in the chamber. "Do I know what I am doing right now? I am casting a vote in support of the death penalty. Do I really want to do this? I really don't know." I stopped thinking and pressed the green button.

The report of the committee on conference was accepted, 85 to 54. Five death penalty opponents, including Marzilli and me, voted in favor; 21 opponents, not wanting to cast an affirmative vote, did not press either button.

Too much was happening too quickly for death penalty supporters to figure out who had switched for the several minutes that the electronic roll call machine was displaying members' votes. Immediately after the closing of the vote, the machine goes blank. After the vote, death penalty proponents on the floor waited anxiously to obtain a paper copy of the roll call to compare it with the October 28 vote. I watched several dozen frantically looking back and forth between the two lists. Finally, they found the switcher: Slattery. Only then did they realize there had been a switch. But the conference report had been accepted, and we were already beginning the debate on enactment. It was too late to go back.

Cellucci came out of his office to rant to reporters: "Speaker Finneran and the House pulled the rug out. . . . Speaker Finneran stole it away," and vowed political revenge against all legislators voting against the bill, first among them, Jack Slattery. Back on the House floor, Slattery addressed a hushed chamber: "To those who think this isn't a difficult vote, you really don't understand how I have struggled over it in the past week."

The final vote on enactment that night was 80 to 80. Because a tie vote is insufficient to pass a bill, the death penalty legislation was dead, not just for 1997 but for 1998 as well because the legislative rules do not permit the same matter to be considered twice during the two-year session.

AFTERMATH

On November 3, 1998, Jack Slattery was easily reelected to his seat in the House of Representatives, having handily defeated opponents in the September Democratic primary as well. Although some accused Slattery of having made a secret deal with Finneran to change his vote in exchange for a prestigious chairmanship, Finneran, in January 1999, gave Slattery low-level committee assignments, sans chairmanship, as he did to all other House rebels. Of the few members defeated for reelection in the fall 1998 contests, none lost because of a death penalty vote, pro or con. Paul Cellucci, running for his first full term as governor in the same election, narrowly defeated anti–death penalty Attorney General Scott Harshbarger, 52 to 48 percent, and promised to continue to press for death penalty restoration. In the spring of 1999, the House again defeated death penalty restoration, this time by a comfortable ten-vote margin, foreclosing further debate until at least 2001.

.   .   .

I wrestled a long while about pairing the conversation-game duality with the death penalty case story. I feared that lighter connotations of the word *game* (amusement, pastime, fun, sport, joke) would suggest to some a lack of respect for the gravity of the issues involved in capital punishment, especially in the context of Jeffrey Curley's vicious murder. But the definition of *game* that fits in this case is not frivolous: "a competitive activity . . . on the part of two or more who play according to a set of rules." Fear of misinterpretation is an occupational hazard in many aspects of life, including writing. I decided to take that risk because I could not find another story that illustrated the conversation-game dynamic in such a compelling way.

Our legislative bodies—federal, state, and local—frequently address issues with life-and-death consequences. Some are obvious—declaration of war, capital punishment, abortion, physician-assisted suicide, provision of bulletproof vests for police—while many others also have life-and-death consequences that are less immediately apparent: public health protection, educational opportunities, toxic waste disposal, and much more. In the course of deliberations on all these issues, legislators use both conversation to persuade and rules to steer outcomes to their preferred results. Each side presumes that the other will take advantage of every appropriate opportunity to defend and advance its respective position. To do anything less suggests that the party is less than serious in of view. If the issue is serious enough, one should ex-

S. Senate and House of Representatives, majority
to thwart passage of legislation holding tobacco
le and liable for decades of deliberate deceit that
_ths of millions of people in the United States, and
_.._ worldwide. Some, myself included, jeered at this outcome, especially because of the way campaign money from the tobacco industry seemed to steer the final result. We have every right to jeer, even a duty to do so if we are sincere in our convictions. But so do the industry, the growers, the sellers, the smokers, and the antitaxers have every right to push their viewpoints and to protect their positions. If my side does its job right, the public indignation will continue to grow to force the kind of policy changes we deem necessary. But it's *our* job to win, not our opponents' to make it easier for us. Our appropriate object of scorn should be the positions and arguments of our opponents, not their right to defend their interests to the hilt.

It is essential to recognize political conflict for what it really is—a conversation *and* a game—and to work as hard as possible on both levels. They both matter, and they are inseparable. Understanding and using both well create victories.

CHAPTER NINE

Concluding Remarks

When the tide is receding from the beach,
it is easy to imagine that one can empty the ocean
by removing water with a pail.

René Dubos

I wrote this book to provide useful tools to empower readers to understand and interact with the political in their lives in a clearer and more productive way. In this final chapter, I provide summarizing and concluding remarks on the models, legislatures, health care, and, of course, politics.

MODELS

It may be useful to summarize for some readers the "take-home" points implicit in the various models described in this book. Here goes.

Politics is the way we decide in society who gets what, when, where, how, and why without resorting to violence. By its very nature, it is universal to government everywhere and intrudes to one extent or another in every other aspect of our lives. The most common alternative to politics is violence, the use of force to get what one wants. Indeed, the collapse of politics is often predecessor to acts of force. Any politicized situation can be immediately understood and analyzed by first asking the question: who is trying to get what, when, where, how, and why? The rest then follows much more easily.

While we can all agree on certain points (e.g., President Bill Clinton was reelected in 1996; cardiovascular disease is the leading cause of mortality in the United States), the meanings we attach to these facts, events, and data are nearly always contested terrain. Meaning is not absolute, handed down from the mountaintop, but tied to the values, beliefs, and opinions of each individual. Indeed, much of policymaking is debates about values masquerading as debates about facts and data. Political actors play with language, symbols, metaphors, and numbers to construct meanings to advance their political goals—in other words, to get whatever they are after. Effective political actors are cautious consumers of others' political constructions and are skilled crafters of their own stories.

Any political dispute of significance triggers conflict. To get something usually means taking something from someone else, whether that involves resources or rights. While many of us are taught to be conflict-averse, conflict is generally a sign of a healthy society where individuals feel free to express their political desires and wants through constructive engagement. Those who find themselves on the losing side of a fight will exhibit some familiar behavior patterns: broadening the scope of conflict to invite others to join their side; changing the site of conflict to a friendlier venue; and appealing to government or other higher authorities for support.

Most commonly, our actions reflect a mix of altruistic and selfish motives. To suggest that everyone acts primarily out of self-interest is as wrong as suggesting that public interest is the universal motivator of human behavior. Nonetheless, the rational choice perspective provides a powerful mechanism and an increasingly sophisticated way to understand better how and why we act. It is always a useful exercise to analyze the self-interest motivations of all parties, major and minor, to a conflict.

Popular views suggest an irreconcilable clash between the duties to represent constituents and to be true to one's conscience. In reality, representation is better understood as a continuum, not a dichotomy. Officials will place themselves at varying points along the continuum depending on their length of service, constituency, personal style and beliefs, ambitions, and more. A more useful construct than representation is relationships, whether between an official and voters, colleagues, leadership, party, other branches of government, media, and more. As in the rest of life, relationships are central to politics and to political success. Individuals engaged in political activity who can develop positive relationships can achieve much, while those who cannot are more often stymied. Relationships between principals and agents—a distinct but common form in politics—are particularly prevalent and important.

Incremental versus comprehensive change is also not an either/or choice. The political system embraces both. Most of the time, incremental change is the order of the day. But times also emerge when the underlying assumptions behind a regulatory-political structure are brought into question and the interests guarding it are fundamentally challenged. Real change can only happen when a new replacement structure—a new *idea*—develops sufficient support and momentum to topple and replace the predecessor regime. Pushing for broad yet unattainable systemic change when real incremental progress can be achieved is foolishness. Pushing for small, incremental advances when broader, fundamental change can happen is tragedy.

While the policy change process appears random and unpredictable, whether observed close up or from afar, more structure exists than is apparent. Change—incremental or comprehensive—happens when three streams or dynamics move at the same time and at the necessary level of intensity: 1. The problem stream, the sense among those with the power to act that a real problem needs to be addressed; 2. The policy stream, the existence of an implementable program to address the problem; and 3. The political stream, the shared sense that the policy change is consistent with public opinion and other key elements in the political environment. When all three streams are moving, a window of opportunity opens for change to occur. A policy significantly larger in scope than the sense of the problem usually will not fit through the window. Also, just as windows open, they also close—*carpe diem* (seize the day)!

Real politics involves both conversational and game elements. The conversation is a vitally important dynamic where shared meaning is created, arguments are honed, and compromises/adjustments are made. The game is an essential element as well because all policy and political processes have rules subject to interpretation and manipulation. To treat politics as a conversation and to ignore the game is reckless; to treat politics as a game and to ignore the conversation is shortsighted.

.　　　.　　　.

While most of the concepts and models in this volume are presented individually in their respective chapters, it is worth emphasizing that they are by no means mutually exclusive. In fact, they can be most helpful when used in combination with each other or with other political models not discussed here. This is most evident in reviewing several of the case stories.

Every story in this book meets the basic test of who gets sential threshold of the political: the X-Men seeking con Egleston Square; advocates trying to win protections for condominium conversions; citizens seeking to pass a new ing campaign finance and ethics requirements for public officials—if a story fails this test, it doesn't belong in this volume. Similarly, each involves the use of language, the manipulation of symbols and numbers, and the construction of stories to create meanings helpful to attaining political objectives: the competing synecdoches of Jeffrey Curley and Bobby Joe Leaster in the death penalty story; the symbol of the golden screw used by Chet Suhoski to defeat changes in Medicaid nursing home eligibility rules in 1990; the struggle over the meaning of numbers in the 1996 campaign for children's health insurance expansion. The use and misuse of language, numbers, and symbols are universal.

Conflict is not just a theme for tenants and landlords: my challenging Jimmy Craven's hold on the state representative seat in 1984 was picking a fight (he understood this far better than I did); Common Cause instigated conflict by gathering 80,000 signatures to place its Act for Accountable Politics on the state ballot in 1994; Paul Cellucci begged for a fight with any legislator who opposed reimposition of the death penalty in 1997. Self-interest versus public interest is a political theme by no means confined to the fiscal crisis of 1989 and 1990: my perceived political self-interest led me to do whatever I could to eliminate obstacles to economic development in Egleston Square, even standing on street corners on Friday evenings; that same self-interest led me to push obsessively for expanded health care access. Both of these controversies involved a strong public interest motivation on my part, but there is no denying the self-interested components as well.

Representation is a compelling dynamic in more than the campaign finance story. The Massachusetts fiscal crisis placed many legislators in a serious personal conflict between reflecting their districts and fulfilling their sense of public duty. Representation was also an important dynamic in the death penalty fight—not just for Jack Slattery but for other legislators fearful of the electoral consequences. Relationships also mattered hugely in each of the stories: the bond I was able to establish with my district during the 1984 campaign; the relationships between me and interest groups; the relationships between me and other legislators— George Keverian, Charlie Flaherty, Tom Finneran, Carmen Buell, Jim Marzilli, Mark Montigny, Stan Rosenberg—for better or worse! The trust that builds from positive relationships is a powerful force.

The dynamics of the two formal models in this book—punctuated equilibrium and agenda setting—are also in evidence throughout. In the condominium conversion fight, tenant activists sought comprehensive change and had to settle for incrementalism, while rent control opponents, who in earlier days would have settled for smaller adjustments, eventually eliminated an entire regulatory superstructure. The broad ambitions of Massachusetts health reformers in 1988 to create universal health insurance coverage in one state culminated in substantial yet incremental expansions in 1996. Finally, windows of opportunity appear throughout, sometimes serendipitously (my chance to run for office in 1984, my appointment as election laws chairman in 1994) and sometimes deliberately (the landlords' initiative to repeal rent control, the creation of the campaign finance reform package, both in 1994).

Both the conversation and the game are perpetually in play in every story. Our efforts in Egleston Square to disorganize the X-Men began as a conversation with them. Finding a winnable campaign finance package required incessant conversation among Stan Rosenberg, Nathan Gibson, and me, as well as with our respective principals. Incessant conversation was necessary to grapple with the realities of the 1989–90 fiscal crisis, however clumsily. And the game: Jimmy Craven's and my efforts to manipulate the shape of the candidate field; sending the "warchest" provision to the state's highest court for an advisory opinion in order to thwart a floor amendment; manipulating the budget process in 1996 to prevent an amendment to repeal the 1988 employer mandate. The conversation and the game are both everywhere.

·   ·   ·

Having elevated each of these ways of understanding politics, I should also acknowledge their limitations. No single model or combination— in this volume or elsewhere—can predict with certainty the outcome of a political confrontation. Using these constructs can enlighten and lead to better results. But all of them veer toward aiding the political artist more than the political scientist. The individual's contribution remains paramount.

That is how it should be. If an ingenious political scientist ever constructed the all-purpose predictive model to be used with certainty to predict the outcome of any political conflict, that would be tragic. Any serious political actor, at one time or another, takes on a fight in which all the "smart money" is wagered against him or her. Lots of times, smart money wins; but lots of times it loses, hands down. Those are magic moments when a political actor's commitment and intensity outweigh all the resources and clout of well-heeled establishment opponents. Even substantial losses can often open unexpected paths for future accomplishments and victories. We must never lose the potential for magic in our political lives. The perfect model, if ever devised, could have the unfortunate effect of draining spontaneity from our politics. I am not holding my breath waiting for its arrival.

Take these models for their intended purposes—as tools to help build political victories or as directional aids: signposts, maps, compasses to guide the traveler through unimaginable and provocative terrains. Enjoy the trip!

.   .   .

I have one final thought relative to the political-policy models. In my time in the Massachusetts legislature, I had the pleasure and opportunity to work with a good number of academic researchers, many of them political scientists, engaged in various forms of health services research. Thus, it was a surprise to me to recognize how unaware most professional politicians and government officials—as well as citizens—are of these useful ways to understand the political. I humbly suggest that the political science community needs to develop ways to connect more immediately and helpfully with those making policy and political decisions on the ground. The disconnect is unfortunate. Both sides, political scientists and public officials, could benefit from more robust and consistent exchange.

LEGISLATURES

There are many places in which one can fully participate in politics. Legislative bodies—federal, state, county, municipal—represent only one. They just happen to be my personal favorite. More than anyplace else in the public sphere, legislatures are the collecting points for a broad array of perspectives, ideas, biases, values, and much more. We each participate in the selection of our own representative and then watch as he or she attempts to make a difference in a body composed of other committed individuals pursuing their ideas and priorities. Somehow, they all have to figure out how to make a go of it.

Most people who have never served or worked in a legislative body are baffled by them. This is unfortunate because of the vitally important role played by these institutions in all our lives. The breadth of what legislators do is simply astounding, far beyond what most citizens understand. Traditional ways that experiences are translated to broad publics have not worked to explain the legislative experience and reality. One important way experiences are translated in our culture is through art.

Literature, cinema, painting—these and other art forms give us the ability to imagine experiences of which we will never partake. Climbing Mt. Everest, fighting a fire, caring for a disabled child, experiencing discrimination, cross-examining a hostile witness, performing a dangerous medical operation—most of us experience these and other activities only through art.

In art, though, the political experience is most often expressed through the eyes of chief executives: presidents, governors, mayors, the individuals with vast administrative powers. The legislative experience receives short shrift by comparison. My friend former California Assemblyman Phil Isenberg referred me to a wonderful novel, *The Gay Place,* a trio of stories about Texas politics in the 1950s written by a former aide to then U.S. Senator Lyndon Baines Johnson.[1] The first story is an engrossing tale about a state legislator. Yet, even here, only a handful of pages involve the process of making laws, the consuming passion for real-life legislators, and bring readers inside the legislative chamber. Nearly all the novels and films I have encountered that touch on the legislative experience do so in comic book fashion. Either they ignore the experience and process of lawmaking or they use it as a foil to play on the easy themes of political corruption or sexual indiscretion. In most of our fiction, opponents do not operate from differing values or principles—they're just on the take or in the tank. From *Mr. Smith Goes to Washington* onward, it's the same old story.

All of this misses the drama and the passion experienced on a daily basis by many thousands of men and women who serve in our nation's varied legislative bodies. William M. Bulger, one of the most skilled political leaders I have met, served seventeen years as President of the Massachusetts Senate. He wrote in his 1996 memoir:

> When it all began for me—I realize now—I was almost totally innocent of any understanding of the life I had chosen. I expected to create great legislation without knowledge of the process; to be effective with no awareness of the anatomy of political power; to continue in office with only a rudimentary grasp of politics. . . . I have learned a bit. . . . To make law, to make what you believe is *good* law, to see laws you have sponsored or effectively supported improve the happiness of people, is the ultimate satisfaction.[2]

I believe the vast majority of individuals who serve and who have served in our legislative assemblies would agree firmly with this sentiment. It is the crafting of good law, correctly mixing appropriate portions of needed policy and sensible compromise, that drives most legislators.

Do we have villains, neanderthals, and scoundrels who find their way into our assemblies? Absolutely. Are their numbers substantial? Absolutely not. And there is one more thing about them: every one of them was chosen as representative and sent to serve by voters, not by the other members of their respective legislative bodies. One thing over which legislators have no control is the selection of their colleagues. We are thrust into legislative assemblies with individuals, rules, customs, and structures already predetermined. Within that framework, we endeavor to find our individual ways to make a difference, to leave a mark, to sing out to anyone who cares to listen that we were there. Many individuals who have served regard their service as the greatest experience of their lives. It is an invigorating challenge from which many fall short. Few would deny, though, that it was worth the effort.

We need better ways to translate the legislative experience for each other and for the citizens we serve. This book is one such attempt. I sincerely hope it encourages other current and former legislators to come forward with their experiences as well. I know the stories are out there. I have heard too many firsthand to believe otherwise.

HEALTH CARE

My chief passion, for thirteen years in the Massachusetts House of Representatives and beyond, has been health: public health, health care access, health care quality, health care cost control. It is often noted that access, quality, and costs are the three legs of the health care stool, and we are advised in crafting policy proposals to "pick any two" because you can't have all three. Sometimes you can. Improving child immunization rates, for example, improves quality and access and lowers costs. Reducing medical errors—an epidemic in U.S. medical practice—improves quality and reduces costs without harming access. Those victories, though, tend to be rare. Most of the time, we try to improve one or two legs without doing heavy damage to the third.

I entered the Massachusetts House ignorant of most realities pertaining to health care and health policy. Like William Bulger, "I have learned a bit." My consuming commitment throughout has been to health care access. In 1985, as I discovered the system for the first time, it made no sense to me that about thirty million Americans lacked any health insurance coverage; as I write this, the number is heading toward forty-five million. I have traveled the gamut in the search for solutions, from incremental steps, to employer mandates, to single payer, back to mandates, and back to incrementalism. For a time, I worshiped at the perpetual shrine of the single payer but eventually turned agnostic. I see many routes to universal coverage and just want one that can do the job, win legislative approval, and actually be implemented. It is a dark stain on our nation—not on our health system—that we permit this shame to continue. As I write, federal and state governments enjoy unprecedented surpluses; additionally, billions in new dollars are being poured into the states from the national tobacco settlement. Yet the voices pushing to devote a share of these dollars to the needs of uninsured Americans are few and far between. By the time many read these words, many of the surpluses and tobacco settlement funds will be gone and a historic opportunity lost. This demonstrates that it will take more than dollars to achieve this goal. Foremost, it requires determined political will.

We will not accidentally stumble upon the road to universal health coverage for all Americans. It will instead be a deliberate and considered political choice, a "who gets what . . ." of historic proportions. I have watched the policy process long enough now to believe in waves and tides. Phony issues, left unaddressed, fade from the scene. Real issues, left unresolved, find their way back to the front of the public's consciousness through the persistent labors of those who don't give up, regardless of current fashions and trends. So it will be with the uninsured. America has a date with them, one we will not be able to avoid. The longer we wait, the more expensive the price will be.

For the past several years, the dominant issue in health care policy has been regulation of managed-care plans, particularly health maintenance organizations. I was initially stunned, in the mid-1990s, when I first observed legislators who did not give a fig about more than 600,000 uninsured citizens in my state and yet were fully prepared to go all out to secure unlimited choice and privileges for the well insured. I shared concerns about the aggressive practices of some managed-care plans, particularly the for-profit variety that report to shareholders on a quarterly basis. Before I stepped down as Health chair in Massachusetts, I initiated the process to establish a broad-based patients' bill of rights. But I have been skeptical of those who define the access challenge as one focused on fully insured individuals, with no attention to nearly forty-five million uninsured Americans. I also question the judgment of those who define the quality challenges facing our health system as reining in the practices of managed-care plans.

Aside from my access obsession, the key event shaping my perception was the immense cost crisis facing our system in the late 1980s and early 1990s, when costs for public and private payers were growing by 20 percent or more in a single year while overall public budgets were in decline (described in chapter 4). To me and to others who endured that period, managed care is not a dirty word, particularly if the alternative is un-managed care. The outrageous practices of some HMOs need to be curbed and/or prohibited, but the continuing effort to rationalize our health system must go on—we have no alternative.

By far, the most serious quality challenges facing the U.S. health sys-tem have nothing to do with one's enrollment in a managed-care or fee-for-service arrangement. The overwhelming challenge is the epidemic of error, inexplicable variation, overuse of unnecessary treatments, and un-deruse of necessary services. I have seen no data indicating the human price of managed-care practices in terms of lives lost. But we have siz-able and growing evidence of the human burden of these other forms of poor quality.

This is an immense challenge requiring relentless attention from all parts of the health system: public and private, provider, plan, consumer, employer and government. Progress on this front is already being made by innovative and creative leaders, people such as Dr. Donald Berwick, Dr. Lucian Leape, and Dr. Mark Chaissen. But this effort has only be-gun and has a long way to go. To achieve the kind of progress needed requires rethinking traditional behavior patterns, moving away from a litigious, blaming pattern in response to error and toward new models of practice both for the medical community and for government regula-tors. To achieve success, we can't afford to dismantle managed care; we need to transform it to focus on genuine quality improvement, disease prevention and health promotion, and public health.

We live in an era of outrageous contradictions: supreme progress in the midst of calamitous decline. We can make real progress in many ways to improve our health system. We can't do it without the involvement of the political system. Enlightened political engagement is not the only route to health system reform, but it is an essential part. Like it or not, our health and political systems are intimately intertwined, now and forever. We need to make the best of this.

POLITICS

If pressed to cite a single goal for this book, it would be to challenge the relentless negativity that imbues attitudes toward our nation's politics today. While a small segment of society participates with gusto, the vast majority—growing larger every day—tunes out the conversation and everything else that goes with it. Those who carry messages similar to mine are derided as naïve or insincere pollyannas (if you have never read *Pollyanna*, by the way, check it out—that little girl had guts!). How can anyone compliment a system that gives us PACs, lobbying scandals, scandal-scandals, soft money, and the rest? Who can cite a time when our political system was so crass, so openly up for sale, so morally bankrupt, so reprehensible?

I can. Here are just three examples:

In the latter part of the nineteenth century the U.S. political system gradually came to adopt the Australian secret ballot. Why? Prior to the secret ballot, political bosses across the nation herded voters to balloting stations with different colored ballots for each candidate or party so bosses could make sure voters cast the boss's preferred choice.

In the early part of the twentieth century, the U.S. Constitution was amended to provide for the direct election of members of the U.S. Senate. Why? Under the prior arrangement in which senators were elected by their respective state legislatures, the going price for a railroad or other industrialist to purchase the vote of a state legislator in the frontier states for a favored candidate was estimated at about $2,000.

In the 1960s and 1970s, the federal and state governments began to adopt laws requiring the disclosure of campaign contributors as well as donation limits and other controls. Why? Under the prior arrangements, most of our campaign system operated on a cash basis, often forwarded in suitcases with zero oversight or accountability.

For every columnist's quip about the degradation of our political standards, about the corrupting influence of lobbyists and campaign cash, there are equally damning contemporary statements from every decade of the past 200 years. Frank Baumgartner and Beth Leech point out: "In virtually every decade of the [twentieth] century, observers have noted the increasing numbers of lobbyists in the nation's capital." They quote one 1927 account: "[N]ever before have legislative bodies been subjected to such a continuous and powerful bombardment from private interests as at present."[3]

Yes, there are serious problems in our political system in need of correction. Smartly done public financing of elections, to me, would represent a vast improvement. But the "hell-in-a-handbasket" hypothesis so freely disseminated by some journalists, ambitious pols, and others in order to spice up their stories and legislative proposals simply cannot stand up to serious analysis. Much worse, I fear it contributes mightily to disengagement from politics by many, when positive reform cannot

succeed in the long run without massive engagement by those same
people.

Veterans and old-timers often see the past through rose-colored glasses
and decry the absence of prior statesmen, forgetting yesterday's forgettable scoundrels. Ambition and crudeness always appear to be on the
rise. Chris Matthews, in his useful and enjoyable book *Hardball,* puts
this in perspective:

> Climb aboard *Air Force One,* and you will find a world not all that different
> from your own workplace. People are jockeying for position, all the while
> keeping an eye on the competition across the aisle. Spend some time in the
> Oval Office and you will find it much like any other office, much as the Con-
> gress is like other large, complex organizations. There are friends and ene-
> mies, deals and reputations being made. And there are gladiators, people who
> keep score by the body count around them. Once you learn the rules, you will
> have the street smarts not only to survive the world of everyday politics, but
> to thrive in it.[4]

Whatever the prevailing corruption–influence peddling climate, each
generation spawns leaders who attempt to summon the best in us, who
seek to use politics for the improvement of society, and who keep their
gaze firmly fixed on the opportunities to improve social and economic
justice. Many times, they fall short and fail. At other times, they create
the civil rights and women's rights revolution, public education, Social
Security, workers' compensation, child labor laws, unemployment insurance, Medicare and Medicaid, and so much more.

Politics is by no means the only mechanism at our disposal for the improvement of society and individuals. But it is a mightily important one.
We need to pay it more respect.

Notes

INTRODUCTION

1. Data from 1989 found that 51 percent of women and 67 percent of men could name one of their U.S. senators, 32 percent of women and 43 percent of men could name their U.S. representative, and 18 percent of women and 22 percent of men could name their state representative. The male-female discrepancy was found to evaporate when the elected official in question was female. Verba, Sidney, Nancy Burns, and Kay Schlozman. "Knowing and Caring about Politics: Gender and Political Engagement." *Journal of Politics* 59, no. 4 (1997): 1051–72.

2. Quoted in Boorstin, Daniel. *The Seekers*. New York: Random House, 1998: 49.

3. Allison, Graham. *The Essence of Decision*. Boston: Little, Brown, 1971.

4. Nelson, Barbara. "Public Policy and Administration: An Overview." In *A New Handbook of Political Science*, edited by Goodin, Robert, and Hans-Dieter Klingemann. New York: Oxford University Press, 1996: 569.

5. Longest, Beaufort. *Health Policymaking in the United States*, 2d ed. Chicago: Health Administration Press, 1998: 56.

6. Rosenthal, Alan. *The Decline of Representative Democracy*. Washington, D.C.: CQ Press, 1998.

7. Loftus, Tom. *The Art of Legislative Politics*. Washington, D.C.: CQ Press, 1994.

CHAPTER ONE

1. De Waal, Frans. *Chimpanzee Politics: Power and Sex among Apes*. Baltimore: Johns Hopkins University Press, 1989.

2. Lasswell, Harold. *Politics: Who Gets What, When and How?* New York: World, 1958.

3. Arendt, Hannah. *The Human Condition.* Chicago: University of Chicago Press, 1958.

4. Center for Political Studies. *American National Election Studies.* Ann Arbor, Mich.: Center for Political Studies, 1996.

5. Machiavelli, Niccolò. "The Discourses." In *The Portable Machiavelli,* edited by Bondanella, Peter, and Mark Mosa. New York: Penguin, 1979: 193.

6. Mao Tse-tung. "On Protracted War." May 1938. In Baker, Daniel. *Power Quotes.* Detroit: Visible Ink, 1992: 238.

7. Clausewitz, Karl von. "On War." 1833. In *The Oxford Dictionary of Quotations,* 3d ed. Oxford: Oxford University Press, 1979: 152.

CHAPTER TWO

1. Stone, Deborah. *Policy Paradox: The Art of Political Decision Making.* New York: Norton, 1997.

2. Two contemporary books, one right and one left, nicely exemplify the normative outlook in their titles: Rush Limbaugh's *The Way Things Ought To Be* and James Carville's *We're Right, They're Wrong.*

3. Alinsky, Saul. *Rules for Radicals.* New York: Vintage, 1972: 17.

4. Lakoff, George, and Mark Johnson. *Metaphors We Live By.* Chicago: University of Chicago Press, 1980.

5. Stone, 9.

6. Annas, George. "Reframing the Debate on Health Care Reform by Replacing Our Metaphors." *New England Journal of Medicine* 332, no. 11 (March 16, 1995): 744–47.

7. *Boston Globe,* March 6, 1994.

CHAPTER THREE

1. Machiavelli, Niccolò. *The Portable Machiavelli.* Edited by Bondanella, Peter, and Mark Musa. New York: Penguin, 1979.

2. Machiavelli, 290.

3. Machivelli, 183, 184, 193, 295.

4. Weart, Spencer R. *Never at War: Why Democracies Will Not Fight One Another.* New Haven, Conn.: Yale University Press, 1998.

5. Madison, James. *The Federalist Papers,* No. 10. New York: New American Library, 1961: 77.

6. Madison, 78.

7. Madison, 81.

8. Madison. *The Federalist Papers,* No. 51, 322.

9. Schattschneider, E. E. *The Semisovereign People: A Realist's View of Democracy in America.* Fort Worth, Tex.: Harcourt Brace Jovanovich College, 1975.

10. Schattschneider, 36–37.

11. Schattschneider, 34.

12. Schattschneider, 30.

13. Schattschneider, 37.

14. Schattschneider, 40.

15. Van Horn, Carl, Donald Baumer, and William Gormley. *Politics and Public Policy.* Washington, D.C.: Congressional Quarterly Press, 1992.

16. The classic essay on policy networks is Heclo, Hugh. "Issue Networks and the Executive Establishment." In *Public Policy: The Essential Readings,* edited by Theodoulou, Stella, and Matthew Cahn. Englewood Cliffs, N.J.: Prentice Hall, 1995: 46–57.

17. Most discussion of the SPOA is taken from Moncreiff, Robert. "The Repeal of Rent Control in Cambridge." *New England Journal of Public Policy* 12, no.1 (fall/winter 1996): 117–40.

18. Van Horn, Baumer, and Gormley.

19. Moncreiff, 131–32.

20. *Boston Globe,* December 7, 1994.

21. *Boston Globe,* December 10, 1994.

22. *Boston Globe,* December 20, 1994.

23. *Boston Globe,* December 28, 1994.

24. *Boston Globe,* December 29, 1994.

25. *Boston Globe,* December 30, 1994.

26. *Boston Herald,* December 30, 1994.

CHAPTER FOUR

1. Feldstein, Paul. *The Politics of Health Legislation.* Ann Arbor, Mich.: Health Administration Press, 1988.

2. Feldstein, 3.

3. The duality of concentrated versus diffuse interests was developed by James Q. Wilson. See his *Political Organizations.* Princeton, N.J.: Princeton University Press, 1995

4. For a rich discussion of the history of self-interest in politics, on which much of this section is based, see Mansbridge, Jane. "The Rise and Fall of Self Interest in the Explanation of Political Life." In *Beyond Self Interest,* edited by Mansbridge, Jane. Chicago: University of Chicago Press, 1990.

5. In Boorstin, Daniel. *The Creators.* New York: Random House, 1992: 62.

6. In Mansbridge, 5–8.

7. Schumpeter, Joseph. *Capitalism, Socialism and Democracy.* New York: Harper and Row, 1962: 56–64.

8. Arrow, Kenneth. *Social Choice and Individual Values.* New York: Wiley. 1951.

9. Downs, Anthony. *An Economic Theory of Democracy.* New York: Harper and Row, 1957: 3–35.

10. Buchanan, James, and Gordon Tullock. *The Calculus of Consent.* Ann Arbor: University of Michigan Press, 1962.

11. Mayhew, David. *Congress: The Electoral Connection.* New Haven, Conn.: Yale University Press, 1974. Also Fiorina, Morris. *Congress: Keystone of the Washington Establishment.* New Haven, Conn.: Yale University Press, 1977: 977.

12. Stigler, George. "The Theory of Economic Regulation." In *Chicago Studies in Political Economy,* edited by Stigler, George. Chicago: University of Chicago Press, 1988: 209–33.

13. Mansbridge, 12.

14. Fenno, Richard. *Congressmen in Committees.* Boston: Little, Brown, 1973.

15. Derthick, Martha, and Paul Quirk. *The Politics of Deregulation.* Washington, D.C.: Brookings Institution, 1985.

16. In Mansbridge, 15.

17. Meier, Kenneth. *Regulation: Politics, Bureaucracy and Economics.* New York: St. Martin's Press, 1985: 19.

18. Kelman, Stephen. "Congress and the Public Spirit: A Commentary." In *Beyond Self Interest,* edited by Mansbridge, Jane. Chicago: University of Chicago Press, 1990: 206.

19. Green, Donald, and Ian Shapiro. *Pathologies of Rational Choice Theory: A Critique of Applications in Political Science.* New Haven, Conn.: Yale University Press, 1994: 202–4.

20. See, for example, Reich, Robert, ed. *The Power of Public Ideas.* Cambridge, Mass.: Ballinger, 1988.

21. Buchanan, James. "Then and Now, 1961–1986: From Delusion to Dystopia." Paper presented at the Institute for Humane Studies, Arlington, Virginia, 1986. Quoted in Mansbridge, "The Rise and Fall of Self-Interest in the Explanation of Political Life," 21.

22. Becker, Gary. *The Economic Way of Looking at Behavior.* Essays in Public Policy. Stanford, Calif.: Hoover Institution on War, Revolution and Peace, Stanford University, 1996.

23. Feldstein, 19.

24. Mansbridge, 17.

CHAPTER FIVE.

1. Pitkin, Hanna. *The Concept of Representation.* Berkeley: University of California Press, 1967: 165.

2. Rosenthal, Alan. *The Decline of Representative Democracy.* Washington, D.C.: CQ Press, 1998: 10.

3. Kingdon, John. *Congressmen's Voting Decisions,* 3d ed. Ann Arbor: University of Michigan Press, 1989: 7–22, 242.

4. Rosenthal, 11–22.

5. Fenno, Richard. *Home Style.* Boston: Little, Brown, 1978.

6. Pitkin, 232–33.

7. Eisenhardt, Kathleen M. "Agency Theory: An Assessment and Review." *Academy of Management Review* 14, no. 1 (1989): 57–74.

8. Pitkin, 232–33.

CHAPTER SIX

1. Lindblom, Charles. "The Science of Muddling Through." *Public Administration Review* 19 (1959): 79–88.

2. Kuhn, Thomas. *The Structure of Scientific Revolutions.* Chicago: University of Chicago Press, 1962.

3. Kuhn, 92–93.

4. For a useful overview of reactions to Kuhn, see Gutting, Gary, ed. *Paradigms and Revolutions: Appraisals and Applications of Thomas Kuhn's Philosophy of Science.* Notre Dame, Ind.: University of Notre Dame Press, 1980.

5. Eldredge, Niles, and Stephen Jay Gould. "Punctuated Equilibria: An Alternative to Phyletic Gradualism." In *Models in Paleobiology,* edited by Scoph, T. J. San Francisco: Freeman Cooper, 1972.

6. Tushman, Michael, and Elaine Romanelli. "Organizational Evolution: A Metamorphosis Model of Convergence and Reorientation." In *Research in Organizational Behavior,* edited by Cummings, L., and B. Staw. Greenwich, Conn.: JAI Press, 1985.

7. Grove, Andrew. *Only the Paranoid Survive.* New York: Doubleday, 1996.

8. Baumgartner, Frank, and Bryan Jones. *Agendas and Instability in American Politics.* Chicago: University of Chicago Press, 1993.

9. Kuhn, 77.

10. Lindblom, Charles. "The Science of Muddling Through." *Public Administration Review* 19 (1959): 79 88. And Van Horn, Carl, Donald Gaumer, and William Gormley. *Politics and Public Policy,* 2d ed. Washington, D.C.: CQ Press, 1992.

11. Riker, William. *Liberalism against Populism.* Prospect Heights, Ill.: Waveland Press, 1982.

12. I give a more complete—though less personal—account of the fate of hospital rate setting in four key states, Maryland, Massachusetts, New Jersey, and New York, in my prior book, *Interests, Ideas, and Deregulation: The Fate of Hospital Rate Setting.* Ann Arbor: University of Michigan Press, 1997.

13. Annas, George. "Reframing the Debate on Health Care Reform by Replacing Our Metaphors." *New England Journal of Medicine* 332, no. 11 (March 16, 1995): 744–47.

14. Eby, C. L., and D. R. Cohodes. "What Do We Know about Rate Setting?" *Journal of Health Politics, Policy and Law* 10, no. 2 (1985): 299–327.

15. Goldsmith Jeff. "Death of a Paradigm: The Challenge of Competition." *Health Affairs* 3, no. 3 (1984): 5–19.

16. Robinson, James, and Harold Luft. "Competition, Regulation, and Hospital Costs, 1982 to 1986." *Journal of the American Medical Association* 260, no. 18 (1988): 2676–81.

CHAPTER SEVEN

1. Kingdon, John. *Agendas, Alternatives and Public Policies,* 2d ed. New York: HarperCollins College, 1995.

2. The best narrative description of the Clinton health reform fiasco can be found in Johnson, Haynes, and David Broder. *The System: The American Way of Politics at the Breaking Point.* Boston: Little, Brown, 1996.

3. Kingdon, 109.

4. Reich, Robert. *Locked in the Cabinet.* New York: Knopf, 1997: 166.

5. Kluger, Richard. *Ashes to Ashes.* New York: Knopf, 1996.

CHAPTER EIGHT

1. Frederking, Brian. "Teaching Metaphors of Politics to Overcome Students' Dislike of Politics." *PS: Political Science & Politics,* June 1997: 157.

2. Lee, Emery. "Representation, Virtue, and Political Jealousy in the Brutus-Publius Dialogue." *Journal of Politics* 59, no. 4 (November 1997): 1073–95.

3. Schattschneider, E. E. *The Semisovereign People: A Realist's View of Democracy in America.* Fort Worth, Tex.: Harcourt Brace Jovanovich College, 1975: 31.

4. Fein, Ellen, and Sherrie Schneider. *The Rules: Time Tested Secrets for Capturing the Heart of Mr. Right.* New York: Warner, 1996.

5. Urdang, Laurence. *The Random House Dictionary of the English Language.* New York: Random House, 1968: 542.

6. *Boston Globe,* October 9, 1997.

7. Details of the history of the death penalty in Massachusetts from Burns, K. "A History of the Massachusetts Death Penalty." *Massachusetts Bar Association Criminal Justice Section News,* December 1997 and May 1998.

8. *Boston Globe,* October 23, 1997.

9. *Boston Globe,* October 27, 1997.

CHAPTER NINE

1. Brammer, Billy Lee. *The Gay Place.* Austin: University of Texas Press, 1989.

2. Bulger, William M. *While the Music Lasts: My Life in Politics.* Boston: Houghton Mifflin, 1996: 316.

3. Baumgartner, Frank, and Beth Leech. *Basic Interests: The Importance of Groups in Politics and in Political Science.* Princeton, N.J.: Princeton University Press, 1998: 100.

4. Matthews, Christopher. *Hardball: How Politics Is Played, Told by One Who Knows the Game.* New York: HarperPerennial, 1988: 16.

Select Bibliography

Alinsky, Saul. *Rules for Radicals*. New York: Vintage Books, 1972.

Allison, Graham. *The Essence of Decision*. Boston: Little, Brown, 1971.

Annas, George. "Reframing the Debate on Health Care Reform by Replacing Our Metaphors." *New England Journal of Medicine* 332, no. 11 (March 16, 1995): 744–47.

Arrow, Kenneth. *Social Choice and Individual Values*. New York: Wiley, 1951.

Baumgartner, Frank, and Bryan Jones. *Agendas and Instability in American Politics*. Chicago: University of Chicago Press, 1993.

Baumgartner, Frank, and Beth Leech. *Basic Interests: The Importance of Groups in Politics and in Political Science*. Princeton, N.J.: Princeton University Press, 1998.

Becker, Gary. *The Economic Way of Looking at Behavior*. Essays in Public Policy. Stanford, Calif.: Hoover Institution on War, Revolution and Peace, Stanford University, 1996.

Boorstin, Daniel. *The Seekers*. New York: Random House, 1998.

Brammer, Billy Lee. *The Gay Place*. Austin: University of Texas Press, 1989.

Buchanan, James. "Then and Now, 1961–1986: From Delusion to Dystopia." Paper presented at the Institute for Humane Studies, Arlington, Va., 1986.

Buchanan, James, and Gordon Tullock. *The Calculus of Consent*. Ann Arbor: University of Michigan Press, 1962.

Bulger, William M. *While the Music Lasts: My Life in Politics*. Boston: Houghton Mifflin, 1996.

Burns, K. "A History of the Massachusetts Death Penalty." *Massachusetts Bar Association Criminal Justice Section News*, December 1997 and May 1998.

Center for Political Studies. *American National Election Studies*. Ann Arbor, Mich.: Center for Political Studies, 1996.

De Waal, Frans. *Chimpanzee Politics: Power and Sex among Apes*. Baltimore: Johns Hopkins University Press, 1989.

Derthick, Martha, and Paul Quirk. *The Politics of Deregulation.* Washington, D.C.: Brookings Institution, 1985.

Downs, Anthony. *An Economic Theory of Democracy.* New York: Harper and Row, 1957.

Eby, C. L., and D. R. Cohodes. "What Do We Know about Rate Setting?" *Journal of Health Politics, Policy and Law* 10, no. 2 (1985): 299–327.

Eisenhardt, Kathleen M. "Agency Theory: An Assessment and Review." *Academy of Management Review* 14, no. 1 (1989): 57–74.

Eldredge, Niles, and Stephen Jay Gould. "Punctuated Equilibria: An Alternative to Phyletic Gradualism." In *Models in Paleobiology,* edited by Scoph, T. J. San Francisco: Freeman Cooper, 1972.

Fein, Ellen, and Sherrie Schneider. *The Rules: Time Tested Secrets for Capturing the Heart of Mr. Right.* New York: Warner, 1996.

Feldstein, Paul. *The Politics of Health Legislation.* Ann Arbor, Mich.: Health Administration Press, 1988.

Fenno, Richard. *Congressmen in Committees.* Boston: Little, Brown, 1973.

———. *Home Style.* Boston: Little, Brown, 1978.

Fiorina, Morris. *Congress: Keystone of the Washington Establishment.* New Haven, Conn.: Yale University Press, 1977.

Frederking, Brian. "Teaching Metaphors of Politics to Overcome Students' Dislike of Politics." *PS: Political Science & Politics,* June 1997: 157.

Goldmith, Jeff. "Death of a Paradigm: The Challenge of Competition." *Health Affairs* 3, no. 3 (1984): 5–19.

Green, Donald, and Ian Shapiro. *Pathologies of Rational Choice Theory: A Critique of Applications in Political Science.* New Haven, Conn.: Yale University Press, 1994.

Grove, Andrew. *Only the Paranoid Survive.* New York: Doubleday, 1996.

Gutting, Gary, ed. *Paradigms and Revolutions: Appraisals and Applications of Thomas Kuhn's Philosophy of Science.* Notre Dame, Ind.: University of Notre Dame Press, 1980.

Heclo, Hugh. "Issue Networks and the Executive Establishment." In *Public Policy: The Essential Readings,* edited by Theodoulou, Stella, and Matthew Cahn. Englewood Cliffs, N.J.: Prentice Hall, 1995: 46–57.

Johnson, Haynes, and David Broder. *The System: The American Way of Politics at the Breaking Point.* Boston: Little, Brown, 1996.

Kelman, Stephen. "Congress and the Public Spirit: A Commentary." In *Beyond Self Interest,* edited by Mansbridge, Jane. Chicago: University of Chicago Press, 1990.

Kingdon, John. *Congressmen's Voting Decisions,* 3d ed. Ann Arbor: University of Michigan Press, 1989.

———. *Agendas, Alternatives and Public Policies,* 2d ed. New York: HarperCollins College, 1995.

Kluger, Richard. *Ashes to Ashes.* New York: Knopf, 1996.

Kuhn, Thomas. *The Structure of Scientific Revolutions.* Chicago: University of Chicago Press, 1962.

Lasswell, Harold. *Politics: Who Gets What, When and How?* New York: World, 1958.

Lee, Emery. "Representation, Virtue, and Political Jealousy in the Brutus-Pub-
   lius Dialogue." *Journal of Politics* 59, no. 4 (November 1997): 1073–95.
Lindblom, Charles. "The Science of Muddling Through." *Public Administration
   Review* 19 (1959): 79–88.
Longest, Beaufort. *Health Policymaking in the United States,* 2d ed. Chicago:
   Health Administration Press, 1998.
Machiavelli, Niccolò. *The Portable Machiavelli.* Edited by Bondanella, Peter, and
   Mark Musa. New York: Penguin, 1979.
Madison, James. *The Federalist Papers.* New York: New American Library, 1961.
Mansbridge, Jane. "The Rise and Fall of Self-Interest in the Explanation of Po-
   litical Life." In *Beyond Self Interest,* edited by Mansbridge, Jane. Chicago:
   University of Chicago Press, 1990.
Matthews, Christopher. *Hardball: How Politics Is Played, Told by One Who
   Knows the Game.* New York: HarperPerennial, 1988: 16.
Mayhew, David. *Congress: The Electoral Connection.* New Haven, Conn.: Yale
   University Press, 1974.
McDonough, John. *Interests, Ideas, and Deregulation: The Fate of Hospital Rate
   Setting.* Ann Arbor: University of Michigan Press, 1997.
Meier, Kenneth. *Regulation. Politics, Bureaucracy and Economics.* New York:
   St. Martin's Press, 1985.
Moncreiff, Robert. "The Repeal of Rent Control in Cambridge." *New England
   Journal of Public Policy* 12, no. 1 (fall/winter 1996): 117–40.
Nelson, Barbara. "Public Policy and Administration: An Overview." In *A New
   Handbook of Political Science,* edited by Goodin, Robert, and Hans-Dieter
   Klingemann. New York: Oxford University Press, 1996.
Pitkin, Hanna. *The Concept of Representation.* Berkeley: University of Califor-
   nia Press, 1967.
Reich, Robert, ed. *The Power of Public Ideas.* Cambridge, Mass.: Ballinger, 1988.
———. *Locked in the Cabinet.* New York: Knopf, 1997.
Riker, William. *Liberalism against Populism.* Prospect Heights, Ill.: Waveland
   Press, 1982.
Robinson, James, and Harold Luft. "Competition, Regulation, and Hospital
   Costs, 1982 to 1986." *Journal of the American Medical Association* 260, no.
   18 (1988): 2676–81.
Rosenthal, Alan. *The Decline of Representative Democracy.* Washington, D.C.:
   Congressional Quarterly Press, 1998.
Schattschneider, E. E. *The Semisovereign People: A Realist's View of Democ-
   racy in America.* Fort Worth, Tex.: Harcourt Brace Jovanovich College,
   1975.
Schumpeter, Joseph. *Capitalism, Socialism and Democracy.* New York: Harper
   and Row, 1962.
Stigler, George. "The Theory of Economic Regulation." In *Chicago Studies in
   Political Economy,* edited by Stigler, George. Chicago: University of Chicago
   Press, 1988: 209–33.
Stone, Deborah. *Policy Paradox: The Art of Political Decision Making.* New York:
   Norton, 1997.
Tushman, Michael, and Elaine Romanelli. "Organizational Evolution: A Meta-

morphosis Model of Convergence and Reorientation." In *Research in Organizational Behavior,* edited by Cummings, L., and B. Staw. Greenwich, Conn.: JAI Press, 1985.

Urdang, Laurence. *The Random House Dictionary of the English Language.* New York: Random House, 1968.

Van Horn, Carl, Donald Baumer, and William Gormley. *Politics and Public Policy.* Washington, D.C.: Congressional Quarterly Press, 1992.

Verba, Sidney, Nancy Burns, and Kay Schlozman. "Knowing and Caring about Politics: Gender and Political Engagement." *Journal of Politics* 59, no. 4 (1997): 1051–72.

Weart, Spencer R. *Never at War: Why Democracies Will Not Fight One Another.* New Haven, Conn.: Yale University Press, 1998.

Wilson, James Q. *Political Organizations.* Princeton, N.J.: Princeton University Press, 1995.

Index